# Best of Five MCQs for the European Specialty Examination in Gastroenterology and Hepatology

T0177711

# Best of Five MCQs for the European Specialty Examination in Gastroenterology and Hepatology

**Second edition**

*Edited by*

**Dr Thomas Marjot** BSc (Hons), MBBS, MRCP(UK)
*Specialist Registrar, Translational Gastroenterology Unit, Nuffield Department of Experimental Medicine, University of Oxford, Oxford, UK*

**Dr Colleen G C McGregor** BSc (Hons), MBBS, MRCP(UK)
*Specialist Registrar, Translational Gastroenterology Unit, Nuffield Department of Experimental Medicine, University of Oxford, Oxford, UK*

**Dr Tim Ambrose** BSc (Hons), MBChB, MRCP(UK), DPhil
*Consultant Gastroenterologist, Translational Gastroenterology Unit, Nuffield Department of Experimental Medicine, University of Oxford, Oxford, UK*

*Consultant Editors*

**Dr Aminda N De Silva** BSc (Hons), MBBS, FRCP
*Consultant Gastroenterologist, Royal Berkshire NHS Foundation Trust, Reading, UK*

**Dr Jeremy Cobbold** MA, PhD, FRCP
*Consultant Hepatologist, Oxford Liver Unit, Department of Gastroenterology and Hepatology, Oxford University Hospitals NHS Foundation Trust, Oxford, UK*

**Professor Simon Travis** DPhil, FRCP, MA (Hon)
*Professor of Clinical Gastroenterology, Translational Gastroenterology Unit, Nuffield Department of Experimental Medicine, University of Oxford, Oxford, UK*

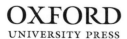
OXFORD
UNIVERSITY PRESS

# OXFORD
## UNIVERSITY PRESS

Great Clarendon Street, Oxford, OX2 6DP,
United Kingdom

Oxford University Press is a department of the University of Oxford.
It furthers the University's objective of excellence in research, scholarship,
and education by publishing worldwide. Oxford is a registered trade mark of
Oxford University Press in the UK and in certain other countries

First Edition published in 2013
Second Edition published in 2021

Published in the United States of America by Oxford University Press
198 Madison Avenue, New York, NY 10016, United States of America

British Library Cataloguing in Publication Data

Data available

Library of Congress Control Number: 2020945295

ISBN 978–0–19–883437–3

DOI: 10.1093/oso/9780198834373.001.0001

Printed and bound by
CPI Group (UK) Ltd, Croydon, CR0 4YY

*Dedicated to Professor Satish Keshav—clinician, academic, mentor, and friend. He taught us all how to think outside the box.*

# FOREWORD

For many trainees and colleagues, the European Specialty Examination in Gastroenterology and Hepatology (ESEGH) will represent the last in a seemingly endless series of formal examinations required to navigate a career in Medicine. It will also appear a particularly daunting task, with the ESEGH designed to cover the full range and breadth of gastrointestinal and liver pathology. Furthermore, the exam's 'best of five' multiple choice questions are notoriously difficult, pushing candidates to pick the most correct answer from a series of plausible options. To survive the examination and emerge victorious therefore requires a combination of composure, experience, clinical problem-solving, and a solid grasp of first principles. Therefore, the value of a comprehensive, tailor-made resource such as this textbook cannot be overstated.

This book has been compiled by Specialist Registrars affiliated with Oxford University Hospitals NHS Trust, who are no strangers to the rigors of post-graduate exams. The authors have drawn on this collective experience to produce the first dedicated textbook to assist candidates in their preparation for the ESEGH. The book has been meticulously assembled to ensure that all relevant domains of the curriculum are covered and that the weighting of questions on each topic precisely matches the proportions found in the examination itself. The questions are engaging, being based on real-life clinical scenarios which have all required specialist input and decision making. Some questions are relatively straight forward, but many I found challenging! However, each answer helpfully includes a summary of the key learning points, alongside a concise explanation that walks the reader through the necessary background information. In addition, the book has clearly been written for the broad European audience, with all the answers rooted in the most up-to-date European guidelines.

Writing a textbook is a mammoth undertaking, which is why as a former President both of the British Society of Gastroenterology and of the Royal College of Physicians, it is particularly satisfying to see Specialist Registrars work together to produce such a high-quality resource, for the wider benefit of their trainee colleagues.

I have no doubts that you will find this book an extremely useful and enjoyable read, and I wish you all the best, both in the examination and in your future careers as Specialists in Gastroenterology and Hepatology. You will not regret your career choice (or indeed your use of this book!)

Sir Ian Gilmore

Former President of Royal College of Physicians of London
Former President of British Society of Gastroenterology
Director, Liverpool Centre for Alcohol Research
Chairman, Alcohol Health Alliance UK

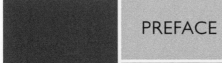

# PREFACE

In 2018, the European Specialty Examination in Gastroenterology & Hepatology (ESEGH) came into force, merging the Specialty Certificate Examination (SCE) in the UK with the European Section and Board of Gastroenterology and Hepatology Examination (ESBGH). This aimed to unify and improve standards of practice across Europe, and completing the exam now demonstrates that sufficient knowledge has been acquired to fulfil the requirements of a specialist in gastroenterology and hepatology according to a curriculum agreed upon across the continent. The exam involves 200 'Best of Five' multiple-choice questions, meaning that several of the choices may be plausible but only one is the best answer. Successfully answering this type of question is challenging and requires synthesis of basic knowledge, experience, data analysis, and clinical problem solving. Practice, as always, is crucial and we therefore aimed to produce a valuable tool for all trainees revising for the exam, as well as international reference material for other professionals working in gastroenterology and hepatology.

This is the first question book specifically designed to help prepare for the ESEGH. It contains 300 original 'Best of Five' multiple-choice questions covering the breath of the European curriculum. Furthermore, the composition of the book exactly matches the proportion of questions for each curriculum area found in the exam. For example, the ESEGH contains 20% questions on hepatology, 10% on small intestinal disorders, 8% on pancreatic disorders, and so on, and therefore the same proportions of questions for each topic area are reflected in the book. Each question is accompanied by an answer, a set of succinct bullet points of key 'take-home' messages and a short summary of the relevant background, evidence base and up-to date European guidelines. The book ends with a chapter of 50 questions designed to act as a mock examination for use in the final stages of preparation. Questions have been contributed by 15 UK specialty trainees in Oxford, many of whom have successfully passed the former UK Specialty Certificate Examination or the ESEGH itself. All questions were scrutinized by senior editors, Professor Simon Travis, Dr Aminda de Silva, and Dr Jeremy Cobbold who deserve particular thanks for their invaluable advice and guidance throughout the writing and editing process. We would also like to thank the broader gastroenterology and hepatology consultant body at the John Radcliffe Hospital who have supported trainees in their question contributions, and the radiology and histology department team who have sourced many of the images included in the book.

We sincerely hope that you find reading this book and answering the questions both interesting and helpful in your exam preparations. Good luck!

Dr Thomas Marjot
Dr Colleen McGregor
Dr Tim Ambrose

# CONTENTS

# CONTRIBUTORS

**Khansa Adam**
LAS Gastroenterology, Royal Berkshire NHS Foundation Trust
Reading, UK

**Sophie Arndtz**
Specialist Registrar, Royal Berkshire NHS Foundation Trust
Reading, UK

**Homira Ayubi**
Clinical Fellow, Milton Keynes University Hospital NHS Foundation Trust
Milton Keynes, UK

**Vincent T. F. Cheung**
Clinical Research Fellow, Translational Gastroenterology Unit, John Radcliffe Hospital
Oxford, UK

**Emma L. Culver**
Consultant Hepatologist, Translational Gastroenterology Unit, John Radcliffe Hospital
Oxford, UK

**Michael FitzPatrick**
Clinical Research Fellow, Translational Gastroenterology Unit, Nuffield Department of
   Experimental Medicine, University of Oxford
Oxford, UK

**David J. Harman**
Specialist Registrar, Oxford University Hospitals NHS Foundation Trust
Oxford, UK

**Omar Herman**
Specialist Registrar, Royal Berkshire NHS Foundation Trust
Reading, UK

**Arif Hussenbux**
Specialist Registrar, Oxford University Hospitals NHS Foundation Trust
Oxford, UK

**Kate Lynch**
Clinical Research Fellow, Translational Gastroenterology Unit, Nuffield Department of
   Experimental Medicine, University of Oxford
Oxford, UK

**Charis D. Manganis**
Specialist Registrar, Oxford University Hospitals NHS Foundation Trust
Oxford, UK

**Rory Peters**
Clinical Research Fellow, Translational Gastroenterology Unit, John Radcliffe Hospital
Oxford, UK

**Rahul P. Ravindran**
Academic Clinical Fellow, Translational Gastroenterology Unit, John Radcliffe Hospital
Oxford, UK

**Emmanuel A. Selvaraj**
Clinical Research Fellow, Oxford University Hospitals NHS Foundation Trust
Oxford, UK

**Shahana Shahid**
Specialist Registrar, Oxford University Hospitals NHS Foundation Trust
Oxford, UK

# ABBREVIATIONS

| | |
|---|---|
| 5-ASA | 5-aminosalicylate |
| 5-HT$_4$ | 5-hydroxytryptamine type 4 receptor |
| A1ATD | alpha-1-antitrypsin deficiency |
| Ach | acetylcholine |
| ADM | adenomyomatosis |
| AE | adverse event |
| AF | atrial fibrillation |
| AFLP | acute fatty liver of pregnancy |
| AFP | alpha-fetoprotein |
| AH | alcoholic hepatitis |
| AIDS | acquired immunodeficiency syndrome |
| AIN | anal intraepithelial neoplasia |
| AIP | autoimmune pancreatitis type 1 |
| AKI | acute kidney injury |
| ALD | alcohol related liver disease |
| ALF | acute liver failure |
| ALP | alkaline phosphatase |
| ALT | alanine aminotransferase |
| AMA | antimitochondrial antibody |
| AN | anorexia nervosa |
| ANA | antinuclear antibody |
| ANC | acute necrotic collection |
| ANCA | anti-neutrophil cytoplasmic antibody |
| Anti-TNF | anti-tumour necrosis factor |
| Anti-TTG | anti-tissue transglutaminase antibody |
| APC | argon plasma coagulation |
| APFC | acute peripancreatic fluid collections |
| ARM | anorectal manometry |
| AS | anastomotic |
| ASC | acute severe colitis |
| AST | aspartate transaminase |

| | |
|---|---|
| ASUC | acute severe ulcerative colitis |
| ATN | acute tubular necrosis |
| AWS | alcohol withdrawal syndrome |
| BAM | bile acid malabsorption |
| BCLC | Barcelona clinic liver cancer |
| BFT | biofeedback therapy |
| BMI | body mass index |
| BTI | botulinum toxin injection |
| BWT | bowel wall thickness |
| BZD | benzodiazepine |
| CA | coeliac axis |
| CACRC | colitis-associated colorectal cancer |
| CASR | calcium-sensing receptor |
| CBD | common bile duct |
| CCK | cholecystokinin |
| CD | Crohn's disease |
| CDI | *Clostridioides difficile* infection |
| CE | capsule endoscopy |
| CE | cystic echinococcosis |
| CFTR | cystic fibrosis transmembrane conductance regulator |
| CHB | chronic HBV infection |
| CHD | common hepatic duct |
| CHS | cannabis hyperemesis syndrome |
| CI | confidence interval |
| CLD | chronic liver disease |
| CMV | cytomegalovirus |
| COPD | chronic obstructive pulmonary disease |
| CP | chronic pancreatitis |
| CRC | colorectal cancer |
| CrCl | creatinine clearance |
| CRP | C-reactive protein |
| CSF | cerebrospinal fluid |
| CSPH | clinically significant portal hypertension |
| CTP | Child-Turcotte-Pugh (score) |
| CTZ | chemoreceptor trigger zone |
| CVID | common variable immunodeficiency |
| CYP | cytochrome P450 |
| DAA | direct-acting antiviral |
| DCI | distal contractile integral |

| | |
|---|---|
| DEXA | dual energy x-ray absorptiometry |
| DILI | drug-induced liver injury |
| DOC | dual-operator cholangioscopy |
| DS | dominant strictures |
| EASL | European Association for the Study of the Liver |
| ECCO | European Crohn's and Colitis Organisation |
| ECG | electrocardiogram |
| EDS | early dumping syndrome |
| EEG | electroencephalography |
| EEN | exclusive enteral nutrition |
| EIM | extra-intestinal manifestation |
| ELF | enhanced liver fibrosis |
| ELT | emergency liver transplantation |
| EMR | endoscopic mucosal resection |
| EOE | eosinophilic oesophagitis |
| ERCP | endoscopic retrograde cholangiopancreatography |
| ESBGH | European Section and Board of Gastroenterology and Hepatology Examination |
| ESD | endoscopic submucosal dissection |
| ESEGH | European Specialty Examination in Gastroenterology & Hepatology |
| ESGE | European Society of Gastrointestinal Endoscopy |
| ESMO | European Society of Medical Oncology |
| ESWL | extracorporeal shockwave lithotripsy |
| EUS | endoscopic ultrasound |
| EVL | endoscopic variceal ligation |
| FAP | familial adenomatous polyposis |
| FDR | first-degree relative |
| FE | faecal elastase |
| FENa | fraction of excreted sodium |
| FGP | fundic gland polyps |
| FI | faecal incontinence |
| FNA | fine-needle aspiration |
| GAVE | gastric antral vascular ectasia |
| GC | gastric cancer |
| GDH | glutamate dehydrogenase |
| GI | gastrointestinal |
| GIP | gastric inhibitory polypeptide |
| GIST | gastrointestinal stromal tumour |
| GLP-2 | glucagon-like peptide 2 |
| GORD | gastro-oesophageal reflux disease |

| | |
|---|---|
| GOV | gastro-oesophageal varices |
| GTN | topical glyceryl trinitrate |
| GWAS | genome-wide association studies |
| HA | hepatic artery |
| HAART | highly active antiretroviral therapy |
| HAS | hepatic artery stenosis |
| HAT | hepatic artery thrombosis |
| HBV | hepatitis B virus |
| HCC | hepatocellular carcinoma |
| HCV | hepatitis C virus |
| HDGC | hereditary diffuse gastric cancer |
| HDV | hepatitis D |
| hEDS | hypermobile-type Ehlers-Danlos syndrome |
| HELLP | haemolysis, elevated liver enzymes, and low platelets |
| HFE-HC | HFE haemochromatosis |
| HLA | human leukocyte antigen |
| HNPCC | hereditary non-polyposis colorectal cancer |
| HPS | hepatopulmonary syndrome |
| HPV | human papilloma viruses |
| HR | heart rate |
| HRS–AKI | hepatorenal syndrome–acute kidney injury |
| HVPG | hepatic venous pressure gradient |
| IAP | International Association of Pancreatology |
| IBD | inflammatory bowel disease |
| IBS | irritable bowel syndrome |
| IBS-C | irritable bowel syndrome with predominant constipation |
| ICP | intrahepatic cholestasis of pregnancy |
| IEL | intraepithelial lymphocytes |
| IFX | infliximab |
| IgA TTG | immunoglobin A tissue transglutaminase antibody |
| IgG4-RD | IgG4-related disease |
| IGV | isolated gastric varices |
| IM | intestinal metaplasia |
| IOP | interstitial oedematous pancreatitis |
| IPAA | ileal pouch anal anastomosis |
| IPMN | intraductal papillary mucinous neoplasm |
| IPVD | intrapulmonary vascular dilatations |
| IRP | integrated relaxation pressure |
| ISDE | International Society for Diseases of the Esophagus |

| | |
|---|---|
| IUS | intestinal ultrasound |
| JPS | juvenile polyposis syndrome |
| JVP | jugular venous pressure |
| KF | Kayser–Fleischer |
| LDS | late dumping syndrome |
| LG | lymphocytic gastritis |
| LGV | *chlamydia lymphogranuloma venereum* |
| LHM | laparoscopic Heller myotomy |
| LMWH | low molecular weight heparin |
| LPAC | low-phospholipid associated cholelithiasis |
| LS | lynch syndrome |
| LSM | liver stiffness measurement |
| LT | liver transplantation |
| MAP | MUTYH-associated polyposis |
| MARSIPAN | management of really sick patients with anorexia nervosa |
| MCV | mean corpuscular volume |
| MD | Ménétrier's disease |
| MDMA | 3,4-methyl-enedioxy-methamphetamine |
| MDT | multidisciplinary team |
| MEN | multiple endocrine neoplasia |
| MMR | mismatch repair |
| MMX | multimatrix |
| MPD | main pancreatic duct |
| MRCP | magnetic resonance cholangiopancreatography |
| MSM | men who have sex with men |
| MUST | Malnutrition Universal Screening Tool |
| MYH | MutY human homologue |
| NA | nucleoside analogue |
| NAFLD | non-alcoholic fatty liver disease |
| NAS | non-anastomotic |
| NASH | non-alcoholic steatohepatitis |
| NKT | Natural Killer T |
| NNRTI | non-nucleoside reverse transcriptase inhibitors |
| NOD2 | nucleotide-binding oligomerization domain-containing protein 2 |
| NP | necrotizing pancreatitis |
| NRH | nodular regenerative hyperplasia |
| NRTI | nucleoside reverse transcriptase inhibitors |
| OCA | obeticholic acid |
| OCP | contraceptive pill |

| | |
|---|---|
| OR | odds ratio |
| PAS | periodic-acid Schiff |
| PBC | primary biliary cholangitis |
| pCCA | perihilar cholangiocarcinoma |
| PEG | polyethylene glycol |
| PEP | post-ERCP pancreatitis |
| PET | positron emission tomography |
| PG | pyoderma gangrenosum |
| PH | potential hydrogen |
| PHG | portal hypertensive gastropathy |
| PJS | Peutz-Jeghers syndrome |
| PN | parenteral nutrition |
| p-NET | pancreatic neuroendocrine tumour |
| PNR | primary non-response |
| PPI | proton pump inhibitor |
| PPI-REE | PPI responsive oesophageal eosinophilia |
| PSC | primary sclerosing cholangitis |
| PSC-IBD | primary sclerosing cholangitis-inflammatory bowel disease |
| PUD | peptic ulcer disease |
| RAAS | renin–angiotensin–aldosterone system |
| RBL | rubber band ligation |
| RCT | randomized controlled trial |
| RIG | radiologically inserted gastrostomy |
| rPSC | recurrent PSC |
| RR | relative risk |
| RY-GBP | Roux-en-Y gastric bypass |
| SAAG | serum-ascites albumin gradient |
| SBP | spontaneous bacterial peritonitis |
| SCE | Specialty Certificate Examination |
| SCFA | short-chain fatty acid enemas |
| SG | sleeve gastrectomy |
| SSRI | selective serotonin reuptake inhibitor |
| STK11 | serine/threonine kinase 11 |
| SIBO | small intestinal bacterial overgrowth |
| SIRS | systemic inflammatory response syndrome |
| SMA | superior mesenteric artery |
| SNVA | seronegative villous atrophy |
| SOD | sphincter of Oddi dysfunction |
| SPS | serrated polyposis syndrome |

| | |
|---|---|
| SRUS | solitary rectal ulcer syndrome |
| SS | somatostatin |
| SUSS | Sit Up Squat Stand |
| SVR | sustained virologic response |
| TACE | transarterial chemoembolization |
| TE | transient elastography |
| TIPSS | transjugular intrahepatic portosystemic shunt |
| TNF | tumour necrosis factor |
| TPMT | thiopurine methyltransferase |
| TSH | thyroid-stimulating hormone |
| UC | ulcerative colitis |
| UDCA | ursodeoxycholic acid |
| ULN | upper limit of normal |
| VCE | video capsule endoscopy |
| VH | variceal haemorrhage |
| VIP | vasoactive intestinal peptide |
| VTE | venous thromboembolism |
| WCC | white cell count |
| WD | Wilson's disease |
| WHO | World Health Organization |
| WON | walled-off necrosis |
| ZES | Zollinger–Ellison syndrome |

# NORMAL RANGES

## Haematology

| | |
|---|---|
| haemoglobin | |
| males | g/L (130–180) |
| females | g/L (115–165) |
| red cell count | |
| males | × $10^{12}$/L (4.3–5.9) |
| females | × $10^{12}$/L (3.5–5.0) |
| haematocrit | |
| males | (0.40–0.52) |
| females | (0.36–0.47) |
| mean corpuscular volume | fL (80–96) |
| mean corpuscular haemoglobin | pg (28–32) |
| mean corpuscular haemoglobin concentration | g/dL (32–35) |
| white cell count | × $10^9$/L (4.0–11.0) |
| neutrophil count | × $10^9$/L (1.5–7.0) |
| lymphocyte count | × $10^9$/L (1.5–4.0) |
| monocyte count | × $10^9$/L (< 0.8) |
| eosinophil count | × $10^9$/L (0.04–0.40) |
| basophil count | × $10^9$/L (< 0.1) |
| platelet count | × $10^9$/L (150–400) |
| reticulocyte count | × $10^9$/L (25–85) |
| reticulocyte count | % (0.5–2.4) |
| CD4 count | × $10^6$/L (430–1690) |
| | |
| erythrocyte sedimentation rate | |
| under 50 years of age: | |
| males | mm/1st hour (< 15) |
| females | mm/1st hour (< 20) |
| over 50 years of age: | |
| males | mm/1st hour (< 20) |
| females | mm/1st hour (< 30) |
| | |
| plasma viscosity (25°C) | mPa/second (1.50–1.72) |

## Coagulation screen

| | |
|---|---|
| prothrombin time | seconds (11.5–15.5) |
| international normalized ratio | (< 1.4) |
| activated partial thromboplastin time | seconds (30–40) |
| thrombin time | seconds (15–19) |

Fibrinogen g/L (1.8–5.4)
bleeding time minutes (3.0–8.0)

### Coagulation factors

factors II, V, VII, VIII, IX, X, XI, XII IU/dL (50–150)
von Willebrand factor antigen IU/dL (45–150)
von Willebrand factor activity IU/dL (50–150)
protein C IU/dL (80–135)
protein S IU/dL (80–120)
Antithrombin IU/dL (80–120)
activated protein C resistance (2.12–4.00)
fibrin degradation products mg/L (< 100)
D-dimer mg/L (< 0.5)

### Haematinics

serum iron µmol/L (12–30)
serum iron-binding capacity µmol/L (45–75)
serum ferritin µg/L (15–300)
serum transferrin g/L (2.0–4.0)
serum vitamin $B_{12}$ ng/L (160–760)
serum folate µg/L (2.0–11.0)
red cell folate µg/L (160–640)
serum haptoglobin g/L (0.13–1.63)
zinc protoporphyrin:haemoglobin ratio µmol/mol haemoglobin (< 70)

Haemoglobinopathy screen:
    haemoglobin A % (> 95)
    haemoglobin $A_2$ % (2–3)
    haemoglobin F % (< 2)
    haemoglobin S % (0)
transferrin saturations % (20–50)
methaemoglobin % (< 1)

## Chemistry

### Blood

serum sodium mmol/L (137–144)
serum potassium mmol/L (3.5–4.9)
serum chloride mmol/L (95–107)
serum bicarbonate mmol/L (20–28)
anion gap mmol/L (12–16)
serum urea mmol/L (2.5–7.0)
serum creatinine µmol/L (60–110)
estimated glomerular filtration rate (MDRD) mL/minute (> 60)
serum corrected calcium mmol/L (2.20–2.60)
serum ionized calcium mmol/L (1.13–1.32)
serum phosphate mmol/L (0.8–1.4)
serum total protein g/L (61–76)
serum albumin g/L (37–49)

serum globulin                                          g/L (24–27)
serum total bilirubin                                   µmol/L (1–22)
serum conjugated bilirubin                              µmol/L (< 3.4)
serum alanine aminotransferase                          U/L (5–35)
serum aspartate aminotransferase                        U/L (1–31)
serum alkaline phosphatase                              U/L (45–105)
serum gamma glutamyl transferase
    males                            U/L (< 50)
    females                          U/L (4–35)
serum lactate dehydrogenase                             U/L (10–250)
serum acid phosphatase                                  U/L (2.6–6.2)
serum creatine kinase
    males                            U/L (24–195)
    females                          U/L (24–170)
serum creatine kinase MB fraction                       % (< 5)
serum troponin I                                        µg/L (< 0.1)
serum troponin T                                        µg/L (< 0.01)
fasting plasma glucose                                  mmol/L (3.0–6.0)
haemoglobin A1$_c$                                      % (4.0–6.0); mmol/mol (20–42)
serum $\alpha_1$-antitrypsin                            g/L (1.1–2.1)
serum copper                                            µmol/L (12–26)
serum caeruloplasmin                                    mg/L (200–350)
serum aluminium                                         µg/L (< 10)
blood lead                                              µmol/L (< 0.5)
serum magnesium                                         mmol/L (0.75–1.05)
serum zinc                                              µmol/L (6–25)
serum urate
    males                            mmol/L (0.23–0.46)
    females                          mmol/L (0.19–0.36)
plasma lactate                                          mmol/L (0.6–1.8)
plasma ammonia                                          µmol/L (12–55)
serum angiotensin-converting enzyme                     U/L (25–82)
plasma fructosamine                                     µmol/L (< 285)
serum amylase                                           U/L (60–180)
plasma osmolality                                       mosmol/kg (278–300)
plasma osmolar gap                                      mosmol (< 10)
thiopurine methyltransferase                            U/L (> 25)

## Urine

glomerular filtration rate                              mL/minute (70–140)
24-hour urinary total protein                           g (< 0.2)
24-hour urinary albumin                                 mg (< 30)
24-hour urinary creatinine                              mmol (9–18)
24-hour urinary calcium                                 mmol (2.5–7.5)
24-hour urinary copper                                  µmol (0.2–0.6)
24-hour urinary urate                                   mmol (< 3.6)
24-hour urinary oxalate                                 mmol (0.14–0.46)
24-hour urinary urobilinogen                            µmol (1.7–5.9)
24-hour urinary coproporphyrin                          nmol (< 300)

24-hour urinary uroporphyrin     nmol (6–24)
24-hour urinary δ-aminolevulinate     μmol (8–53)
24-hour urinary 5-hydroxyindoleacetic acid     μmol (10–47)
urinary osmolality     mosmol/kg (350–1000)
urinary osmolality after dehydration     mosmol/kg (> 750)
urinary albumin:creatinine ratio
    males     mg/mmol (< 2.5)
    females     mg/mmol (< 3.5)
urinary protein:creatinine ratio     mg/mmol (< 30)
urine microscopy:
    white cells     /μL (< 10)

### Faeces

stool weight (non-fasting)     g (< 200)
24-hour faecal nitrogen     mmol (70–140)
24-hour faecal urobilinogen     μmol (50–500)
24-hour faecal coproporphyrin     μmol (0.018–1.200)
faecal coproporphyrin     mmol/g dry weight (0.46)
24-hour faecal protoporphyrin     μmol (< 4)
faecal protoporphyrin     nmol/g dry weight (< 220)
faecal total porphyrin
    ether soluble     nmol/g dry weight (10–200)
    ether insoluble     nmol/g dry weight (< 24)
24-hour faecal fat (on normal diet)     mmol (< 20)
osmolality     mosmol/kg (300)
osmolar gap [300 − 2 × (faecal Na + K)]     mosmol/kg (< 100)
faecal calprotectin     μg/g (< 50)
faecal elastase     μg/g (> 200)
faecal $\alpha_1$-antitrypsin     μg/g (< 300)

### Body mass index

body mass index     kg/m$^2$ (18–25)

### Lipids and lipoproteins

serum cholesterol     mmol/L (< 5.2)
serum LDL cholesterol     mmol/L (< 3.36)
serum HDL cholesterol     mmol/L (> 1.55)
fasting serum triglycerides     mmol/L (0.45–1.69)

### Arterial blood gases, breathing air

$PO_2$     kPa (11.3–12.6)
$PCO_2$     kPa (4.7–6.0)
pH     (7.35–7.45)
$H^+$     nmol/L (35–45)
bicarbonate     mmol/L (21–29)
base excess     mmol/L (±2)
lactate     mmol/L (0.5–1.6)
carboxyhaemoglobin:
    non-smoker     % (< 2)
    smoker     % (3–10)

oxygen saturations      % (94–99)
methaemoglobin      % (< 1)

## Endocrinology

### Adrenal steroids (blood)

plasma renin activity
    (after 30 minutes supine)      pmol/mL/hour (1.1–2.7)
    (after 30 minutes upright)      pmol/mL/hour (3.0–4.3)

plasma aldosterone (normal diet)
    (after 30 minutes supine)      pmol/L (135–400)
    (after 4 hours upright)      pmol/L (330–830)
plasma aldosterone:renin ratio      (< 25)
plasma angiotensin II      pmol/L (5–35)

serum cortisol (09.00 hours)      nmol/L (200–700)
serum cortisol (22.00 hours)      nmol/L (50–250)

overnight dexamethasone suppression test (after 1 mg dexamethasone):
    serum cortisol      nmol/L (< 50)

low-dose dexamethasone suppression test (2 mg/day for 48 hours):
    serum cortisol      nmol/L (< 50)

high-dose dexamethasone suppression test (8 mg/day for 48 hours):
    serum cortisol      nmol/L (should suppress to < 50%
    of day 0 value)

short tetracosactide (Synacthen®) test (250 micrograms):
    serum cortisol (30 minutes after tetracosactide)      nmol/L (> 550)

plasma 11-deoxycortisol      nmol/L (24–46)
serum dehydroepiandrosterone (09.00 hours)      nmol/L (7–31)
serum dehydroepiandrosterone sulphate
    males      μmol/L (2–10)
    females      μmol/L (3–12)
serum androstenedione
    males      nmol/L (1.6–8.4)
    females      nmol/L (0.6–8.8)
    post-menopausal      nmol/L (0.9–6.8)
serum 17-hydroxyprogesterone
    males      nmol/L (1–10)
    females
        follicular      nmol/L (1–10)
        luteal      nmol/L (10–20)
serum oestradiol
    males      pmol/L (< 180)
    females
        post-menopausal      pmol/L (< 100)
        follicular      pmol/L (200–400)
        mid-cycle      pmol/L (400–1200)
        luteal      pmol/L (400–1000)

serum progesterone
    males                                                nmol/L (< 6)
    females
        follicular                        nmol/L (< 10)
        luteal                               nmol/L (> 30)
serum testosterone
    males                                                nmol/L (9–35)
    females                                      nmol/L (0.5–3.0)
serum dihydrotestosterone
    males                                                nmol/L (1.0–2.6)
    females                                      nmol/L (0.3–9.3)
serum sex hormone binding protein
    males                                                nmol/L (10–62)
    females                                      nmol/L (40–137)

### Adrenal steroids (urine)

24-hour urinary aldosterone                     nmol (14–53)
24-hour urinary free cortisol                  nmol (55–250)

### Pancreatic and gut hormones

oral glucose tolerance test (75 g)
    2-hour plasma glucose                mmol/L (< 7.8)
plasma gastrin                                  pmol/L (< 55)
plasma or serum insulin
    overnight fasting after hypoglycaemia     pmol/L (< 186)
    (plasma glucose < 2.2 mmol/L)          pmol/L (< 21)
serum C-peptide                              pmol/L (180–360)
plasma glucagon                              pmol/L (< 50)
plasma pancreatic polypeptide           pmol/L (< 300)
plasma vasoactive intestinal polypeptide   pmol/L (< 30)

### Anterior pituitary hormones

plasma adrenocorticotropic hormone (09.00 hours)     pmol/L (< 18)
plasma follicle-stimulating hormone
    males                                           U/L (1.0–7.0)
    females
        follicular                       U/L (2.5–10.0)
        mid-cycle                     U/L (25–70)
        luteal                          U/L (0.32–2.10)
        post-menopausal           U/L (> 30)

plasma growth hormone
    basal, fasting and between pulses        μg/L (< 0.4)
    2 hours after glucose tolerance test (75 g)   μg/L (< 1)

insulin-induced hypoglycaemia (blood glucose < 2.2 mmol/L):
    plasma growth hormone              μg/L (> 3)
    serum cortisol                         nmol/L (> 580)

plasma luteinizing hormone
    males                                                U/L (1.0–10.0)
    females
        follicular                         U/L (2.5–10.0)
        mid-cycle                      U/L (25–70)
        luteal                             U/L (1.0–13.0)
        post-menopausal        U/L (> 30)
plasma prolactin                         mU/L (< 360)
plasma thyroid-stimulating hormone     mU/L (0.4–5.0)

### Posterior pituitary hormones

plasma antidiuretic hormone             pmol/L (0.9–4.6)

### Thyroid hormones

plasma thyroid-binding globulin         mg/L (13–28)
plasma T4                               nmol/L (58–174)
plasma free T4                       pmol/L (10.0–22.0)
plasma T3                               nmol/L (1.07–3.18)
plasma free T3                       pmol/L (3.0–7.0)

serum thyroid-stimulating hormone receptor antibodies U/L (< 7)
serum anti-thyroid peroxidase antibodies     IU/mL (< 50)
serum thyroid-receptor antibodies       U/L (< 10)
technetium-99m scan of thyroid (20-minute uptake)   % (0.4–3.0)

### Catecholamines (blood)

(Plasma recumbent with venous catheter in place for 30 minutes before collection of sample)
plasma adrenaline                     nmol/L (0.03–1.31)
plasma noradrenaline                nmol/L (0.47–4.14)

### Catecholamines (urine)

24-hour urinary vanillylmandelic acid      μmol (5–35)
24-hour urinary dopamine            nmol (< 3100)
24-hour urinary adrenaline           nmol (< 144)
24-hour urinary noradrenaline        nmol (< 570)

### Others

plasma parathyroid hormone           pmol/L (0.9–5.4)
plasma calcitonin                     pmol/L (< 27)
serum cholecalciferol (vitamin D3)     nmol/L (60–105)
serum 25-OH-cholecalciferol         nmol/L (45–90)
serum 1,25-(OH)2-cholecalciferol       pmol/L (43–149)
serum insulin-like growth factor 1
    13–20 years                  nmol/L (9.3–56.0)
    21–40 years                  nmol/L (7.5–37.3)
    41–60 years                  nmol/L (5.6–23.3)
    > 60 years                   nmol/L (3.3–23.3)
serum IGF1:IGF2 ratio                (< 10)

## *Immunology/Rheumatology*

| | |
|---|---|
| serum complement C3 | mg/dL (65–190) |
| serum complement C4 | mg/dL (15–50) |
| total serum haemolytic complement activity CH50 | U/L (150–250) |
| serum C-reactive protein | mg/L (< 10) |
| serum immunoglobulin G | g/L (6.0–13.0) |
| serum immunoglobulin A | g/L (0.8–3.0) |
| serum immunoglobulin M | g/L (0.4–2.5) |
| serum immunoglobulin E | kU/L (< 120) |
| serum immunoglobulin D | mg/L (20–120) |
| serum immunoglobulin G4 | g/L (0.08–1.30) |
| serum β2-microglobulin | mg/L (< 3) |
| serum mast cell tryptase (1 hour post-reaction) | μg/L (2–14) |

## *Autoantibodies*

| | |
|---|---|
| anti-acetylcholine-receptor antibodies | |
| anti-adrenal antibodies | (negative at 1:10 dilution) |
| anticentromere antibodies | (negative at 1:40 dilution) |
| anticardiolipin antibodies: | |
|     immunoglobulin G | U/mL (< 23) |
|     immunoglobulin M | U/mL (< 11) |
| anti-cyclic citrullinated peptide antibodies | |
| anti-double-stranded DNA antibodies (ELISA) | U/mL (< 73) |
| anti-glomerular basement membrane antibodies | |
| anti-lactoferrin antibodies | |
| anti-neutrophil cytoplasmic antibodies: | |
|     c-ANCA | |
|     p-ANCA | |
|     PR3-ANCA | U/mL (< 10) |
|     MPO-ANCA | U/mL (< 10) |
| antinuclear antibodies | (negative at 1:20 dilution) |
| extractable nuclear antigen | |
| gastric parietal cell antibodies | (negative at 1:20 dilution) |
| intrinsic factor antibodies | |
| interstitial cells of testis antibodies | (negative at 1:10 dilution) |
| anti-Jo-1 antibodies | |
| anti-La antibodies | |
| antimitochondrial antibodies | (negative at 1:20 dilution) |
| anti-RNP antibodies | |
| anti-Scl-70 antibodies | |
| anti-Ro antibodies | |
| anti-skeletal muscle antibodies | (negative at 1:60 dilution) |
| anti-Sm antibodies | |
| anti-smooth muscle antibodies | (negative at 1:20 dilution) |
| anti-thyroid colloid and microsomal antibodies | (negative at 1:10 dilution) |
| anti-gliadin antibodies | IU/L (< 10) |
| anti-endomysial antibodies | |

anti-tissue transglutaminase antibodies | U/mL (< 15)
rheumatoid factor | kIU/L (< 30)
antistreptolysin titre | IU/mL (< 200)

## Hepatitis virus serology

HBs Ag | IU/mL (lower detection limit 50)
HBV DNA | IU/mL (lower detection limit 250)
Hepatitis B genotype | A–H
HCV RNA | IU/mL (lower detection limit 15)
Hepatitis C genotype | 1–6

### *Tumour markers*

serum α-fetoprotein | kU/L (< 10)
serum carcinoembryonic antigen | µg/L (< 10)
serum neuron-specific enolase | µg/L (< 12)
serum prostate-specific antigen
    males < 40 years of age | µg/L (< 2)
    males > 40 years of age | µg/L (< 4)
serum β-human chorionic gonadotropin | U/L (< 5)
serum CA 125 | U/mL (< 35)
serum CA 19–9 | U/mL (< 33)

### *Viral loads*

cytomegalovirus viral load | copies/mL (lower detection limit 400)
Epstein–Barr viral load | copies/mL (lower detection limit 250)
hepatitis B viral load | IU/mL (lower detection limit 250)
hepatitis C viral load | IU/mL (lower detection limit 15)
HIV viral load | copies/mL (lower detection limit 40)
human herpesvirus-6 viral load | copies/mL (lower detection limit 50)
human herpesvirus-8 viral load | copies/mL (lower detection limit 50)

### *Therapeutic drug concentrations*

plasma carbamazepine | µmol/L (34–51)
blood ciclosporin | nmol/L (100–150)
blood tacrolimus
    ≤12 months following transplant | nmol/L (8–12)
    > 12 months following transplant | nmol/L (5–10)
plasma digoxin (taken at least 6 hours post-dose) | nmol/L (1.0–2.0)
serum gentamicin (peak) | mg/L (5–7)
    pre-dose | mg/L (< 1)
    1 hour post-dose | mg/L (3–5)
serum vancomycin (trough) | mg/L (10–15)
serum lithium | mmol/L (0.5–1.2)
serum phenobarbital | µmol/L (65–172)
serum phenytoin | µmol/L (40–80)
serum primidone | µmol/L (23–55)
plasma theophylline | µmol/L (55–110)

### Cerebrospinal fluid

| | |
|---|---|
| opening pressure | mmH$_2$O (50–180) |
| total protein | g/L (0.15–0.45) |
| albumin | g/L (0.066–0.442) |
| chloride | mmol/L (116–122) |
| glucose | mmol/L (3.3–4.4) |
| lactate | mmol/L (1.0–2.0) |
| cell count | /µL (≤5) |
|     white cell count | /µL (≤5) |
|     red cell count | /µL (0) |
| lymphocyte count | /µL (≤3.5) |
| neutrophil count | /µL (0) |
| immunoglobulin G:albumin ratio | (≤0.26) |
| immunoglobulin index | (≤0.88) |

### Synovial fluid

| | |
|---|---|
| white cell count | /mL (< 200) |

### Pulmonary function

| | |
|---|---|
| transfer factor for CO (TLCO) | % (80–120) mmol/minute/kPa % (100) |
| transfer coefficient (KCO) | mmol/minute/kPa |

### Cardiac pressures

| | |
|---|---|
| mean arterial pressure | mmHg (96) |
| mean right atrial pressure | mmHg (3) |
| mean pulmonary arterial pressure | mmHg (15) |
| mean pulmonary arterial wedge pressure | mmHg (9) L/min (5) |
| mean cardiac output | |

### Hepatic venous pressures

| | |
|---|---|
| portal venous pressure | mmHg (4–8) |
| hepatic venous pressure | mmHg (2–4) |
| hepatic venous pressure gradient | mmHg (< 5) |

### ECG measurements

| | |
|---|---|
| PR interval | ms (120–200) |
| QRS complex | ms (40–120) |

### Ascites

white cell count < 250 cells/mm$^3$

# chapter 1

# GASTROINTESTINAL HAEMORRHAGE

## QUESTIONS

1. **A 52-year-old man presented to the emergency department reporting black, tarry stools. He had a history of gastric bypass surgery seven years ago for obesity but no other comorbidities. He had been using ibuprofen for back pain. Pulse was 110 beats per minute and blood pressure 100/ 58 mmHg.**

   Investigations:

   | | |
   |---|---|
   | Haemoglobin | 95 g/L |
   | Mean corpuscular volume (MCV) | 78 fL |
   | Platelet count | $395 \times 10^9$/L |
   | Serum urea | 14 mmol/L |
   | Serum creatinine | 80 µmol/L |
   | Prothrombin time | 13 seconds |

   **Which of these contributes to the Glasgow-Blatchford score (GBS)?**

   A. Platelet count

   B. Presentation with melaena

   C. Previous gastric bypass surgery

   D. Prothrombin time

   E. Use of non-steroidal anti-inflammatory drugs (NSAIDs)

*Best of Five MCQs for the European Specialty Examination in Gastroenterology and Hepatology.* Thomas Marjot, Colleen G C McGregor, Tim Ambrose, Aminda N De Silva, Jeremy Cobbold, and Simon Travis, Oxford University Press (2021). © Oxford University Press.
DOI: 10.1093/oso/9780198834373.003.0001

2.  **A 23-year-old woman presented after her housemate noticed blood-stained vomit in the bathroom. She had been drinking heavily the night before but was no longer intoxicated. She reported a few episodes of loose, brown stools and nausea, but was able to tolerate oral fluids. Physical examination was unremarkable. She was afebrile with blood pressure of 122/74 mmHg and pulse 86 beats per minute.**

    Investigations:

    | | |
    |---|---|
    | Haemoglobin | 133 g/L |
    | Platelet count | 289 × 10⁹/L |
    | Serum sodium | 143 mmol/L |
    | Serum potassium | 3.6 mmol/L |
    | Serum urea | 5.4 mmol/L |
    | Serum creatinine | 115 µmol/L |

    ### What is the most appropriate management?

    A.  Admit for overnight observation

    B.  Discharge with outpatient gastroscopy

    C.  Intravenous fluids and anti-emetic

    D.  Intravenous proton pump inhibitor (PPI) infusion

    E.  Urgent inpatient gastroscopy

3.  **A 42-year-old man presented to the emergency department with haematemesis and melaena. He had a past medical history of gout and had recently increased his dose of ibuprofen.**

    Investigations:
    　　Gastroscopy　　　　　　　　　　　See Fig. 1.1

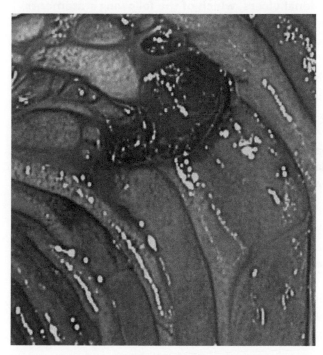

**Fig. 1.1** Endoscopic image of the second part of the duodenum. See also Plate I

**Which Forrest classification best describes this lesion?**

A.  Ia

B.  Ib

C.  IIa

D.  IIc

E.  III

4.  **A 45-year-old man presented with melaena. He smoked 20 cigarettes per day. He was otherwise fit and well, and not taking any regular medication.**

    Investigations:

    Gastroscopy          Duodenal ulcer with a clean base (Forrest III)

    **With regard to duodenal ulcers, which of the following statements is true?**

    A.  Duodenal ulcers are an infrequent cause of gastrointestinal bleeding
    B.  Gastric ulcers have a higher risk of perforation
    C.  PPI infusion given before endoscopy reduces risk of re-bleeding
    D.  Routine follow-up gastroscopy is required because of high risk of malignancy
    E.  Most duodenal ulcers are associated with *Helicobacter pylori*

5.  **A 63-year-old woman underwent urgent gastroscopy for weight loss, dyspepsia, and melaena. She had a history of type 2 diabetes but with good performance status.**

    Investigations:

    | | |
    |---|---|
    | Haemoglobin | 54 g/L |
    | Gastroscopy | Partially obstructing pyloric tumour with active diffuse bleeding |
    | Staging computed tomography (CT) | Not yet performed |

    **How should the bleeding be controlled?**

    A.  Adrenaline injection alone
    B.  Adrenaline injection with placement of multiple clips
    C.  Bipolar coagulation
    D.  Haemostatic powder
    E.  Pyloric stent placement

6. **A 73-year-old man with a history of cirrhosis presented with large-volume haematemesis. Emergency endoscopy revealed three columns of Grade 3 oesophageal varices with active bleeding. Despite band ligation, the patient continued to bleed and was not stable for transfer to his local hepatology unit for consideration of porto-systemic shunting.**

   **Which one of the following statements about management of refractory variceal bleeding is true?**

   A. Balloon tamponade can be safely used for three days

   B. Patients must be kept nil by mouth once a self-expanding metal stent (SEMS) has been inserted and the bleeding controlled

   C. SEMS is as effective and safer than balloon tamponade

   D. SEMS can be useful for managing refractory gastric variceal bleeding

   E. SEMS can only be inserted under direct endoscopic guidance

7. **A 54-year-old man with Hepatitis C virus-related cirrhosis presented with haematemesis and syncope. Following resuscitation, he underwent urgent gastroscopy.**

   Investigations:

   Gastroscopy          Two columns of Grade 2 oesophageal varices, not bleeding, no red spots. Large varix extending from oesophagus into fundus and towards the greater curvature with active bleeding

   **What is the most appropriate next management step?**

   A. Adrenaline injection + clip placement

   B. Cyanoacrylate injection

   C. Insertion of a Sengstaken-Blakemore tube

   D. Transjugular intrahepatic porto-systemic shunt (TIPSS)

   E. Variceal band ligation

8. **A 69-year-old man presented with breathlessness and a one-week history of melaena. He had a background of a metallic mitral valve replacement and was on warfarin. Blood pressure was 110/65 mmHg with pulse 88 bpm. He had a similar presentation two months previously with a normal gastroscopy. Outpatient colonoscopy to the caecum showed minor sigmoid diverticulosis but no cause of bleeding was found. Bowel preparation was excellent.**

Investigations:

| | |
|---|---|
| Haemoglobin | 75 g/L |
| MCV | 69 fL |
| Serum urea | 7.6 mmol/L |
| Serum creatinine | 70 µmol/L |
| INR | 3.2 |
| Repeat gastroscopy | Normal |

**What is the next most appropriate investigation?**

A. CT angiogram

B. CT colonoscopy

C. Magnetic resonance enterography

D. Red cell scintigraphy

E. Video capsule endoscopy (VCE)

9. **An 83-year-old woman presented with symptomatic anaemia. Eight units of red blood cells had been transfused in the past two months. Gastroscopy was normal but colonoscopy revealed bleeding angiodysplasia in her ascending colon, which was treated with argon plasma coagulation.**

**Which of the following investigations would be most important to arrange?**

A. Echocardiogram

B. Factor VIII levels

C. Hepatic elastography

D. HIV test

E. Renal ultrasound

10. **An 81-year-old man presented with large-volume rectal bleeding in the absence of haematemesis. He had a past history of diverticular disease. On examination, he was tender in the left iliac fossa. Dark red blood with clots were identified on digital rectal examination. No melaena was seen. He received 2 litres of intravenous crystalloid and a transfusion of 2 units of red blood cells.**

Investigations (after initial resuscitation):
Heart rate             106 bpm
Blood pressure         99/64 mmHg

**What is the most appropriate next investigation?**

A. Abdominal radiograph

B. Colonoscopy

C. CT angiography

D. Gastroscopy

E. Magnetic resonance angiography

11. **A 19-year-old man presented with recurrent melaena and abdominal pain. Previous gastroscopies and colonoscopies had been normal. His heart rate was 128 bpm and blood pressure 114/58 mmHg.**

Investigations:

CT mesenteric          Aberrant branch of the superior mesenteric artery and active
angiography            contrast extravasation 40 cm upstream of the ileocaecal valve

**Regarding the likely diagnosis, which of the following is true?**

A. Ectopic pancreatic tissue is most commonly identified

B. Nuclear medicine scanning with 99m technetium pertechnetate can be diagnostic

C. Symptomatic disease can usually be managed medically

D. These lesions are usually found in the middle third of the ileum

E. This is a rare congenital malformation with a prevalence of less than 0.01%

12. **An 83-year-old man presented with persistent rectal bleeding and constipation. He had a past medical history of hypertension, type 2 diabetes, atrial fibrillation (on apixaban), and prostate cancer for which he had had external beam radiotherapy two years before.**

    Investigations:

    | | |
    |---|---|
    | Haemoglobin | 129 g/L |
    | Flexible sigmoidoscopy | Pale mucosa with multiple telangiectasia and contact bleeding extending to 13 cm from the anal verge |

    ## What would be your initial management?

    A. Argon plasma coagulation

    B. Optimize bowel function and stool consistency

    C. Rectal formalin

    D. Stop apixaban

    E. Sucralfate enemas

## 1. B. Presentation with melaena

- The GBS is a pre-endoscopy scoring system used to stratify the need for endoscopic intervention as well as predict death in patients presenting with gastrointestinal bleeding
- It is better at predicting need for endoscopic intervention compared with the admission Rockall score

GBS was developed to identify patients presenting with upper gastrointestinal tract bleeding that would require intervention. It incorporates simple clinical and laboratory parameters to identify low-risk patients. In a large study of over 3,000 participants, patients scoring ≤1 on the GBS had a 0.4% mortality rate and 1.4% required endoscopic intervention. The score comprises urea, blood pressure, haemoglobin, pulse, syncope, melaena, history of liver disease, and cardiac failure.

Blatchford O, Murray WR, Blatchford M. A risk score to predict need for treatment for upper gastrointestinal haemorrhage. *Lancet*. 2000;356(9238):1318–1321.

## 2. B. Discharge with outpatient gastroscopy

- Patients with a GBS of ≤1 should be considered for early discharge.

The GBS (see Table 1.1) is a validated pre-endoscopic risk score for predicting the need for intervention in upper gastrointestinal bleeding. Very low-risk patients are unlikely to require intervention and thus are suitable for consideration of early discharge. Very low risk was originally defined in guidance from the United Kingdom's National Institute for Health and Care Excellence as a score of 0. However, more recent European Society of Gastrointestinal Endoscopy guidance recommends ≤1. A 2017 comparison study of >3,000 patients with gastrointestinal bleeding found the GBS to be the most accurate for predicting the need for hospital-based intervention and mortality. Other risk scores include Rockall (pre-endoscopy and full), AIMS65, and Progetto Nazionale Emorragia Digestiva scores. The current case likely has a Mallory-Weiss tear and a GBS of 0, and can therefore be discharged.

Gralnek IM, Dumonceau JM, Kuipers EJ et al. Diagnosis and management of nonvariceal upper gastrointestinal hemorrhage: European Society of Gastrointestinal Endoscopy (ESGE) Guideline. *Endoscopy*. 2015 Oct;47(10):a1–46. doi: 10.1055/s-0034-1393172.

*Best of Five MCQs for the European Specialty Examination in Gastroenterology and Hepatology.* Thomas Marjot, Colleen G C McGregor, Tim Ambrose, Aminda N De Silva, Jeremy Cobbold, and Simon Travis, Oxford University Press (2021). © Oxford University Press. DOI: 10.1093/oso/9780198834373.003.0001

**Table 1.1** The Glasgow-Blatchford score

| Parameter (at presentation) | Score |
| --- | --- |
| **Urea (mmol/L)** | |
| 6.5–7.9 | 2 |
| 8.0–9.9 | 3 |
| 10.0–24.9 | 4 |
| ≥ 25.0 | 6 |
| **Haemoglobin (g/L)** | |
| Men | |
| 120–129 | 1 |
| 100–119 | 3 |
| <100 | 6 |
| Women | |
| 100–119 | 1 |
| <100 | 6 |
| **Systolic blood pressure (mmHg)** | |
| 100–109 | 1 |
| 90–99 | 2 |
| <90 | 3 |
| **Other** | |
| Pulse ≥ 100 bpm | 1 |
| Melaena | 1 |
| Syncope | 2 |
| Hepatic disease | 2 |
| Cardiac failure | 2 |

Stanley AJ, Laine L, Dalton HR et al. Comparison of risk scoring systems for patients presenting with upper gastrointestinal bleeding: international multicentre prospective study. *BMJ*. 2017;356:i6432. Doi:10.1136/bmj.i6432.

## 3. B. Ib

- The Forrest classification grades peptic ulcer haemorrhage in the upper gastrointestinal tract
- It can predict risk of re-bleeding and guide use of endoscopic therapy

The image shows a visible vessel that is oozing blood in the duodenum and corresponds to Forrest classification Ib. Description of peptic ulcers using this classification is helpful for predicting the risk of re-bleeding (see Table 1.2) and the treatment strategy. Other endoscopic features predicting adverse outcomes or endoscopic failure include large ulcers (>2 cm), a large non-bleeding visible vessel, blood in the gastric lumen, a posterior duodenal wall ulcer, and a lesser curvature gastric ulcer.

Forrest Ia, Ib, and IIa lesions require dual endoscopic therapy with adrenaline and a second haemostatic technique (thermal, mechanical, etc.) followed by high-dose intravenous infusion of a PPI for 72 hours. Forrest IIb lesions with an adherent clot may be managed either by removal of the clot and dual endoscopic therapy followed by intravenous PPI therapy for 72 hours, or without clot removal and medical management alone with high-dose intravenous PPI infusion for 72 hours. Forrest IIc and III lesions require medical therapy alone with oral PPI therapy. All patients should be considered for eradication of *Helicobacter pylori*.

**Table 1.2** The Forrest classification

| Forrest classification | Bleeding | Lesion description | Risk of re-bleeding (%) |
|---|---|---|---|
| Ia | Acute haemorrhage | Spurting haemorrhage | 23.6 |
| Ib | | Oozing haemorrhage | 19.0 |
| IIa | Signs of recent haemorrhage | Visible vessel | 19.5 |
| IIb | | Adherent clot | 17.0 |
| IIc | | Haematin on ulcer base | 9.7 |
| III | Lesions without active bleeding | Lesions without signs of recent haemorrhage | 1.1 |

Adapted from Heldwein W et al. Is the Forrest classification a useful tool for planning endoscopic therapy of bleeding peptic ulcers? *Endoscopy*. 1989;21(6):258–262 with permission.
Gralnek IM, Dumonceau JM, Kuipers EJ et al. Diagnosis and management of nonvariceal upper gastrointestinal haemorrhage: European Society of Gastrointestinal Endoscopy (ESGE) guideline. *Endoscopy*. 2015;47:a1–46. Doi:10.1055/s-0034-1393172.

### 4. E. Most duodenal ulcers are associated with *Helicobacter pylori*

- Fifty to seventy-five per cent of peptic ulcers are associated with *Helicobacter pylori*
- The risk of malignancy in duodenal ulcers is low; therefore, routine histology and follow-up endoscopy are not recommended
- Pre-endoscopy PPI use for upper gastrointestinal bleeding does not reduce mortality or risk of re-bleeding

Duodenal ulcers are the most common cause of gastrointestinal haemorrhage. Risk factors include *Helicobacter pylori*, smoking, use of NSAIDS, and alcohol excess. Unlike duodenal ulcers, gastric ulcers are associated with an increased risk of malignancy, and therefore routine biopsy and follow-up endoscopy after 8–12 weeks of acid suppression therapy is recommended. Routine administration of PPIs in patients presenting with gastrointestinal bleeding does not reduce mortality, transfusion requirements, or risk of re-bleeding. Continuous PPI infusion in selected patients following endoscopic therapy does have an impact on re-bleeding rates or mortality.

Lau JY, Leung WK, Wu JC, et al. Omeprazole before endoscopy in patients with gastrointestinal bleeding. *N Engl J Med*. 2007;356(16):1631–1640.

### 5. D. Haemostatic powder

- Haemostatic powder (e.g. Hemospray–Cook Medical, USA) is effective in managing diffuse tumour bleeding
- Good performance status, non-end-stage cancer, and definitive haemostatic therapy are predictors of six-month survival in gastric cancer bleeding

Management of diffuse tumour bleeding is challenging. The usual modalities of adrenaline, clip placement, and bipolar coagulation are rarely successful because there is no single target. Haemostatic powder or argon plasma coagulation may be successful. However, the equipment for the latter may not be widely available. External beam radiotherapy has a well-defined role in the palliative phase of gastric cancer bleeding but can take some days to take effect. Placement of a pyloric stent is not indicated here because the patient is not completely obstructed and this may affect plans for definitive surgery if she is shown to have localized disease.

Pittayanon R, Rerknimitr R, Barkun A. Prognostic factors affecting outcomes in patients with malignant GI bleeding treated with a novel endoscopically delivered hemostatic powder. *Gastrointest Endosc.* 2018;87(4):994–1002. Doi:10.1016/j.gie.2017.11.013.

## 6. C. SEMS is as effective and safer than balloon tamponade

- The Baveno VI consensus report states that a SEMS is as effective and safer than balloon tamponade
- Stents can be left in situ for up to one week pending definitive management of portal hypertension
- A key benefit is that patients can resume oral intake once a SEMS is inserted and the bleeding controlled

A SEMS (e.g. Danis stent, ELLA CS) can be used to manage refractory bleeding from oesophageal varices and may be inserted using endoscopic, radiological, or no guidance. Using this technology avoids the major risk of balloon tamponade, which is perforation secondary to inflation of the gastric balloon in the oesophagus. A SEMS may be left in situ for up to one week but must be removed whether or not definitive management is planned (e.g. TIPSS or liver transplantation). The use of stents allows a focus on oral nutrition alongside management of portal hypertension, and critically does not require the patient to be maintained under general anaesthesia. In contrast, balloon tamponade should only be used for 24–36 hours and does not allow for enteral nutrition. Also, the patient must be cared for in an intensive care unit with tracheal intubation.

National Institute for Health and Care Excellence. Danis stent for acute oesophageal variceal bleeds (Medtech innovation briefing [MIB185]). Available at: https://www.nice.org.uk/advice/mib185/chapter/ Summary Published June 2019. Accessed 11 September 2020.

## 7. B. Cyanoacrylate injection

- Band ligation is recommended for oesophageal varices and gastro-oesophageal varices type 1 (GOV-1)
- Sclerotherapy, usually with cyanoacrylate, is recommended for gastro-oesophageal varices type 2 (GOV-2) and isolated gastric varices (IGV)

Endoscopic management of gastric varices is guided by the Sarin classification (see Table 1.3). GOV-1 should be treated as for oesophageal varices with band ligation. GOV-2 and IGV should be treated with sclerotherapy, most commonly using cyanoacrylate although thrombin is an alternative. If control of bleeding cannot be achieved endoscopically, then insertion of a Sengstaken-Blakemore tube or urgent TIPSS should be considered.

**Table 1.3** Sarin classification of gastric varices

| Variceal type | Description |
| --- | --- |
| GOV-1 | Extend from oesophagus along lesser curvature |
| GOV-2 | Extend from oesophagus into fundus, towards greater curvature |
| IGV-1 | Isolated varices in fundus |
| IGV-2 | Isolated varices elsewhere in stomach |

Tripathi D, Stanley AJ, Hayes PC et al. UK guidelines on the management of variceal haemorrhage in cirrhotic patients. *Gut.* 2015;64(11):1680–1704. Doi:10.1136/gutjnl-2015-309262.

## 8.  E. Video capsule endoscopy

- Obscure (overt or occult) gastrointestinal bleeding describes bleeding that persists or recurs after endoscopic evaluation of the upper and lower gastrointestinal tract fails to identify a cause
- VCE is recommended as the first-line investigation and should ideally be performed within 14 days of bleeding

Obscure gastrointestinal bleeding accounts for 5% of all cases of gastrointestinal bleeding. Commonly arising from the small intestine, aetiologies include angioectasia, NSAID-related enteropathy, small bowel tumours, and Crohn's disease. Small bowel vascular lesions are the most common aetiology in overt bleeding. VCE is recommended as the first-line investigation for small bowel examination in patients with obscure bleeding. It has a diagnostic yield of up to 60% in this patient group and is less invasive than double balloon enteroscopy.

A standard capsule measures 26 × 11 mm and transmits images via radiofrequency to a recording device worn by the patient. Unless bowel obstruction is clinically suspected, cross-sectional imaging or a patency capsule check is not required. The diagnostic yield is highest if the study is performed within 14 days of a bleeding episode. A normal VCE is a good negative predictor for re-bleeding and need for further blood transfusions.

Pennazio M, Spada C, Eliakim R et al. Small-bowel capsule endoscopy and device-assisted enteroscopy for diagnosis and treatment of small-bowel disorders: ESGE clinical guideline. *Endoscopy*. 2015;47(4):352–376. Doi:10.1055/s-0034-1391855.

## 9.  A. Echocardiogram

- Angiodysplasia is the most common cause of bleeding from the small bowel and can be associated with aortic stenosis, particularly in elderly patients
- Gastrointestinal angiodysplasia is also associated with end-stage renal disease, von Willebrand disease, ventricular assist devices, and hereditary haemorrhagic telangiectasia
- Multiple endoscopic and systemic treatment options exist with variable rates of success and high rates of recurrence

The association of aortic stenosis, angiodysplasia, and an acquired coagulopathy (Heyde's syndrome) is well recognized in elderly patients although the aetiology is not completely understood. Angiodysplasia is commonly seen in the ascending colon/caecum but may also be found in the small intestine. Other conditions associated with gastrointestinal angiodysplasia include end-stage renal disease, von Willebrand disease, ventricular assist devices, and hereditary conditions such as hereditary haemorrhagic telangiectasia (Osler-Weber-Rendu syndrome).

Non-bleeding and non-symptomatic lesions do not require therapy. However, in the presence of active bleeding or transfusion dependency, treatment should be considered. Endoscopic management options include argon plasma coagulation, thermocoagulation, and mechanical haemostasis (clips and band ligation). In patients with persistent bleeding despite repeated endoscopic treatment, systemic therapy with hormone therapy, thalidomide, octreotide, and bevacizumab have been tried with variable success. Angiography with embolization or surgery may be required.

Gerson LB, Fidler JL, Cave DR et al. ACG clinical guideline: diagnosis and management of small bowel bleeding. *Am J Gastroenterol*. 2015;110(9):1265–87. Doi:10.1038/ajg.2015.246.

## 10. C. CT angiography

- CT angiography should be offered to patients with lower gastrointestinal bleeding (LGIB) with haemodynamic instability after initial resuscitation and/or signs of active bleeding

LGIB presents a diagnostic challenge, with up to 23% of hospitalized patients being discharged without a diagnosis. The most common cause in the United Kingdom is diverticular disease, followed by benign anorectal pathology such as haemorrhoids, anal ulcers, and fissures. In-hospital mortality ranges from 3.4% up to 20% for those with a blood transfusion requirement of four or more units.

Patients who remain haemodynamically unstable after initial resuscitation, or who show signs of active bleeding, should be offered CT angiography prior to targeted endoscopic or radiological therapy. If no source is identified, the patient should proceed to gastroscopy to exclude upper gastrointestinal bleeding with fast transit. Surgery should only be considered in exceptional cases, usually when radiological and/or endoscopic therapy has failed.

Haemodynamic instability may be quantified using the shock index (heart rate ÷ systolic blood pressure), with a shock index of ≥1 classed as an unstable bleed. An index of <1 is classed as a stable bleed and is unlikely to be associated with active bleeding. Stable patients with major LGIB should have inpatient colonoscopy on the next available list, and patients with minor self-terminating LGIB may be considered for discharge with urgent outpatient investigation.

Oakland K, Chadwick G, East JE et al. Diagnosis and management of acute lower gastrointestinal bleeding: guidelines from the British Society of Gastroenterology. *Gut.* 2019;68(5):776–89. Doi:10.1136/gutjnl-2018-317807.

## 11. B. Nuclear medicine scanning with 99m technetium pertechnetate can be diagnostic

- Meckel's diverticulum is the most common congenital malformation of the gut and represents a persistent remnant of the omphalomesenteric duct
- Bleeding occurs due to a rich blood supply from the vitelline artery and the presence of acid produced by ectopic gastric mucosa
- Surgery is usually required for symptomatic disease

Meckel's diverticulum is a common malformation of the intestine, usually located within 61 cm (2 feet) of the ileocaecal valve. The prevalence is between 0.3% and 2.9% of the general population and higher in males. The presence of ectopic tissue, usually gastric but occasionally pancreatic, is associated with symptoms. Gastrointestinal bleeding may occur secondary to acid secretion from the ectopic gastric mucosa, causing ulceration of the surrounding small bowel mucosa combined with the rich blood supply to the diverticulum. The vitelline artery is a branch of the superior mesenteric artery. Intestinal obstruction and acute abdominal pain are other recognized presentations.

The diagnosis may be made following histopathological examination of a surgical resection specimen in the context of intestinal obstruction. Imaging modalities such as ultrasound, CT, and angiography have low sensitivity and specificity but a visible vitelline artery is pathognomonic. Nuclear scans with 99m technetium pertechnetate can be diagnostic but require functional ectopic gastric mucosa within the diverticulum. A symptomatic Meckel's diverticulum requires surgical resection.

Hansen CC, Søreide K. Systematic review of epidemiology, presentation, and management of Meckel's diverticulum in the 21st century. *Medicine (Baltimore).* 2018;97(35):e12154. Doi:10.1097/MD.0000000000012154.

## 12.  B. Optimize bowel function and stool consistency

- Fifty per cent of patients will experience some degree of rectal bleeding after pelvic radiotherapy
- Radiation proctopathy can present several years after cancer treatment and risk increases with increased dose of radiotherapy
- Endoscopic interventions are not without risk and should not be considered first line

Radiation proctopathy can be acute or chronic. Chronic radiation proctopathy is likely caused by chronic cytokine activation leading to ischaemia, fibrosis, and formation of telangiectasia. Telangiectasia can heal spontaneously but may take many years. Treatment is targeted at controlling bleeding. The initial focus should be on optimizing bowel function and stopping contributory medications, if appropriate. —This patient has a significant thrombotic risk from atrial fibrillation, and apixaban should not be stopped without giving him adequate counselling. Randomized trial evidence exists for sucralfate, metronidazole, vitamin A, and hyperbaric oxygen therapy. Rectal formalin and argon plasma coagulation may also be used but are not without risk.

van de Wetering FT, Verleye L, Andreyev HJ et al. Non-surgical interventions for late rectal problems (proctopathy) of radiotherapy in people who have received radiotherapy to the pelvis. *Cochrane Database Syst Rev.* 2016;4:CD003455. Doi:10.1002/14651858.CD003455.pub2.

# chapter 2

# OESOPHAGEAL DISORDERS

## QUESTIONS

1. **A 71-year-old patient was diagnosed with squamous cell carcinoma of the oesophagus.**

   **Which of the following is a recognized risk factor for this disease?**
   A. Alcohol
   B. Gastro-oesophageal reflux disease (GORD)
   C. *Helicobacter pylori* (*H. pylori*) infection
   D. Non-steroidal anti-inflammatory drugs
   E. Obesity

2. **A 63-year-old man presented to the gastroenterology clinic with progressive dysphagia to solid food. He was assessed as World Health Organization (WHO) performance status of 1.**

   Investigations:

   | | |
   |---|---|
   | Gastroscopy | A malignant-appearing oesophageal tumour is identified at 22 cm from the incisors. |
   | Computed tomography (CT) neck, chest, and abdomen | A 2 cm tumour is localized to the upper thoracic oesophagus. No distant metastases are seen on this scan. |

   **Which investigation(s) would be most appropriate to stage this patient's disease?**
   A. Positron emission tomography (PET)-CT
   B. PET-CT and endoscopic ultrasound (EUS)
   C. PET-CT, EUS, and staging laparoscopy
   D. PET-CT, EUS, and tracheobronchoscopy
   E. PET-CT, EUS, tracheobronchoscopy, and staging laparoscopy

*Best of Five MCQs for the European Specialty Examination in Gastroenterology and Hepatology.* Thomas Marjot, Colleen G C McGregor, Tim Ambrose, Aminda N De Silva, Jeremy Cobbold, and Simon Travis, Oxford University Press (2021). © Oxford University Press.
DOI: 10.1093/oso/9780198834373.003.0002

3.  **A 70-year-old woman with a WHO performance status of 2 and mild inhaler controlled chronic obstructive pulmonary disease (COPD) was found on gastroscopy to have a 45 mm flat adenocarcinoma of the oesophagus at 35 cm, not bordering the gastro-oesophageal junction.**

    Investigations:

    | | |
    |---|---|
    | Endoscopic ultrasound | Tumour invades lamina propria but not submucosa, no regional lymphadenopathy |
    | PET-CT chest, abdomen, pelvis | No evidence of lymphadenopathy, no distant metastases |

    **Which is the next best option in her management?**

    A.  Chemoradiotherapy

    B.  Endoscopic mucosal resection (EMR)

    C.  Palliative care

    D.  Radiofrequency ablation

    E.  Surgical resection

4.  **A 76-year-old man was diagnosed with metastatic oesophageal adenocarcinoma. A self-expanding metal stent (SEMS) was inserted to relieve his dysphagia but he requested this to be removed because of persistent chest discomfort in the absence of oesophageal perforation. His WHO performance status was 3.**

    **Which of the following is a useful option in the palliation of dysphagia for this patient?**

    A.  Botulinum toxin injection

    B.  Brachytherapy

    C.  Calcium channel blockers

    D.  Chemotherapy

    E.  Local ethanol injection

5.  **An 83-year-old man with T4N1M1 oesophageal adenocarcinoma was admitted with progressive dysphagia. He requested to be managed symptomatically and a SEMS had been suggested.**

    **Which of the following statements is true regarding SEMS in malignant oesophageal strictures?**

    A.  Brachytherapy should not be used at the same time as SEMS placement

    B.  Photodynamic therapy is superior to SEMS in the palliation of malignant dysphagia

    C.  SEMS is contraindicated in the presence of a tracheo-oesophageal fistula

    D.  SEMS should be inserted in advance of palliative radiotherapy for dysphagia

    E.  SEMS should not be used as a bridge to definitive surgery

6.  **A 47-year-old man attended for a gastroscopy to investigate persistent hoarseness of voice, cough, and sore throat. He had previously seen the ear, nose, and throat team who had performed flexible nasendoscopy and commented that the laryngeal folds were mildly erythematous. They wondered whether his symptoms were caused by acid reflux.**

Investigations:

Gastroscopy        A salmon-coloured area was seen at 18 cm from the incisors (Fig. 2.1). Otherwise this was a normal endoscopy.

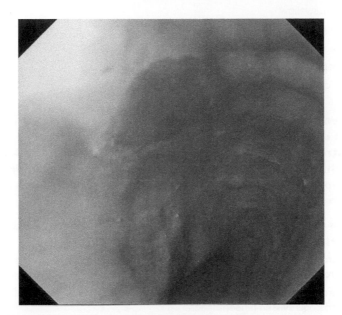

**Fig. 2.1** Endoscopic image of upper oesophagus. See also Plate 2

Image courtesy of Oxford University Hospitals NHS Foundation Trust

## What is the diagnosis?

A. Barrett's oesophagus

B. Candidiasis

C. Cervical inlet patch

D. Squamous cell carcinoma

E. Tracheo-oesophageal fistula

7.  **A 46-year-old man was reviewed in clinic with a two-year history of heartburn and regurgitation. His symptoms persisted despite omeprazole 40 mg twice daily.**

    Investigations:

    | | |
    |---|---|
    | Gastroscopy | No evidence of erosive oesophagitis |
    | Oesophageal histology | Four eosinophils per high-power field |

    **What is the next most appropriate step?**

    A.  Barium swallow

    B.  Fasting gastrin level

    C.  Long-term metoclopramide

    D.  Oesophageal pH/impedence studies

    E.  Trial of swallowed budesonide

8.  **A 53-year-old man was reviewed for persistent heartburn and nocturnal cough despite omeprazole 40 mg twice daily and lifestyle optimization. A gastroscopy two years previously had demonstrated LA Grade C oesophagitis, and recent pH/impedence monitoring confirmed ongoing pathological acid reflux. Manometry was normal. He was keen to explore surgical options to manage his condition.**

    **Which of the following statements about anti-reflux surgery is most accurate?**

    A.  Laparoscopic fundoplication is less effective than open fundoplication at relieving heartburn and regurgitation but has lower mortality

    B.  Laparoscopic magnetic sphincter augmentation results in lower rates of gas bloating than laparoscopic Nissen fundoplication

    C.  Most patients with post-operative dysphagia will require revisional surgery

    D.  Nissen fundoplication is preferred over Toupet fundoplication for patients with oesophageal motility disorders

    E.  Transoral incisionless fundoplication is the operation of choice for most patients

9.  **A 71-year-old woman was reviewed in clinic following a surveillance endoscopy for Barrett's oesophagus.**

    **Which of the following histopathological features best supports a diagnosis of Barrett's oesophagus without dysplasia?**

    A.  Cardiac-type columnar cells bordering squamous mucosa

    B.  Columnar mucosa with nuclear pleomorphism in all cells seen

    C.  Gastric-type mucosa with a similarity in nuclear/cytological appearances between the crypt base cells and those at the surface epithelium

    D.  Increased foci of mitotic activity seen at the gastro-oesophageal junction

    E.  Intestinal metaplastic glandular mucosa with adjacent oesophageal ducts

10. **A 63-year-old man attended for surveillance gastroscopy for Barrett's oesophagus.**

    Investigations:

    Gastroscopy    C3M6 Barrett's oesophagus with no visible lesions

    Histology    Consistent with Barrett's oesophagus with evidence of low-grade dysplasia in two biopsies (confirmed by a second expert gastrointestinal pathologist)

    **How should he be managed?**

    A. Endoscopic resection of Barrett's oesophagus

    B. Laparoscopic oesophagectomy

    C. Radiofrequency ablation

    D. Repeat endoscopy in six months

    E. Repeat endoscopy in 12 months

11. **A 53-year-old man attended for a gastroscopy to investigate persistent reflux symptoms.**

    Investigations:

    Gastroscopy    C5M7 Barrett's oesophagus

    Histology    Consistent with Barrett's oesophagus with intestinal metaplasia (IM) but no evidence of dysplasia

    **The patient is keen for surveillance because he is concerned about the risk of oesophageal cancer. When should he receive his next endoscopy?**

    A. Between two and three years

    B. Between three and five years

    C. Between eight and ten years

    D. No surveillance

    E. Within six months to confirm the diagnosis

12. **A 67-year-old woman with Barrett's oesophagus was found to have an area of high grade dysplasia at recent surveillance endoscopy.**

    **Regarding visible foci of high-grade dysplasia in Barrett's oesophagus, which of the following statements are true?**

    A. Fewer than 5% of patients with a visible dysplastic focus will develop metachronous lesions over the subsequent two years

    B. Once the focus of high-grade dysplasia has been resected, the patient should receive surveillance endoscopy after two years

    C. PET-CT should be performed prior to endoscopic resection of high-grade dysplasia

    D. The 'cap and snare' technique is more effective at resecting visible lesions than band ligation

    E. When endoscopic resection is performed, histological examination of the resection specimen is the most accurate staging technique for Barrett's oesophagus-related early neoplasia

13. **A 75-year-old man presented with a six-month history of non-cardiac chest pain and intermittent dysphagia to solids and liquids.**

    Investigations:

    Gastroscopy              Grade A reflux oesophagitis
    Oesophageal              Average distal peristaltic amplitude >180 mmHg
    manometry

    **What is the diagnosis?**

    A. Achalasia

    B. Diffuse oesophageal spasm

    C. Hypertensive lower oesophageal sphincter

    D. Ineffective oesophageal motility

    E. Nutcracker oesophagus

14. **A 37-year-old Brazilian man with a history of non-cardiac chest pain was referred to the gastroenterology clinic by cardiology. He described a history of episodic dysphagia and occasional regurgitation that persisted despite PPI therapy and a short trial of prokinetics.**

    Investigations:

    Gastroscopy              Normal
    Oesophageal pH studies   DeMeester score 11.3
    Oesophageal motility     Premature contractions in 35% of swallows; normal relaxation
    studies                  of the gastro-oesophageal junction during swallowing. The
                             distal contractile integral never exceeds 8,000 mmHg/cm/s.

    **What is the most likely diagnosis?**

    A. Achalasia

    B. Chagas disease

    C. Distal (diffuse) oesophageal spasm

    D. GORD

    E. Jackhammer oesophagus

15. **A 44-year-old patient presented with a two-year history of progressive dysphagia and occasional retrosternal discomfort. Dysphagia occurred for both solids and liquids. Following a normal upper gastrointestinal endoscopy, the patient underwent high-resolution oesophageal manometry.**

    Investigations:
    High resolution oesophageal manometry (Fig. 2.2)
    Integrated relaxation pressure (IRP) 28 mmHg (normal <15)
    Distal contractile integral (DCI) 90 (normal 450–8,000)
    Distal latency (DL)—not calculated as DCI <450

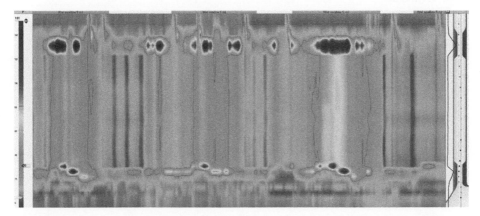

**Fig. 2.2** Pressure topography plot obtained during high resolution oesophageal manometry. See also Plate 3

Image courtesy of Dr Tanya Miller, Principal Clinical Scientist in GI Physiology, Oxford University Hospitals NHS Foundation Trust

## What is the most likely diagnosis?

A. Absent contractility

B. Pseudoachalasia

C. Type I achalasia

D. Type II achalasia

E. Type III achalasia

16. **A 64-year-old Argentinian man presented to the gastroenterology clinic complaining of dysphagia and regurgitation of undigested food. Systemic examination revealed an irregular pulse and pitting oedema of the lower limbs.**

    Investigations:

    Gastroscopy        Grossly dilated oesophagus containing undigested food and fluid. The lower oesophageal sphincter was slow to relax with otherwise normal appearances to the oesophago-gastric junction.

    ## Which of the following investigations would confirm the diagnosis?

    A.  CT thorax

    B.  High-resolution oesophageal manometry

    C.  Thick and thin film microscopy with Giemsa stain

    D.  *Treponema whipplei* serology

    E.  *Trypanosoma cruzi* serology

17. **An 87-year-old man presented with weight loss, one year of worsening dysphagia and regurgitation of both solids and liquids. Past medical history included ischaemic heart disease, hypertension, chronic kidney disease, and recurrent falls.**

Investigations:

| | |
|---|---|
| Gastroscopy | Dilated oesophagus with some food residue, normal stomach and duodenum |
| CT chest, abdomen and pelvis | No extrinisic compression of the gastro-oesophageal junction (Fig. 2.3) |

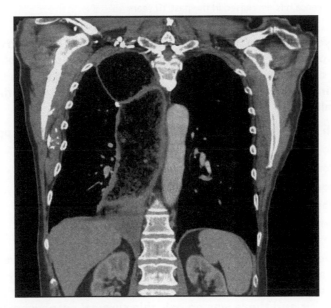

**Fig. 2.3** CT chest and upper abdomen.

Image courtesy of Dr Emma Culver, Consultant Gastroenterologist, Oxford University Hospitals NHS Foundation Trust

## What is the next best treatment approach?

A. Botulinum toxin injection to the lower oesophageal sphincter

B. Laparoscopic Heller myotomy (LHM)

C. Oesophagectomy

D. Peroral endoscopic myotomy

E. Short-acting calcium antagonist

18. **A 21-year-old woman with asthma underwent an endoscopy to investigate dysphagia.**

    **Which statement regarding eosinophilic oesophagitis is correct?**

    A. An empiric six-food elimination diet achieves histologic remission in 10% of patients

    B. Diagnosis requires a two-month trial of a proton pump inhibitor (PPI) with persistence of eosinophilia on oesophageal biopsy

    C. Endoscopic dilation is a safe procedure, with a risk of oesophageal perforation <1%

    D. Male gender is a protective factor

    E. Prevalence has decreased in the past 10 years

19. **A 19-year-old woman was admitted from a local psychiatric hospital four-hours after ingesting a cylindrical battery, a scalpel blade, and three coins. Chest and abdominal radiography suggested the items were in the stomach. She was able to swallow without difficulty and was clinically well.**

    **Which of the following management strategies is most appropriate?**

    A. Endoscopy within six hours with an overtube

    B. Endoscopy within six hours without an overtube

    C. Endoscopy within 24 hours with an overtube

    D. Endoscopy within 24 hours without an overtube

    E. Urgent laparotomy

20. **A 19-year-old woman presented to the emergency department three hours after ingesting approximately 300 ml of car battery fluid following an argument with her partner. Her abdomen was tender but not peritonitic and there was no palpable surgical emphysema. There were no signs of airway compromise.**

    **Which of the following should form part of initial management?**

    A. Broad spectrum antibiotics and corticosteroids

    B. Endoscopy between 12 and 24 hours of ingestion

    C. Intubation and ventilation

    D. Oral ammonia as a neutralizing agent

    E. Oral hypertonic saline to induce vomiting

## 1. A. Alcohol

- Risk factors for squamous cell oesophageal cancer include smoking, alcohol, N-nitroso compounds, and atrophic gastritis
- Alcohol excess is not a risk factor for oesophageal adenocarcinoma

Rates of oesophageal squamous cell carcinoma are highest in Northern Iran, Central Asia and North Central China. Key risk factors include cigarette smoking and alcohol consumption (notably there is no association between alcohol intake and oesophageal adenocarcinoma). Dietary factors that have been implicated include those rich in N-nitroso compounds (e.g. pickled foods), areca nuts, betel quid, and low selenium or zinc intake. Atrophic gastritis increases the risk of oesophageal squamous cell carcinoma as does a previous partial gastrectomy. Human papillomavirus serotypes 16 and 18 may be associated, as may oral bisphosphonates.

GORD and obesity are risk factors for oesophageal adenocarcinoma. Non-steroidal anti-inflammatory drugs may be protective against oesophageal adenocarcinoma, and the impact of *H. pylori* on oesophageal cancer risk is not yet fully understood.

Xie SH, Lagergren J. Risk factors for oesophageal cancer. *Best Pract Res Clin Gastroenterol.* 2018;36–37:3–8. Doi:10.1016/j.bpg.2018.11.008.

## 2. D. PET-CT, EUS, and tracheobronchoscopy

- PET-CT is recommended in all oesophageal carcinoma patients with potentially resectable disease
- EUS should be used to stage the T (tumour) and N (lymph node) categories in oesophageal carcinoma
- Tumours located either within the proximal oesophagus, or at the oesophago-gastric junction, may require additional staging investigations

European Society for Medical Oncology (ESMO) guidelines recommend PET-CT to exclude distant metastases in all potentially resectable oesophageal cancers. EUS has a sensitivity of 81%–92% and specificity of 94%–97% when used for oesophageal tumour staging, and it is therefore recommended for use in staging oesophageal tumours. In the case discussed here, the tumour is located in the upper thoracic oesophagus at 22 cm from the incisors. Because this is above the level of the carina (25 cm), ESMO guidelines additionally recommend tracheobronchoscopy to exclude tracheal invasion. Staging laparoscopy would be an appropriate staging investigation for the locally advanced (T3/4) oesophago-gastric junction tumours in which peritoneal metastases are detected in approximately 15% of patients.

Lordick F, Mariette C, Haustermans K et al. Oesophageal cancer: ESMO Clinical Practice Guidelines for diagnosis, treatment and follow-up. *Ann Oncol.* 2016;27(suppl 5):v50–v57.

*Best of Five MCQs for the European Specialty Examination in Gastroenterology and Hepatology.* Thomas Marjot, Colleen G C McGregor, Tim Ambrose, Aminda N De Silva, Jeremy Cobbold, and Simon Travis, Oxford University Press (2021). © Oxford University Press.
DOI: 10.1093/oso/9780198834373.003.0002

### 3. B. Endoscopic mucosal resection

- Resection is the treatment of choice in limited disease (T1–2, N0, M0)
- Endoscopic therapy is preferred for T1a disease because it is effective and well tolerated
- Chemoradiotherapy is superior to radiotherapy alone for limited disease in patients unfit for resection

Limited oesophageal cancer is defined by disease up to and including T2, in the absence of lymphadenopathy or metastases:

| | |
|---|---|
| T1 | Tumour invades lamina propria or submucosa |
| T1a | Tumour invades mucosa or lamina propria or muscularis mucosae |
| T1b | Tumour invades submucosa |
| T2 | Tumour invades muscularis propria |

This patient has T1a, N0, and M0 oesophageal adenocarcinoma and should be considered for resection. Endoscopic resection, either with EMR or endoscopic submucosal dissection (ESD), is effective for T1a disease. Her mild COPD should not be considered a contraindication to endoscopic intervention. T1b and T2 disease are better served by surgical oesophagectomy (e.g. Ivor Lewis procedure). The evidence for neoadjuvant chemoradiotherapy in addition to resection is uncertain. Chemoradiotherapy with cisplatin/5-fluorouracil and 50.4 Gy radiation, or six cycles of folinic acid/5-fluorouracil/oxaliplatin (FOLFOX) can be used for patients unable or unwilling to undergo resection. This is more effective than radiotherapy alone. There is no role for radiofrequency ablation in the management of oesophageal adenocarcinoma and palliative care would not be the preferred route for this patient for whom curative treatment is possible.

Lordick F, Mariette C, Haustermans K et al. Oesophageal cancer: ESMO Clinical Practice Guidelines for diagnosis, treatment and follow-up. *Ann Oncol.* 2016;27(suppl 5):v50–v57.

### 4. B. Brachytherapy

- Brachytherapy, stent insertion, and chemotherapy all have roles in advanced oesophageal cancer
- Brachytherapy provides better long-term relief of dysphagia with fewer complications than stent insertion
- Chemotherapy should be reserved for patients with a good performance status

Patients with metastatic oesophageal cancer have incurable disease and the focus should be symptom control. A SEMS, inserted either endoscopically or radiologically, is often used to relieve dysphagia but post-procedural chest pain can limit tolerability. Brachytherapy describes intraluminal radiotherapy treatment using a radioactive source (e.g. iridium-192) placed into the oesophagus via a non-radioactive applicator. Brachytherapy can precisely and safely deliver high doses of radiation to the tumour while minimizing unwanted side effects. Therapy may be delivered as a single dose, and has been shown to have fewer complications than stent insertion and result in better long-term relief of dysphagia. Therefore, this is not an option when life expectancy is very short.

Chemotherapy can be used for palliation of patients with oesophageal adenocarcinoma and a good performance status, but it is less successful with squamous cell carcinoma. There is no role for botulinum toxin injections or calcium channel blockers in the management of dysphagia in oesophageal adenocarcinoma. An ethanol injection may exacerbate the dysphagia and pain.

Lordick F, Mariette C, Haustermans K et al. Oesophageal cancer: ESMO Clinical Practice Guidelines for diagnosis, treatment and follow-up. *Ann Oncol.* 2016;27(suppl 5):v50–v57.

## 5. E. SEMS should not be used as a bridge to definitive surgery

- SEMS are recommended for the palliation of malignant dysphagia over photodynamic therapy or oesophageal bypass
- Fully or partially covered SEMS should be used for malignant strictures or tracheo-oesophageal fistulae
- SEMS should not be used as a bridge to surgery, nor concurrently with external beam radiotherapy

Dysphagia is the most common symptom of oesophageal cancer with the aim of stent placement being to improve quality of life and enable oral intake of food and water in patients unfit for surgery or oncological therapies. Covered metal stents are recommended for malignant strictures rather than plastic or uncovered ones. These stents should also be used to seal over malignant fistulae between the airways and oesophagus. In patients being considered for surgery, placement of a feeding tube is preferable over insertion of a stent because of the high incidence of SEMS-related adverse events. Brachytherapy may provide a survival benefit over SEMS placement and should be considered in patients with a longer life expectancy. Relief from dysphagia is less rapid with brachytherapy but similar in magnitude after one month. Palliative external beam radiotherapy may relieve dysphagia after 4–6 weeks. SEMS should not be used prior to radiotherapy because of a high risk of life-threatening complications. A single dose of brachytherapy concurrently with SEMS placement is safe and effective.

Spaander MC, Baron TH, Siersema PD et al. Esophageal stenting for benign and malignant disease: European Society of Gastrointestinal Endoscopy (ESGE) Clinical Guideline. *Endoscopy.* 2016;48(10):939–948. Doi:10.1055/s-0042-114210.

## 6. C. Cervical inlet patch

- Cervical inlet patches (black asterisk in Fig. 2.4) are located in the upper oesophagus, usually just distal to the upper oesophageal sphincter
- It can lead to symptoms of laryngopharyngeal reflux and globus
- Proton pump inhibitors may help symptoms

A cervical inlet patch is a congenital condition whereby islands of heterotopic gastric mucosa form in the upper oesophagus. The pathogenesis is incompletely understood but likely results from incomplete embryonic transformation of the oesophagus from columnar to squamous epithelium. Histologically, it is more common to be fundic mucosa than cardia-type with acid production resulting in laryngo-pharyngeal reflux. Incidence at endoscopy is between 0.1% and 10%, and dependent on the endoscopist's awareness of the condition.

Many patients are asymptomatic, but cough, sore throat, hoarse voice, and throat clearing are not uncommon. In patients presenting with globus, Rome IV criteria recommend exclusion of an inlet patch. Careful endoscopic evaluation of the upper oesophagus, including with narrow band imaging, increases diagnostic yield. Progression to oesophageal adenocarcinoma is rare. Symptomatic patients may derive benefit from PPIs. Limited endoscopic approaches have been described including argon plasma coagulation, endoscopic resection, and radiofrequency ablation.

Barrett's oesophagus does not form in the upper oesophagus although associations with inlet patches have been described. The endoscopic appearance is not consistent with candidiasis, squamous cell carcinoma, or tracheo-bronchial fistula.

Rusu R, Ishaq S, Wong T et al. Cervical inlet patch: new insights into diagnosis and endoscopic therapy. *Frontline Gastroenterol.* 2018;9(3):214–220. Doi:10.1136/flgastro-2017-100855.

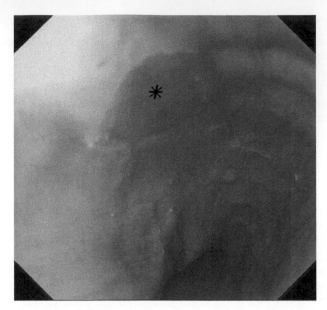

**Fig. 2.4** Endoscopic image of upper oesophagus

Image courtesy of Oxford University Hospitals NHS Foundation Trust

## 7. D. Oesophageal pH/impedence studies

- Patients with symptoms of GORD should receive an empirical trial of PPIs
- Erosive oesophagitis and eosinophilic oesophagitis should be excluded
- Oesophageal pH/impedence studies should be considered for patients with persistent symptoms despite PPI

GORD symptoms are diverse and can be influenced by oesophageal hypersensitivity. In patients with persistent symptoms despite a trial of PPI, and without evidence of erosive oesophagitis endoscopically, oesophageal physiology testing should be considered. Usually, physiology testing should be performed 'off PPI therapy' to maximize symptom/reflux association. The exception is patients with PPI-unresponsive symptoms who have previously had erosive oesophagitis (LA Grade C or D) or positive pH studies, in which case repeat testing can be performed 'on PPI therapy'. PH/impedence allows reflux episodes to be characterized irrespective of acidity (acid vs bile reflux) or contents (liquid vs gas).

The acid exposure time (percentage of total time that oesophageal pH <4) is a critical determinant of pathological reflux with normal <4%, inconclusive 4%–6%, and abnormal >6%. The number of reflux episodes can be used as an adjunct in inconclusive cases. The combination of a positive symptom index and symptom association probability score provides the best evidence of clinically relevant associations between reflux episodes and symptoms.

Barium swallow will not define the diagnosis here although it may visualize an episode of reflux. The symptoms are not suggestive of Zollinger–Ellison syndrome with no peptic ulceration. Long-term metoclopramide should be avoided because of risk of neurological disorders. There is no evidence of eosinophilic oesophagitis in this case and swallowed budesonide cannot be recommended.

Gyawali CP, Kahrilas PJ, Savarino E et al. Modern diagnosis of GERD: the Lyon Consensus. *Gut*. 2018;67:1351–1362. Doi:10.1136/gutjnl-2017-314722.

## 8. B. Laparoscopic magnetic sphincter augmentation results in lower rates of gas bloating than laparoscopic Nissen fundoplication

- Anti-reflux surgery is indicated for PPI-refractory reflux symptoms with endoscopic and/or physiological confirmation of ongoing reflux
- Oesophageal manometry should be encouraged for all patients because it may affect the choice of operation
- Magnetic sphincter augmentation and transoral incisionless fundoplication are emerging techniques although long-term outcomes are not yet known

Anti-reflux surgery should be considered in patients with recurrent, refractory, or persistent reflux disease despite optimization of medical therapy. This includes patients with complications such as erosive oesophagitis or peptic strictures, and in situations of medication intolerance or patient choice not to take lifelong medications. Surgery may also be beneficial for patients with respiratory symptoms linked to reflux (such as nocturnal cough, hoarseness, or laryngitis) who also have typical reflux symptoms.

Laparoscopic and open fundoplication are equally effective at relieving symptoms, with the former resulting in shorter duration of hospital stay and lower mortality. Post-operative dysphagia may be more common with laparoscopic fundoplication, perhaps due to challenges in confirming how tight the wrap is—intra-operative oesophageal bougies are sometimes used, around which to construct the wrap. Toupet fundoplication (posterior 270° wrap) is usually preferred in patients with oesophageal dysmotility and results in lower rates of dysphagia than Nissen fundoplication (360° wrap).

Most patients experience a degree of post-operative dysphagia that often alleviates after two to three months, but may require dilatation. Five to ten per cent of patients will need revisional surgery, potentially converting to a partial fundoplication. Gas bloating is another recognized complication with lower rates in patients receiving magnetic sphincter augmentation than laparoscopic Nissen fundoplication, although long-term follow-up of magnetic sphincter augmentation is not yet known. Transoral incisionless fundoplication is a novel technique and results in lower rates of dysphagia and gas bloating, but it is not yet clear whether durability is as good as surgery.

Mermelstein J, Chait Mermelstein A, Chait MM. Proton pump inhibitor-refractory gastroesophageal reflux disease: challenges and solutions. *Clin Exp Gastroenterol.* 2018;(11):119–134. Doi:10.2147/CEG. S121056.

## 9. E. Intestinal metaplastic glandular mucosa with adjacent oesophageal ducts

Barrett's oesophagus can be defined as an oesophagus in which any part of the normal distal squamous epithelium has been replaced with metaplastic columnar epithelium, clearly visible at least 1 cm above the gastro-oesophageal junction and confirmed histopathologically. The distinction between columnar-lined oesophagus and IM at the cardia can only be definitively made when columnar mucosa with or without IM is seen adjacent to native oesophageal structures (e.g. submucosal glands, gland ducts). Multi-layered epithelium is pathognomonic of Barrett's oesophagus, and squamous islands may suggest the diagnosis. However, native structures are only seen in a minority of cases and so the final diagnosis relies on endoscopic and histological correlation.

The presence of columnar mucosa, without IM, bordering squamous epithelium alone may represent a sampling error and does not necessarily support a diagnosis of Barrett's oesophagus. The remaining answers are all features of dysplasia in Barrett's oesophagus.

Fitzgerald RC, di Pietro M, Ragunath K et al. British Society of Gastroenterology guidelines on the diagnosis and management of Barrett's oesophagus. *Gut.* 2014;63(1):7–42. Doi:10.1136/gutjnl-2013-305372.

## 10. D. Repeat endoscopy in six months

- The identification of low-grade dysplasia on random biopsies requires confirmation by a second expert gastrointestinal pathologist
- Early surveillance at six months to confirm low-grade dysplasia is recommended rather than endoscopic resection

The risk of progression to cancer in patients with non-dysplastic Barrett's oesophagus is about 0.3% per year. However, it is much greater in the presence of dysplasia. Any degree of dysplasia identified in a patient with Barrett's oesophagus should be confirmed by a second expert pathologist. Both patients with 'indefinite for dysplasia' or low-grade dysplasia should have a further endoscopy at six months. Approximately 30% of patients will not have evidence of low-grade dysplasia at follow-up. If low-grade dysplasia is confirmed, endoscopic ablation should be offered, usually with radiofrequency ablation. Visible dysplastic lesions in Barrett's oesophagus should be removed by endoscopic resection, either EMR or ESD.

Weusten B, Bisschops R, Coron E et al. Endoscopic management of Barrett's esophagus: European Society of Gastrointestinal Endoscopy (ESGE) Position Statement. *Endoscopy.* 2017;49(2):191–198. Doi:10.1055/s-0042-122140.

## 11. A. Between two and three years

- The length of Barrett's used to determine need and interval of surveillance is taken from the Maximum (M) extent rather than the Circumferential (C) extent of the Prague classification
- Histologically confirmed Barrett's with IM but without dysplasia requires surveillance every two to three years for segments longer than 3 cm, or three to five years for shorter segments
- Segments of 1 cm or less should be considered an irregular Z-line and no surveillance is necessary

Non-dysplastic Barrett's oesophagus is associated with a risk of high-grade dysplasia and oesophageal adenocarcinoma (0.2%–0.3% per year). Outcomes are improved if the disease is identified at an earlier stage. The presence of IM is an important histological feature as this is associated with a greater risk of cancer. Patients with short (less than 3 cm) Barrett's oesophagus without IM (confirmed on two separate endoscopies) have a low risk of cancer and do not require surveillance. If IM is confirmed, surveillance should take place every three to five years. For longer segment disease (greater than 3 cm) surveillance should take place every two to three years. European guidelines suggest segments longer than 10 cm require referral to a dedicated Barrett's centre for discussion on management. Usually surveillance should cease at the age of 75 years, if the patient develops other comorbidities which would preclude treatment for high-grade dysplasia or cancer, or at the patient request.

Weusten B, Bisschops R, Coron E et al. Endoscopic management of Barrett's esophagus: European Society of Gastrointestinal Endoscopy (ESGE) Position Statement. *Endoscopy.* 2017;49(2):191–198. Doi:10.1055/s-0042-122140.

## 12. E. When endoscopic resection is performed, histological examination of the resection specimen is the most accurate staging technique for Barrett's oesophagus-related early neoplasia

- Twenty per cent of patients with high-grade dysplasia on biopsies will not have a visible abnormality using high-resolution endoscopy
- More than 20% of patients with visible dysplasia will develop metachronous lesions within two years and so ablation of residual Barrett's oesophagus is essential
- Both 'cap and snare' and band ligation are equally effective techniques

All patients with high-grade dysplasia should be referred for expert high-resolution endoscopy where 80% will have a visible lesion. Patients should be reviewed at a multidisciplinary meeting and then have treatment options discussed with them. Endoscopic therapy, rather than oesophagectomy or surveillance, is desirable for management of high-grade dysplasia. Neither CT, PET-CT, nor EUS is required prior to endoscopic resection for either high-grade dysplasia or suspected T1 cancer. The endoscopic resection specimen provides the most accurate means of staging disease and aids planning of subsequent therapy. 'Cap and snare' and band ligation have similar success rates at resecting visible lesions (85%–98%). Once all visible lesions have been resected, residual Barrett's should be treated using radiofrequency ablation because the risk of metachronous cancer in the subsequent two years is more than 20%. After successful ablation, surveillance should be three-monthly for the first year and then annually.

Fitzgerald RC, di Pietro M, Ragunath K et al. British Society of Gastroenterology guidelines on the diagnosis and management of Barrett's oesophagus. *Gut.* 2014;63(1):7–42. Doi:10.1136/gutjnl-2013-305372.

## 13. E. Nutcracker oesophagus

- Nutcracker oesophagus is defined by peristaltic amplitude >180 mmHg on manometry
- Sildenafil and calcium channel blockers may improve symptoms

Nutcracker oesophagus is a benign condition that occurs most commonly in the sixth and seventh decades of life. It is a form of oesophageal dysmotility characterized by hypertensive peristalsis. The smooth muscle of the oesophagus contracts in a normal sequence but at an excessive amplitude or for a longer duration. Symptoms include non-cardiac chest pain and intermittent dysphagia to both solids and liquids. It is defined by peristaltic amplitude of >180 mmHg identified with oesophageal manometry.

Patients with nutcracker oesophagus have a loss of inhibitory innervation to the oesophagus and lower oesophageal sphincter. They also have thickening of the muscularis propria and greater muscle mass in the distal compared with the proximal oesophagus. Sildenafil, a phosphodiesterase 5 inhibitor, decreases contractile amplitude by more than 70% with effects lasting more than eight hours. Calcium channel blockers (such as diltiazem) or nitrates may be of benefit, but can be associated with unacceptable side effects.

Mittal RK, Bhalla V. Oesophageal motor functions and its disorders. *Gut.* 2004;53(10):1536–1542.

## 14. C. Distal (diffuse) oesophageal spasm

- Diffuse oesophageal spasm has been renamed 'distal oesophageal spasm'
- It is one of the major disorders of oesophageal peristalsis
- Treatment options include nitrates, calcium channel blockers, botulinum toxin, or endoscopic myotomy

Distal (diffuse) oesophageal spasm results in dysphagia and regurgitation, and can be a cause of non-cardiac chest pain. It is one of the major disorders of peristalsis along with jackhammer oesophagus and absent contractility. The recent Chicago classification has redefined the manometric findings in this condition—premature contractions in at least 20% of swallows in conjunction with normal relaxation of the gastro-oesophageal junction. A premature contraction is a swallow with a distal latency (time from relaxation of upper oesophageal sphincter to contractile deceleration point) of less than 4.5 seconds. Treatment is aimed at reducing oesophageal spasm, with calcium channel blockers and nitrates usually used. Emerging therapies include botulinum toxin injection and per-oral endoscopic myotomy.

The normal DeMeester score excludes GORD. Normal relaxation of the gastro-oesophageal junction excludes achalasia and pseudoachalasia caused by Chagas' disease. Jackhammer oesophagus is a hypercontractile oesophageal disorder with an elevated distal contractile integral (>8,000 mmHg/cm/s) in more than 20% of swallows on manometry.

Kahrilas PJ, Bredenoord AJ, Fox M et al. The Chicago Classification of esophageal motility disorders, v3.0. *Neurogastroenterol Motil.* 2015;27(2):160–174. Doi:10.1111/nmo.12477.

## 15. D. Type II achalasia

- The cardinal manometric features of achalasia are loss of normal peristalsis and elevated lower oesophageal sphincter pressure
- Following an upper gastrointestinal endoscopy, high-resolution oesophageal manometry is the investigation of choice for diagnosis and classification of suspected achalasia (Table 2.1)

**Table 2.1** Classification of achalasia

| Achalasia subtype | Distinguishing features |
| --- | --- |
| Type I (classical) | No pan-oesophageal pressurization (oesophageal pressures <30 mmHg [pale/dark blue on manometry trace]) |
| Type II (with oesophageal compression) | Pan-oesophageal pressurization (green/yellow/red on manometry trace) in >20% of swallows |
| Type III (spastic) | >20% of swallows with premature contraction (distal latency <4.5 seconds) with a distal contractile integral >450 |

The manometry trace demonstrates achalasia evidenced by vertical (rather than diagonal) bands of pressurization indicating a loss of normal peristalsis, and by failed relaxation of the lower oesophageal sphincter indicated by an abnormally elevated IRP.

Pseudoachalasia is a possible but less likely diagnosis because of the long duration of symptoms, the patient's young age (<50) and normal endoscopic appearances. Absent contractility is diagnosed by failed peristalsis and normal IRP.

Rohof WOA, Bredenoord AJ. Chicago classification of esophageal motility disorders: lessons learned. *Curr Gastroenterol Rep.* 2017;19(8):37. Doi:10.1007/s11894-017-0576-7.

## 16. E. *Trypanosoma cruzi* serology

- Chagas disease is a rare cause of gastrointestinal dysmotility, usually oesophageal and/or colonic, encountered in patients from endemic areas of South and Central America
- Cardiomyopathy is the most common sequel of chronic infection and a diagnosis of Chagas disease should prompt cardiology referral
- Treatment is symptomatic. Benznidazole is licensed in the USA for treatment of Chagas disease in children. Clinical benefits in adults with chronic disease are unproven

The patient has achalasia secondary to Chagas disease, which can be detected by *Trypanosoma cruzi* serology. High-resolution oesophageal manometry could be used to characterize the oesophageal dysmotility and CT thorax would be advisable to exclude pseudoachalasia, but neither would be diagnostic in this case.

Chagas disease is a parasitic infection usually acquired from the infected faeces of a triotamine vector. Animal vectors are endemic to areas of South and Central America. Acute infection causes a usually self-limiting febrile illness during which time the trypomastigotes can be detected using thick and thin film microscopy with Giemsa stain. Most patients develop a chronic infection that persists lifelong, and up to 30% will develop cardiac or gastrointestinal manifestations. Cardiac disease manifests as Chagas cardiomyopathy, which is highly arrhythmogenic, while the gastrointestinal manifestations cause dysmotility most commonly seen in the oesophagus and colon. In severe cases, this leads to mega-oesophagus and mega-colon.

Bern C. Chagas disease. *N Engl J Med.* 2015;373(5):456–466. Doi:10.1056/NEJMra1410150.

## 17. A. Botulinum toxin injection to the lower oesophageal sphincter

- Pharmacological management of achalasia is ineffective
- Pneumatic dilation, LHM, and peroral endoscopic myotomy (POEM) are all potential first-line treatment options for achalasia
- Botulinum toxin injection is an effective short-term treatment with an excellent safety profile but it has no role in patients <50 years and a high rate of symptom recurrence

The diagnosis here is achalasia with megaoesophagus (see white asterisk in Fig. 2.5). In an elderly patient with worsening dysphagia and weight loss, upper gastrointestinal endoscopy and cross-sectional imaging are particularly important to exclude pseudoachalasia. Furthermore, patients with achalasia for >10 years are at increased risk of oesophageal squamous cell carcinoma.

2018 International Society for Diseases of the Esophagus (ISDE) guidelines found no convincing evidence for medical treatment (e.g. nitrates, calcium antagonists, phosphodiesterase inhibitors) for treatment of achalasia and recommend against their use. Graded pneumatic dilatation is an effective treatment for achalasia but up to a third will need a repeat procedure within five years and therefore patients wishing longer-term remission may opt for LHM or POEM. Because of technical difficulties and lack of evidence, the ISDE makes no recommendation for pneumatic dilatation in cases of megaoesophagus (diameter >6 cm and sigmoid shaped) when LHM is preferred. Given that the patient in this case is not a candidate for surgery or advanced endoscopy, botulinum toxin injection to the lower oesophageal sphincter would be most appropriate. Botulinum toxin injection is an effective short-term treatment for achalasia and has an excellent safety profile. However, it has little benefit in patients <50 years and carries a high rate of recurrence with two-thirds having a return of symptoms after two years.

Zaninotto G, Bennett C, Boeckxstaens G et al. The 2018 ISDE achalasia guidelines. *Dis Esophagus.* 2018;31(9). Doi:10.1093/dote/doy071.

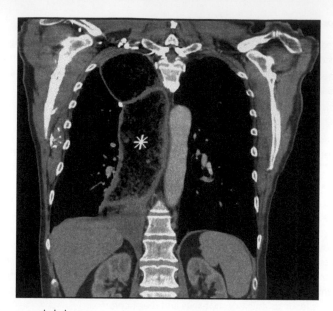

**Fig. 2.5** CT thorax and abdomen

Image courtesy of Dr Emma Culver, Consultant Gastroenterologist, Oxford University Hospitals NHS Foundation Trust

## 18. C. Endoscopic dilation is a safe procedure, with a risk of oesophageal perforation <1%

- Eosinophilic oesophagitis (EoE) and GORD are not mutually exclusive conditions
- Lack of response to trial of a PPI is no longer required in the diagnosis of EoE
- Topical steroids, an empirical six-food elimination diet, and oesophageal dilatation for stricturing disease are all safe and effective treatment modalities in EoE

EoE represents a chronic, immune-mediated oesophageal disease, characterized clinically by symptoms of oesophageal dysfunction and histologically by eosinophil-predominant inflammation (>15 eosinophils per high-power field). EoE should be suspected when rings, exudates, strictures, or crepe paper mucosa are identified endoscopically. Fifty per cent of patients presenting with food bolus obstruction will have EoE. Prevalence is 28/100,000, which has quadrupled over the past 10 years, and those with EoE are twice as likely to be male. Traditional dogma stated that EoE and GORD were mutually exclusive: it is now recognized that their relationship is complex and bidirectional. Previous guidelines recommended a trial of PPI in patients with symptoms and mucosal eosinophilia. Those who responded were classed as PPI-responsive oesophageal eosinophilia (PPI-REE) and those who did not were classed as EoE. Evidence now suggests that PPI-REE is clinically, histologically, and genetically indistinguishable from EoE, and that PPIs are better classified as a treatment for oesophageal eosinophilia that may be due to EoE rather than as a diagnostic criterion. Topical corticosteroids are effective for induction and maintenance of histological remission in EoE although data regarding clinical benefit is limited because of the lack of validated symptom-scoring tools. An empiric six-food elimination diet induces histologic remission in three-quarters of patients with EoE. Endoscopic dilatation for stricturing disease leads to clinical improvement in 75% of patients with the overall risk of oesophageal perforation <1%, comparable with risk of dilatation in other oesophageal disorders.

Lucendo AJ, Molina-Infante J, Arias Á et al. Guidelines on eosinophilic esophagitis: evidence-based statements and recommendations for diagnosis and management in children and adults. *United European Gastroenterol J.* 2017;5(3):335–358. Doi:10.1177/2050640616689525.

## 19. C. Endoscopy within 24 hours with an overtube

- Emergency endoscopy (within two to six hours) is required for foreign bodies causing complete oesophageal obstruction or for sharp-pointed objects and batteries in the oesophagus (Table 2.2)
- Urgent endoscopy (within 24 hours) is required for most at risk objects in the stomach
- The use of an overtube should be considered when removing sharp objects from the stomach, to reduce the risk of oesophageal damage

**Table 2.2** Timing of endoscopy for removal of ingested foreign bodies

| Timing of endoscopy | Type of foreign body |
| --- | --- |
| Emergency (within 2–6 hours) | Complete oesophageal obstruction<br>Sharp-pointed objects and batteries in the oesophagus |
| Urgent (within 24 hours) | All other oesophageal foreign bodies<br>Magnets, sharp-pointed objects, batteries, large objects in the stomach |
| Routine (within 72 hours) | All other objects in the stomach |
| Monitor only | Blunt objects in stomach <2 cm diameter and <5 cm length—allow to pass naturally, weekly radiographs, extract endoscopically if not passed after four weeks. |

Data from Birk M, Bauerfeind P, Deprez PH et al. Removal of foreign bodies in the upper gastrointestinal tract in adults: European Society of Gastrointestinal Endoscopy (ESGE) Clinical Guideline. *Endoscopy*. 2016;48:1–8. Doi:10.1055/s-0042-100456.

Most ingested foreign bodies pass spontaneously; the remainder require endoscopic retrieval or, in 1%, surgery. In patients with oesophageal foreign bodies, especially food boluses, the site of discomfort does not often correlate with the site of impaction. Increased salivation and inability to swallow saliva or liquids suggests complete oesophageal obstruction. Radiography can help localize the site of foreign bodies within the upper gastrointestinal tract but materials such as wood, plastic, glass, and fish/chicken bones are not readily seen. Overtubes should be considered when extracting sharp objects to reduce the risk of oesophageal damage. Generally, objects with a diameter of more than 2 cm will not pass the pylorus or ileocaecal valve, and those longer than 5 cm will not pass through the duodenum due to angulation. Eighty-five per cent of batteries will pass through the intestines within 72 hours once past the duodenum.

Birk M, Bauerfeind P, Deprez PH et al. Removal of foreign bodies in the upper gastrointestinal tract in adults: European Society of Gastrointestinal Endoscopy (ESGE) Clinical Guideline. *Endoscopy*. 2016;48:1–8. Doi:10.1055/s-0042-100456.

## 20. B. Endoscopy between 12 and 24 hours of ingestion

- Neutralization or forced emesis should be avoided
- There is no good evidence for antibiotics or steroids
- Endoscopic staging of oesophageal damage should be performed between 12 and 24 hours after ingestion and a nasogastric tube inserted for feeding if needed

Caustic agents can broadly be divided into strong acids with pH <2 (e.g. sulphuric acid [battery fluid], hydrochloric acid), strong alkalis with pH >12 (ammonia, sodium hydroxide) or oxidating agents with variable pH values (sodium hypochlorite [bleach], hydrogen peroxide). The oesophagus is more at risk of damage than the stomach. The priority in ingestion of caustic material is to protect the airway if there is evidence of compromise. Neutralization should be avoided because of the risk of causing an exothermic injury and worsening oesophageal damage. There is no evidence that antibiotics reduce stricture formation or infection rates. Similarly, there is no good evidence for steroids. Urgent cross-sectional abdominal imaging and consideration of surgery is needed when there is evidence of perforation or peritonitis.

Endoscopic evaluation should be delayed until 12–24 hours after ingestion to stage the initial damage (Grades 1–3). Oesophageal stricturing will occur in 80% and 50% of those with grade 3 and grade 2 damage respectively. A nasogastric tube should be inserted to provide a route for feeding in patients with early stricturing. Endoscopy should be avoided between days 2 and 15 after ingestion because of increased risk of oesophageal perforation. After this time, dilatation, or oesophageal stenting may be needed.

Lupa M, Magne J, Guarisco JL et al. Update on the diagnosis and treatment of caustic ingestion. *Ochsner J.* 2009;9(2):54–9.

# chapter 3

## STOMACH AND DUODENAL DISORDERS

### QUESTIONS

1.  **A 66-year-old woman with a history of peptic ulcer disease (PUD) and ischaemic heart disease was diagnosed with rheumatoid arthritis. She was prescribed regular ibuprofen (400 mg three times daily) and methotrexate.**

    **In view of her history of peptic ulcer disease, which of the following is the most appropriate precaution to take?**

    A. Add Omeprazole 20 mg od

    B. Commence *Helicobacter pylori* (*H. pylori*) eradication therapy

    C. Gastroscopy

    D. Switch to celecoxib

    E. Urea breath test

2.  **A 33-year-old woman of Indian descent was referred with dyspepsia. This had been resistant to omeprazole 20 mg daily and metoclopramide 10 mg three times daily, which she was taking at the time of her gastroscopy. She was on no other medications.**

    Investigations:

    | | |
    |---|---|
    | Gastroscopy | Antral erosions and three large duodenal ulcers in D1 (Forrest class III) |
    | Antral rapid urease test | Negative |
    | Haemoglobin | 138 g/L |
    | Plasma viscosity | 1.70 mPa/s |
    | Serum C-reactive protein (CRP) | 8 mg/L |
    | Plasma gastrin | 90 pmol/L |

    **Which of the following is the most likely diagnosis?**

    A. Crohn's disease

    B. *H. pylori* infection

    C. Human immunodeficiency virus (HIV)

    D. Tuberculosis

    E. Zollinger–Ellison syndrome (ZES)

*Best of Five MCQs for the European Specialty Examination in Gastroenterology and Hepatology.* Thomas Marjot, Colleen G C McGregor, Tim Ambrose, Aminda N De Silva, Jeremy Cobbold, and Simon Travis, Oxford University Press (2021). © Oxford University Press.
DOI: 10.1093/oso/9780198834373.003.0003

3.  **A 53-year-old woman was referred to gastroenterology with ongoing dyspepsia despite adequate treatment. She had required *H. pylori* eradication therapy twice before.**

    **Which of the following is not a factor related to *H. pylori* treatment failure?**

    A.  Acid suppression
    B.  Host IL-1β polymorphism
    C.  Low body mass index (BMI)
    D.  Smoking
    E.  Treatment duration

4.  **A 75-year-old man with coffee ground vomiting was referred for a gastroscopy. His notes stated that he had had a Billroth II procedure 20 years before.**

    **Which of the following most accurately describes his surgery?**

    A.  Division of the vagus nerve and a gastrojejunostomy
    B.  Division of the vagus nerve and lateral division of the pylorus, followed by longitudinal resuturing
    C.  Formation of a gastric pouch; small bowel divided at the duodenojejunal junction; anastomosis of the jejunum to the gastric pouch; anastomosis of the duodenum to the small bowel distal to the jejunal anastomosis
    D.  Longitudinal division of the pylorus
    E.  Resection of the gastric antrum, formation of a gastrojejunostomy, and closure of the first part of the duodenum and gastric outflow

5.  **A 65-year-old man who underwent a Billroth I partial gastrectomy 20 years ago for recurrent gastric ulcers was seen in the gastroenterology clinic.**

    **Which of the following deficiencies is he most likely to suffer from?**

    A.  Calcium
    B.  Folate
    C.  Iron
    D.  Vitamin $B_{12}$
    E.  Vitamin D

6. **A 55-year-old man, originally from China, had a gastroscopy to investigate epigastric discomfort unresponsive to omeprazole. The gastroscopy showed mild erythema in the body and biopsies were taken.**

Investigations:
   Histology (stomach body): See Fig. 3.1

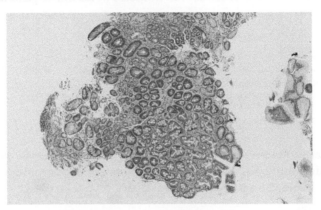

**Fig. 3.1** Histology specimen from stomach body. See also Plate 4

Image courtesy of Dr Eve Fryer, Consultant Histopathologist, Oxford University Hospitals NHS Foundation Trust

**Which of the following intervals is the most appropriate surveillance strategy for this man based on the histological findings?**

A. One year

B. Two years

C. Three years

D. Five years

E. No surveillance

7. **A 57-year-old woman with dyspepsia and weight loss was referred for a gastroscopy. Her medications included omeprazole and ranitidine.**

Investigations:

   Gastroscopy          Multiple fundic gland polyps, largest measuring 1.5 cm. Targeted biopsies taken.

**What is the appropriate next step?**

A. Repeat the gastroscopy in a year's time

B. Repeat the gastroscopy with chromoendoscopy

C. Repeat the gastroscopy with excision of polyps >1 cm

D. Request a *H. pylori* breath test

E. Request colonoscopy to screen for colonic polyps

8. **A 63-year-old librarian with pernicious anaemia was referred for a gastroscopy. This demonstrated features of atrophic gastritis. Performed without sedation, the procedure was poorly tolerated and only one biopsy was taken.**

    **What is the correct protocol for biopsies in atrophic gastritis?**

    A. Biopsies of two topographic sites (antrum and corpus, at the lesser and greater curvature)

    B. Biopsies of two topographic sites (antrum and corpus, at the lesser and greater curvature) in the same vial

    C. Biopsies of two topographic sites (antrum and corpus, at the lesser and greater curvature) plus additional biopsies of suspicious lesions

    D. Targeted biopsies of suspicious lesions only

    E. Two gastric biopsies every 4 cm

9. **A 60-year-old woman presented to the gastroenterology clinic with abdominal pain and nausea. An abdominal examination was unremarkable. She had some investigations performed.**

    Investigations:

    | | |
    |---|---|
    | Haemoglobin | 108 g/L |
    | Mean corpuscular varices | 75 fL |
    | Serum ferritin | 9 ng/ml |
    | Transferrin saturation | 7% |
    | Serum C-reactive protein | 9 mg/L |
    | Serum gastrin | 300 pmol/L |
    | Serum B12 | 88 ng/L |
    | Antibodies to intrinsic factor | Positive |
    | Gastroscopy | 5 mm red lesion on the lesser curve of the body of the stomach (Fig. 3.2) and biopsies were taken |
    | Histology | Gastric mucosa showing infiltration by a tumour composed of sheets, cribriform islands, and glandular structures. The tumour cells are relatively uniform, with a small amount of eosinophilic cytoplasm and stippled chromatin. Positive immunostaining for chromogranin and synaptophysin, with dot-like positivity for pan-cytokeratin. Ki-67 proliferation rate is 2%. The adjacent mucosa shows chronic atrophic gastritis with focal intestinal metaplasia. |
    | Computed tomography (CT) chest, abdomen, and pelvis | No metastatic disease |

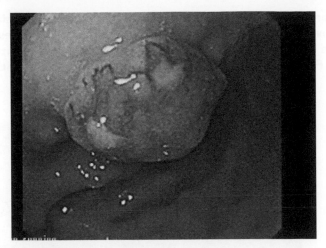

**Fig. 3.2** Endoscopic image of lesion in stomach. See also Plate 5

Courtesy of Oxford University Hospitals NHS Foundation Trust

## What is the most likely diagnosis?

A.  Gastrointestinal stromal tumour (GIST)

B.  Grade 1 neuroendocrine tumour (NET)

C.  Grade 2 NET

D.  Grade 3 NET

E.  Leiomyoma

10. **A 50-year-old man was referred for investigation of dyspepsia.**
    **A gastroscopy showed a gastric lesion in the fundus. Biopsies were taken**
    **from the lesion and immunohistochemistry showed positivity for CD117**
    **(c-KIT). Fig. 3.3 shows a retroflexed view of the stomach with the fundal**
    **lesion.**

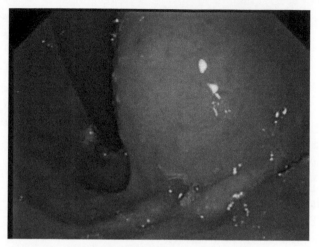

**Fig. 3.3** Endoscopic view of stomach in retroflexion. See also Plate 6
Courtesy of Oxford University Hospitals NHS Foundation Trust

## What is the most appropriate next step of management?

A. CT scan

B. Endoscopic ultrasound

C. *H. pylori* eradication and repeat gastroscopy in 12 months

D. Refer for genetic counselling

E. Repeat gastroscopy in three years' time

11. **An 82-year-old woman was referred for a gastroscopy to investigate dyspepsia and normocytic anaemia. A lesion was identified in the gastric antrum.**

    Investigations:
    Gastroscopy                    Fig. 3.4

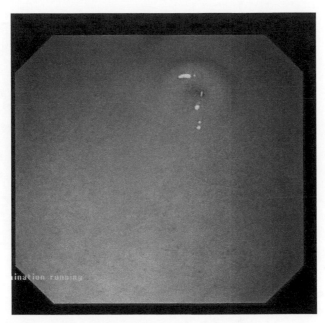

**Fig. 3.4** Endoscopic image of gastric antrum. See also Plate 7

Image courtesy of Dr Tim Ambrose, Oxford University Hospitals NHS Foundation Trust

### What is the most appropriate next step in investigating and managing this lesion?

A. CT thorax, abdomen, and pelvis

B. Endoscopic ultrasound (EUS)

C. No further action required

D. Repeat the gastroscopy after six weeks high-dose proton pump inhibitor (PPI) therapy

E. Test and treat for *H. pylori*

12. **A 45-year-old man was referred by his GP for investigation of epigastric discomfort that had not resolved despite an adequate trial of PPI therapy. A gastroscopy showed a lesion in the antrum. An EUS examination was performed to further characterize the lesion.**

    **The endoscopic ultrasonographic appearance of the lesion is shown in Fig. 3.5.**

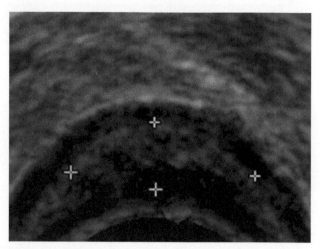

**Fig. 3.5** Endoscopic ultrasound image of gastric lesion

**In which layer of the stomach does the lesion lie?**

A. Interface

B. Mucosa

C. Muscularis propria

D. Serosa

E. Submucosa

13. **A 76-year-old man was referred by his GP for endoscopy complaining of a six-month history of dyspepsia, despite adequate trials of PPI treatment. His *H. pylori* breath test was negative. His stepmother had died from gastric carcinoma.**

    **Among patients who are referred for gastroscopy for alarm features, the prevalence of gastric cancer (GC) is most appropriately described as:**

A. 0.8%

B. 4%

C. 16%

D. 28%

E. 32%

14. **A 27-year-old secretary was referred by her GP with heartburn, abdominal pain, and diarrhoea. Her symptoms had persisted despite high doses of omeprazole. She denied the use of non-steroidal anti-inflammatory drugs (NSAIDs) and was a non-smoker. She reported that her father had a 'pancreas tumour'.**

Investigations:

Gastroscopy        Severe peptic ulcer disease. Predominant ulceration in distal duodenum with multiple small ulcers. Large gastric folds.

**What is the next appropriate investigation?**

A. CLO test

B. Fasting serum gastrin

C. Magnetic resonance (MR) pancreas

D. Secretin stimulation test

E. Serum calcium

15. **A 46-year-old woman was recently diagnosed with gastric adenocarcinoma. She enquired about her son's risk of developing GC.**

**Which is the weakest independent risk factor for gastric adenocarcinoma?**

A. Age

B. Family history

C. Female sex

D. *H. pylori* infection

E. Smoking

16. **A 69-year-old retired builder was recently diagnosed with a diffuse T2N gastric adenocarcinoma. Imaging and laparoscopy excluded occult and distant metastatic disease. He had no significant past medical history of note.**

**Which is the most appropriate treatment option?**

A. Chemoradiotherapy

B. Endoscopic resection

C. Pre-operative chemotherapy and radical gastrectomy

D. Radical gastrectomy

E. Subtotal gastrectomy

17. **A 34-year-old woman presented with nausea, intermittent vomiting, bloating, and 5kg weight loss over three months. She had gastro-oesophageal reflux disease, for which she took omeprazole, but no other past medical history. Examination revealed epigastric distension and a succussion splash.**

Investigations:

| | |
|---|---|
| Haemoglobin | 130 g/L |
| Creatinine | 67 µmol/L |
| Thyroid stimulating hormone | 1.16 munit/L |
| Fasting glucose | 4.5 mmol/L |
| Gastroscopy | Normal |
| MR enterography | Normal |

**What is the most appropriate investigation to make a diagnosis?**

A. $^{13}$C breath testing

B. Barium follow through

C. Scintigraphic gastric emptying at two hours

D. Scintigraphic gastric emptying at four hours

E. Wireless capsule motility testing

18. **A 68-year-old man with Parkinson's disease on levodopa was admitted with vomiting and abdominal pain.**

**Which of the following anti-emetics is the first-line treatment for nausea and vomiting in patients with Parkinson's disease?**

A. Domperidone

B. Haloperidol

C. Metoclopromide

D. Ondansetron

E. Prochlorperazine

19. **A 45-year-old woman attended her general practitioner with recurrent nausea and vomiting associated with travel. She had tried cyclizine to no effect.**

**What is the next choice of medication for her motion sickness?**

A. Betahistine

B. Hyoscine

C. Metoclopromide

D. Ondansetron

E. Prochlorperazine

20. **A 56-year-old man was referred for a gastroscopy with symptoms of dyspepsia and upper abdominal pain. His history included coeliac disease (CD) for which he maintained a gluten-free diet.**

    Investigations:
    Gastroscopy                                    Fig. 3.6
    Urease breath test                             Negative

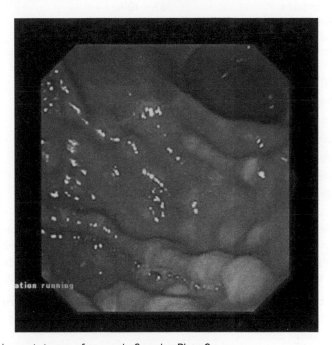

**Fig. 3.6** Endoscopic image of stomach. See also Plate 8

Image courtesy of Dr Tim Ambrose, Oxford University Hospitals NHS Foundation Trust

## What is the most likely diagnosis?

A. Granulomatous gastritis

B. Haemorrhagic gastritis

C. *H. pylori*-associated gastritis

D. Lymphocytic gastritis

E. Upper GI Crohn's disease

21. **A 56-year-old man was referred to the gastroenterology clinic with epigastric pain, anorexia, and weight loss. Abdominal examination was unremarkable. He had peripheral oedema to the mid shins.**

    Investigations:

    | | |
    |---|---|
    | Haemoglobin | 130 g/L |
    | White cell count | $9.0 \times 10^9$/L |
    | Platelet count | $387 \times 10^9$/L |
    | Albumin | 28 g/L |
    | C-reactive protein | 9 mg/L |
    | Gastroscopy | Markedly thickened gastric folds primarily of the body and fundus. Gastric biopsies taken. |
    | Histology | Foveolar hyperplasia |

    **What is the most likely diagnosis?**

    A. Chronic gastritis

    B. Gastric adenocarcinoma

    C. Lymphoma

    D. Ménétrier's disease

    E. Zollinger–Ellison syndrome

22. **A patient had undergone a gastroscopy to investigate iron-deficiency anaemia. Their GP had received the duodenal histology result showing 'intraepithelial lymphocytosis and normal villous architecture', and asked whether this meant that the patient had coeliac disease.**

    **In which other condition can duodenal intraepithelial lymphocytosis be present?**

    A. All the listed options

    B. Crohn's disease

    C. Giardiasis

    D. NSAID enteropathy

    E. Small intestinal bacterial overgrowth

23. **A 69-year-old man was referred for a gastroscopy and colonoscopy to investigate iron deficiency anaemia. He denied any symptoms. His background included ischaemic heart disease and hypertension.**

Investigations:

| | |
|---|---|
| Gastroscopy | A mass was seen in the second part of the duodenum (Fig. 3.7) |
| Histology (duodenal mass) | Small tubular glands lined by eosinophilic absorptive epithelium with pseudostratified hyperchromatic nuclei; no evidence of dysplasia. CD10 and CDX positive |
| Colonoscopy | Sigmoid diverticulae only |

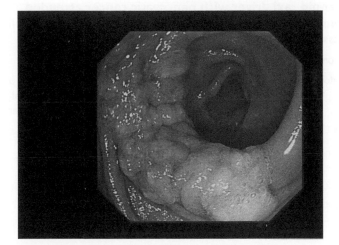

**Fig. 3.7** Endoscopic image of second part of duodenum. See also Plate 9

Image courtesy of Dr Tim Ambrose, Oxford University Hospitals NHS Foundation Trust

### What is the most likely diagnosis?

A. Coeliac disease

B. Crohn's disease

C. Duodenal adenocarcinoma

D. Duodenal adenoma

E. Duodenal lymphoma

24. **At the latest endoscopy user group meeting, the key performance measures for upper GI endoscopy are published for each endoscopist.**

    **Which of the following is a key performance measure for gastroscopy?**

    A. Accurate documentation of indications after therapeutic upper gastrointestinal (UGI) endoscopy

    B. Accurate photo documentation of anatomical landmarks and abnormal findings

    C. Documentation of distance from incisors to gastro oesophageal junction (GOJ), in centimetres

    D. Documentation of patient comfort score

    E. Minimum seven-minute procedure time for index gastroscopy

25. **A 57-year-old taxi driver with pancreatic cancer attended the emergency department with profuse vomiting and metabolic alkalosis. A succussion splash was elicited on examination.**

    Investigations:

    | CT abdomen and pelvis | Distended stomach with evidence of gastric outlet obstruction secondary to duodenal obstruction from locally advanced pancreatic cancer |
    |---|---|

    **What is the most appropriate immediate next step?**

    A. Decompression with large-bore nasogastric tube

    B. Gastrojejunostomy

    C. Gastroscopy and duodenal stent insertion

    D. Gastroscopy and nasojejunal tube insertion

    E. Parenteral nutrition

## 1. E. Urea breath test

- NSAIDs and *H. pylori* are independent risk factors for PUD
- Routine testing and treating of *H. pylori* prior to starting NSAIDs is indicated in those with a history of PUD

NSAIDs and *H. pylori* are independent risk factors for PUD. However, both can have additive effects on the risk of peptic ulcer bleeding. Studies have shown that *H. pylori* eradication is associated with a reduced incidence of peptic ulcer in new NSAID users but not in chronic users. A test and treat strategy is not recommended in all patients prior to starting NSAIDs. However, it is justifiable in those with a history of PUD.

Full-dose PPIs in high-risk patients (age >60, past history of PUD, concomitant oral steroids or oral anticoagulants, comorbidity, and requirement for prolonged use of NSAIDs) is recommended. COX–2 inhibitors, such as celecoxib, have fewer GI side effects. However, their use has to be balanced against the recognized risk of cardiovascular events.

Malfertheiner P, Megraud F, O'Morain CA et al. (on behalf of the European Helicobacter and Microbiota Study Group and Consensus panel). Management of *Helicobacter pylori* infection—the Maastricht V/Florence Consensus Report. *Gut.* 2017 Jan;66(1):6–30. Doi: 10.1136/gutjnl-2016-312288.

## 2. B. *H. pylori* infection

- Rapid urease testing may give false negative results in patients on PPI therapy
- PPI therapy is associated with an elevated serum gastrin

Rapid urease testing (e.g. a CLO test) sensitivity is well recognized as being compromised by acid-suppressing therapy, and patients should ideally withhold these medications for two weeks prior to testing. If patients are still taking their medication at the time of endoscopy, there is a risk of obtaining false negative results. PPI treatment is also associated with an elevated serum gastrin due to the interruption of the normal negative feedback loop.

The most likely diagnosis is of a false negative rapid urease test in a patient with *H. pylori* infection, and this patient should be offered non-invasive *H. pylori* testing off PPI treatment.

ZES is a cause of peptic ulceration in 0.1%–1% of cases. Features suggestive of ZES include:

- severe or resistant ulceration in the absence of NSAIDs or *H. pylori* infection
- unusual sites of ulceration (e.g. D2 or more distally)
- diarrhoea

*Best of Five MCQs for the European Specialty Examination in Gastroenterology and Hepatology.* Thomas Marjot, Colleen G C McGregor, Tim Ambrose, Aminda N De Silva, Jeremy Cobbold, and Simon Travis, Oxford University Press (2021). © Oxford University Press. DOI: 10.1093/oso/9780198834373.003.0003

- large gastric folds
- fasting serum gastrin levels >1,000 pg/ml (off PPI treatment)

Fasting serum gastrin levels can be intermediate in ZES so, if there is strong suspicion clinically, the next step would be a secretin provocation test. Other causes of intermediate elevated fasting serum gastrin levels include atrophic gastritis, pernicious anaemia, gastric outlet obstruction (GOO), renal failure, and small bowel resection.

HIV infection predisposes to cytomegalovirus (CMV) and herpes simplex virus, which can cause ulcers resistant to standard treatment. Crohn's disease is characterized by transmural ulceration, although this is uncommon in the upper GI tract. Tuberculosis is a rare cause of ulceration. The normal blood tests make these diagnoses less likely.

Malfertheiner P, Megraud F, O'Morain CA et al. (on behalf of the European Helicobacter and Microbiota Study Group and Consensus panel). Management of *Helicobacter pylori* infection—the Maastricht V/Florence Consensus Report. *Gut.* 2017 Jan;66(1):6–30. Doi: 10.1136/gutjnl-2016-312288.

## 3. C. Low body mass index

- Failure of first-line *H. pylori* eradication regimens occurs in at least 20% of patients
- Insufficient gastric acid suppression contributes significantly to treatment failure
- Raised BMI and active smoking confer lower eradication rates due to reduced drug bioavailability

Failure of first-line treatment regimens occurs in more than 20% of patients. Contributory factors are multifactorial: host genetic factors, *H. pylori* virulence factors, antimicrobial resistance, compliance with therapy, and duration of therapy.

Factors associated with treatment failure are discussed below:

- *Primary antimicrobial resistance* is increasing worldwide. Resistance patterns vary between regions because of differing antibiotic usage, treatment regimens, and disease prevalence. Amoxicillin rates are low in Europe, the US, Japan, and China in contrast to significantly higher rates in South Korea and Iran. Clinicians must bear in mind the primary antimicrobial resistance patterns for their local population before deciding on empirical treatment.
- *Acid suppression* studies show that higher-dose twice-daily PPI regimens are associated with a higher eradication rate when compared with standard regimens. Intra-gastric acid suppression enables *H. pylori* to enter its growth phase, thereby increasing its vulnerability to antibiotics targeting its replicative cycle.
- *Virulence factors of* H. pylori: certain *H. pylori* strains produce highly immunogenic CagA protein and VacA toxin, both of which result in more severe gastric inflammation. Studies significantly correlate severe gastric inflammation with treatment success. It is postulated that severe inflammation increases drug bioavailability through increased mucosal perfusion.
- *Host IL-1β polymorphism*: eradication rates are significantly better in patients with the *IL-1β*-511 T/T genotype compared with the C/C and C/T genotypes.
- *BMI and smoking*: an elevated BMI (>25kg/m$^2$) and smoking are associated with lower eradication rates, thought to be due to lower drug bioavailability.
- *Treatment duration*: a longer treatment duration (10–14 days) is more efficacious than a seven-day regimen, with eradication rates increased by 4%–6%.

Song M, Ang T. Second and third line treatment options for *Helicobacter pylori* eradication. *World J Gastroenterol.* 2014 Feb 14; 20(6): 1517–1528. Doi:10.3748/wjg.v20.i6.1517.

**4. E. Resection of the gastric antrum, formation of a gastrojejunostomy, and closure of the first part of the duodenum and gastric outflow**

A. Is as described

B. Is a vagotomy and pyloroplasty

C. Is a Roux-en-Y gastric bypass

D. Is a pyloromyotomy.

Fig. 3.8 shows both the Billroth I and Billroth II gastrectomy.

**Billroth I gastrectomy for gastric ulcer**

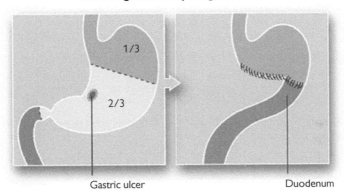

**Billroth II gastrectomy for duodenal ulcer**

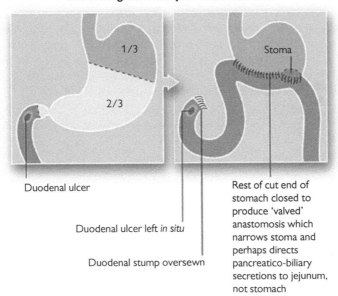

**Fig. 3.8** Billroth I and Billroth II gastrectomy

Burkitt HG, Quick CGR, *Essential Surgery Problems, Diagnosis and Management*, 3rd edition, 2001, Elsevier.

### 5. C. Iron

- Anaemia post gastrectomy may be multifactorial – iron, $B_{12}$, or folate deficiency
- Hypochlorhydria post gastrectomy results in reduced iron absorption
- Folate deficiency is exacerbated by $B_{12}$ deficiency

Iron deficiency is the most common vitamin deficiency post gastrectomy, and occurs approximately 10 years before the onset of vitamin $B_{12}$ deficiency (because the body has substantial reserves of $B_{12}$). Gastric acid is required for the solubilization of ferric iron to form ferrous iron. Therefore, hypochlorhydria post gastrectomy results in reduced iron absorption. Vitamin $B_{12}$ deficiency occurs because of the reduction in intrinsic factor, which is secreted by the parietal cells of the stomach. Folate deficiency has also been documented, and may be exacerbated by vitamin $B_{12}$ deficiency because the latter is required to convert inactive methyltetrahydrofolic acid to the active tetrahydrofolic acid. Vitamin D deficiency with subsequent osteoporosis has also been implicated.

Following partial gastrectomy, 30%–40% of patients experience long-term side effects. The risk of malignant change in the gastric remnant is 3% over 15 years. Dumping syndrome tends to present within three months of surgery, but can resolve within one year post-operatively. It occurs in 25%–50% of patients, but causes significant symptoms in 5%–10%.

A Billroth II gastrectomy is the surgical procedure of choice for a duodenal ulcer, whereas the Billroth I is used for a gastric ulcer.

Rogers C. Postgastrectomy nutrition. *Nutr Clin Pract*. 2011;26:126–136. Doi: 10.1177/0884533611400070.

### 6. C. Three years

- Extensive atrophic gastritis and intestinal metaplasia (IM) are precancerous conditions because they constitute the background in which dysplasia and intestinal-type gastric adenocarcinoma develop
- For adequate staging and grading, at least four non-targeted biopsies of two topographic sites should be taken; additional targeted biopsies of lesions should also be taken
- *Helicobacter pylori* eradication is important to slow progression to cancer

The histopathological slide (Fig. 3.9) demonstrates gastric body mucosa with an almost complete absence of specialized gastritis glands, extensive intestinal metaplasia, and focal pyloric metaplasia. No *H. pylori* organisms are seen.

High-risk features predisposing to GC include the following:

- Membership of a high-risk ethnic population (e.g. East Asian ethnicity)
- Residence in, or migration from, a high-risk geographic location
- Family history of GC
- Dysplasia on biopsy
- Extensive IM on biopsies; the extent of IM is probably more important than the metaplastic subtype
- Operative Link on Gastritis Assessment (OLGA) or Operative Link on Gastric Intestinal Metaplasia (OLGIM) Stage III or IV

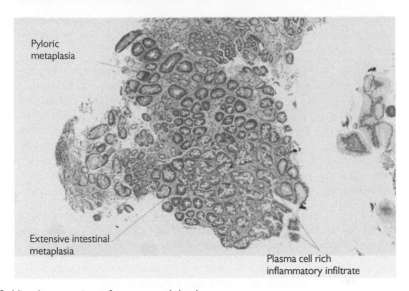

**Fig. 3.9** Histology specimen from stomach body

Image courtesy of Dr Eve Fryer, Consultant Histopathologist, Oxford University Hospitals NHS Foundation Trust

The European Society of Gastrointestinal Endoscopy (ESGE) recommends that patients with extensive atrophy and/or intestinal metaplasia should receive follow-up oesophago-gastro-duodenoscopy assessment every three years after diagnosis. There is no specific treatment for atrophic gastritis or IM. However, *H. pylori* eradication may lead to partial regression of atrophic gastritis. Although it does not reverse intestinal metaplasia, it may slow progression to neoplasia.

Dinis-Ribeiro M et al. Management of precancerous conditions and lesions in the stomach (MAPS). *Endoscopy.* 2012;44:74–94. Doi: 10.1055/s-0031-1291491.

**7. C. Repeat the gastroscopy with excision of polyps >1 cm**

- Fundic gland polyps are the most prevalent type of gastric epithelial polyp
- The number, location and size of the largest polyp should be clearly documented
- Adenomatous polyps should be resected, when appropriate, because of the significant malignant potential

Gastric epithelial polyps can be classified as three types: fundic gland polyps (FGPs), hyperplastic polyps, and adenomatous polyps. FGPs are the most prevalent type of epithelial polyp. They are typically small (<1 cm), multiple, and located in the fundus and body. Their colour is usually the same as the surrounding mucosa. They are not usually associated with an increased risk of cancer unless in the context of familial adenomatous polyposis (FAP). However, larger polyps (>1 cm) have been shown to be dysplastic in approximately 2% of patients. Routine tissue sampling of FGPs (<1 cm) is not required. Unlike hyperplastic and adenomatous polyps, there is no association with *H. pylori* infection. FGPs are associated with long-term PPI use, however, and regress once PPI treatment is stopped. One should question the diagnosis of FGPs if they appear ulcerated, >1 cm, or are in an antral location. Such atypical features warrant excision.

Hyperplastic polyps are typically small, single, or few in number. They are red, dome-shaped, and smooth. Associated with *H. pylori* infection, gastric atrophy and gastric intestinal metaplasia, these polyps regress on eradication of *H. pylori*. Hyperplastic polyps are potentially pre-malignant – diagnosis and absence of dysplasia should be confirmed histologically. Polyps >1 cm, pedunculated or symptomatic, should be endoscopically resected, provided *H. pylori* has been successfully eradicated.

Adenomatous polyps usually affect the antrum and incisura, and are single in number and small (<2 cm) in size. With a velvety pink appearance, they may be sessile or pedunculated. Synchronous gastric adenocarcinoma has been found in up to 30%. Gastric adenomas carry a significant malignant potential and should be resected when appropriate. Endoscopic resection is the preferred mode of treatment. Follow-up endoscopy should be performed at 6–12 months with annual surveillance thereafter.

Banks M, Graham D et al. British Society of Gastroenterology guidelines on the diagnosis and management of patients at risk of gastric adenocarcinoma. *Gut.* 2019;68:1545–1575. Doi: 10.1136/gutjnl-2018-318126.

### 8. C. Biopsies of two topographic sites (antrum and corpus, at the lesser and greater curvature) plus additional biopsies of suspicious lesions

- Chronic atrophic gastritis or intestinal metaplasia increases the risk of gastric adenocarcinoma
- Intestinal metaplasia is the most reliable marker of gastric atrophy
- Sufficient biopsies from at least two topographic sites are required for adequate staging and grading

GC is ranked third for cancer-related mortality worldwide. Although early recognition is possible, many are diagnosed at a late stage with resultant poor prognosis. European guidance, published in 2019, mandates the sampling and management of epithelial precancerous conditions and lesions in the stomach.

Patients with chronic atrophic gastritis or intestinal metaplasia are at risk for developing gastric adenocarcinoma. Intestinal metaplasia confirmed histologically is the most reliable marker of atrophy in gastric mucosa. For adequate staging of gastric precancerous conditions, an index gastroscopy should include gastric biopsies both for *H. pylori* infection diagnosis and for identification of advanced stages of atrophic gastritis.

Biopsies should be taken of at least two topographic sites (both the antrum and the corpus, at the lesser and greater curvature of each). Samples should be clearly labelled in two separate vials. Additional biopsies of any suspicious lesions (for high-grade dysplasia or neoplasia) should be taken.

Pimentel-Nunes P, Libanio D et al. Management of epithelial precancerous conditions and lesions in the stomach (MAPS II): European Society of Gastrointestinal Endoscopy (ESGE), European Helicobacter and Microbiota Study Group (EHMSG), European Society of Pathology (ESP), and Sociedade Portuguesa de Endoscopia Digestiva (SPED) guideline update 2019. *Endoscopy.* 2019;51:365–388. Doi: 10.1055/a-0859-1883.

### 9. B. Grade 1 neuroendocrine tumour (NET)

- See Fig. 3.10. Type 1 NETs constitute most gastric NETs, have low proliferation index, and are associated with atrophic gastritis and $B_{12}$ deficiency (Table 3.1)
- GISTs and leiomyomas (benign) are other intramural gastric tumours with the former having malignant potential
- Gastric NETs are rare, comprising 0.1%–0.6% of all GCs and 7%–8% of all NETs

Delle FG et al. ENETS consensus guidelines update for gastroduodenal neuroendocrine neoplasms. *Neuroendocrinology.* 2016;103–102):119–124. Doi: 10.1159/000443168.

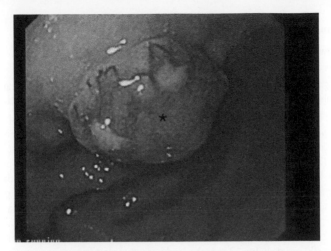

**Fig. 3.10** Endoscopic image of NET (black asterisk) in body of stomach

Courtesy of Oxford University Hospitals NHS Foundation Trust

**Table 3.1** Highlights the features between the different types of neuroendocrine tumours (NETs)

|  | Type 1 | Type 2 | Type 3 |
|---|---|---|---|
| Proportion of all NETs | 75% | 5% | 20% |
| Chance of progression to metastases | <2% | Intermediate | 65% have local or hepatic metastases |
| Appearance | Small reddish nodule, can be multiple | Small and multiple | Solitary and usually >1 cm |
| Associated conditions | Chronic atrophic gastritis, B12 deficiency (pernicious anaemia) | MEN type I, Zollinger-Ellison syndrome | None, sporadic |
| Gastrin levels | May be raised | Usually raised | Normal |
| Enterochromaffin-like cells | Present | Present | Not present |
| Ki-67 index | ≤3% | 3–20% | >20% |
| Presentation with carcinoid syndrome | No | No | Yes, if hepatic metastases |
| Management | Endoscopic resection usually but consider surgery in those >2 cm, extensive gastric wall involvement (increased risk of adenocarcinoma) and emergent bleeding | Endoscopic resection or consider surgery if multiple and large | Partial or total gastrectomy with local lymph node resection |
| Survival at five years | 75%–80% | 80%–90% | 90%–95% |

Data from Delle FG et al. ENETS Consensus Guidelines Update for Gastroduodenal Neuroendocrine Neoplasms. *Neuroendocrinology.* 2016;103(2):119–124. Doi: 10.1159/000443168.

### 10. A. CT scan

- GISTs are rare and account for 1%–2% of gastric neoplasms
- Most GISTs are positive for marker CD117 (c-KIT), CD34, and/or DOG-1
- CT enterography is the best imaging modality for diagnosis and staging, and can be used alongside histology to guide treatment with resection with or without imatinib

See Fig 3.11. GISTs are rare neoplasms of the GI tract associated with high rates of malignant transformation, particularly if found outside the stomach. Many present asymptomatically and are identified incidentally on cross-sectional imaging. GISTs can have three different histologic findings: spindle (70%), epithelioid (20%), or mixed type (10%) and most will stain positive for CD117 (C-KIT), CD34, and/or DOG-1. CT enterography is the best imaging modality for diagnosis staging and can identify tumour location, invasion into nearby structures, perforation, or metastasis (usually to liver, omentum, or mesentery). Several scoring systems have been developed to help risk stratify GISTs to determine optimal treatment modality. Low-risk tumours should be laparoscopically resected, high-risk and metastatic tumours should be resected with adjuvant imatinib 400 mg daily for 12 months, and unresectable tumours can become amenable to surgery with neoadjuvant imatinib. *H. pylori* eradication and repeat upper GI endoscopy is the recommended treatment for gastric MALT lymphomas. Genetic counselling is not indicated for patients with GISTs.

Parab et al. Gastrointestinal stromal tumors: a comprehensive review. *J Gastrointest Oncol.* 2019 Feb;10(1):144–154. Doi: 10.21037/jgo.2018.08.20.

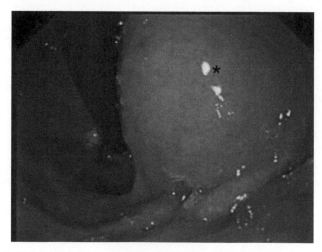

**Fig. 3.11** Retroflexed view of the stomach showing fundal GIST (black asterisk)
Courtesy of Oxford University Hospitals NHS Foundation Trust

### 11. C. No further action required

- Pancreatic rests (ectopic pancreas, heterotopic pancreas) are benign congenital lesions that are rarely symptomatic
- Further investigation is only required if the pathology is uncertain

This lesion (Fig. 3.12) is a pancreatic rest (also known as an 'ectopic' or 'heterotopic' pancreas). They are typically found incidentally during investigation for other symptoms and they are benign,

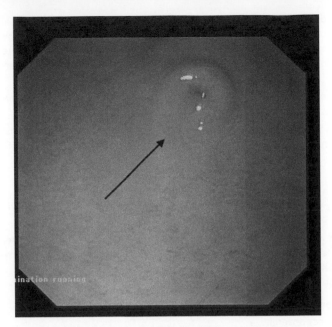

**Fig. 3.12** Endoscopic image of pancreatic rest (black arrow)

Image courtesy of Dr Tim Ambrose, Oxford University Hospitals NHS Foundation Trust

congenital lesions. Most patients are asymptomatic but some may develop abdominal pain, GI obstruction, or even pancreatitis. The typical endoscopic features are of a submucosal lesion with central umbilication and usually <2 cm in size. They are commonly found in the gastric antrum but may be seen anywhere in the foregut and proximal midgut. Biopsy is not necessary if the diagnosis can be confidently made endoscopically. Further investigation, with EUS initially, should be considered if the diagnosis is unclear or the endoscopic appearances suggest a differential, including a GIST.

Masoodi I, Al-Lehibi A et al. *Pancreatic rest—An unusual cause of dyspepsia: a case report with literature review. Saudi J Med Med Sci.* 2016 Sep–Dec;4(3):225–228. Doi: 10.4103/1658-631X.188261.

## 12. E. Submucosa

- A pancreatic rest appears endosonographically as hypoechoic or as intermediate echogenic heterogeneous lesions with indistinct borders
- EUS views of the stomach appear as five distinct layers

The five distinct layers alternate between hyperechoic (bright) and hypoechoic (dark) layers. From the layer closest to the lumen and therefore the probe, they are as follows:

- Interface: bright layer between the probe and the mucosa
- Mucosa (superficial and deep): dark
- Submucosa: bright
- Muscularis propria: dark
- Serosa: bright

This man had an area of ectopic pancreas or pancreatic rest. These are rare submucosal tumours that consist of endocrine and/or exocrine cells. A pancreatic rest is most often seen in the distal stomach, duodenum, or proximal jejunum. Complications of ectopic pancreas are rare, but can lead to ulceration, gastric outflow obstruction, and (rarely) malignancy. They appear endosonographically as hypoechoic or intermediate echogenic (as in this case) heterogeneous lesions with indistinct borders. The diagnosis is made histologically and management is guided by the symptoms.

Asymptomatic lesions can be followed expectantly. Symptomatic lesions can be removed by snare or surgically.

Attwell A, Sams S, Fukami N. Diagnosis of ectopic pancreas by endoscopic ultrasound with fine-needle aspiration. *World J Gastroenterol*. 2015;21(8):2367–2373. Doi:10.3748/wjg.v21.i8.2367.

### 13. B. 4%

- Dyspepsia in individuals >55 despite adequate PPI treatment and/or *H. pylori* eradication should be considered for endoscopy

Not all patients who present with dyspepsia require endoscopy. Alarm features (see the following list) are an indication for urgent endoscopy. However, among those who are referred, the prevalence of GC is around 4%.

Alarm features:

- Weight loss
- Iron-deficiency anaemia
- Gastrointestinal bleeding
- Persistent vomiting
- Dysphagia
- Epigastric mass
- Abnormal barium imaging

Those patients who have truly resistant symptoms, despite best medical therapy, may require a specialist gastroenterology opinion and/or an endoscopy. NICE 2019 guidance attempted to identify a further specific subset of patients who should be offered endoscopy.

Patients over the age of 55 years who have persistent symptoms of dyspepsia despite adequate acid suppression and eradication of *H. pylori* should be considered for endoscopy if there is:

- a previous gastric ulcer
- previous gastric surgery
- continuing need for NSAID treatment
- anxiety about cancer
- increased risk of GC

Family history, gastric ulcers, polyps or polyposis syndromes, Lynch syndrome, previous gastric surgery, Ménétrier's disease, and pernicious anaemia are all associated with an increased risk of gastric carcinoma. Lifestyle factors associated with GC are alcohol excess, smoking, and social deprivation.

National Institute for Health and Care Excellence. Gastro-oesophageal reflux disease and dyspepsia in adults: investigation and management [Internet]. [London]: NICE; 2014 [updated October 2019]. (Clinical guideline [CG184]). Available at: https://www.nice.org.uk/guidance/cg184

## 14. B. Fasting serum gastrin

- Fasting serum gastrin levels >1000 pg/ml are diagnostic of ZES
- 50% of patients with MEN1 develop ZES
- If ZES is suspected, one should screen for MEN1 with a serum calcium, parathyroid hormone and prolactin

Zollinger-Ellison Syndrome (ZES) is comprised of severe PUD, gastro-oesophageal reflux disease and chronic diarrhoea secondary to a gastrin-secreting tumour of the duodenum or pancreas. Gastrinomas are a functional ectopic neuroendocrine tumour that secretes excess gastric acid with resultant GI mucosal ulceration. Gastrinomas causing ZES occurs sporadically in 80% of cases or as part of multiple endocrine neoplasia type 1 (MEN1) in 20%. Inherited in an autosomal dominant pattern, 50% of patients with MEN1 develop ZES.

Symptoms commonly include abdominal pain, diarrhoea and heartburn. Diarrhoea occurs due to malabsorption from hypersecretion of acid. Patients will report ongoing symptoms despite negative *H. pylori* testing and PPI therapy.

Findings suggestive of ZES endoscopically include:

- prominent gastric folds (trophic effect of excess gastrin)
- unusual sites of ulceration (e.g. D2 or more distally)

PPI should be stopped one week before testing for ZES. Initial testing involves measuring fasting serum gastrin levels; this has a 99% sensitivity and is diagnostic if levels are >1,000 pg/ml. Secretin stimulation test measures evoked gastrin levels. Secretin inhibits gastrin release from G cells, therefore failure to suppress gastrin level (>200 pg/ml) following administration is diagnostic. CT or MRI imaging has a role for detecting primary tumours or to evaluate any metastases. If ZES is suspected, one should also consider screening for MEN1 with serum calcium, parathyroid hormone level and prolactin.

Treatment includes high dose PPI or H2-receptor antagonists and surgical resection of the underlying gastrinoma.

Cho MS, Kasi A. Zollinger Ellison Syndrome. [Updated 2019 Jun 4]. In: StatPearls [Internet]. Treasure Island (FL): StatPearls Publishing; 2020 Jan–. Available at: https://www.ncbi.nlm.nih.gov/books/NBK537344/

## 15. C. Female sex

- GC is the fifth most common cause of cancer worldwide
- Risk factors are different for cancers arising from the cardia and non-cardia regions
- Males have a two- to three-fold increased risk of GC

As well as being the fifth most common cause of cancer, GC is the third most common cause of cancer death. The highest incidence rates are observed in East Asia, East Europe and South America. The overall five-year survival rate remains poor at approximately 20%. GC is a multifactorial disease with both environmental and genetic factors at play. Most of the risk factors are modifiable and may be different for cancers arising from the cardia and non-cardia regions of the stomach.

- *Age:* The incidence rate of GC increases with advancing age.
- *Family history:* A significant family history (first-degree relative) of GC increases an individual's risk. Inherited syndromes, such as hereditary diffuse gastric cancer (HDGC), FAP and Peutz-Jeghers syndrome (PJS) account for 1%–3% of GC cases.

- *Sex*: Rates of GC are two- to three-fold higher in men than women, for both cardia and non-cardia GC. Oestrogens may play a protective role against the development of cancer.
- *H. pylori* infection: This is a major risk factor for only non-cardia GC with a relative risk of 6. It accounts for 65%–80% of all GCs. The mechanism by which *H. pylori* causes GC is not fully elucidated.
- *Smoking*: Tobacco smoking is a risk factor for both cardia and non-cardia GC. A meta-analysis of cohort studies demonstrated a significant increased risk of GC by 60% in male smokers and 20% in female smokers compared with never smokers.

Karimi P, Islami F et al. Gastric cancer: descriptive epidemiology, risk factors, screening, and prevention. *Cancer Epidemiol Biomarkers Prev.* 2014;23(5):700–713. Doi: 10.1158/1055-9965.EPI-13-1057.


## 16. C. Pre-operative chemotherapy and radical gastrectomy

- Surgical resection, in very early stages, is potentially curative in GC
- Endoscopic resection should be considered in tumours confined to mucosa, well differentiated, non-ulcerated, and ≤2 cm
- Pre-operative chemotherapy is recommended in Stage IB resectable GC

This patient has Stage IIB GC.

Very early stage GC (T1a) may be amenable to endoscopic resection, endoscopic mucosal resection (EMR), or endoscopic submucosal dissection (ESD). Criteria for endoscopic resection include tumour confined to the mucosa, well differentiated, ≤2 cm, and non-ulcerated. T1 tumours not meeting these criteria for endoscopic resection require surgery. Surgical resection is potentially curative in GC. Most patients still relapse following resection. Therefore, the standard of treatment for Stage IB is combined modality therapies.

For Stage IB to III cancer, radical gastrectomy is indicated. If a macroscopic proximal margin of 5 cm can be achieved between the tumour and the GOJ, a subtotal gastrectomy may be achieved. Otherwise, total gastrectomy plus pre-operative chemotherapy is indicated. The extent of nodal dissection is debated.

Perioperative (pre- and post-) chemotherapy with a platinum/fluoropyrimidine combination is recommended for patients with Stage IB resectable GC. The UK Medical Research Council (MRC) MAGIC trial demonstrated a significant improvement in five-year survival rate in patients who received perioperative chemotherapy versus surgery alone for Stage II and III GCs (36% vs 23%). Chemotherapy naïve patients who undergo gastrectomy for Stage IB GC benefit from post-operative chemoradiotherapy.

Inoperable and metastatic (Stage IV) disease should be considered for palliative chemotherapy or best supportive care if deemed unfit for systemic treatment.

Smyth EC, Verheij M et al. Gastric cancer: ESMO Clinical Practice Guidelines for diagnosis, treatment and follow-up. 2016. *Ann Oncol.* 27(5);38–49. Doi. 10.1093/annonc/mdw350.


## 17. D. Scintigraphic gastric emptying at 4 hours

- Gastroparesis is defined by proven delayed gastric emptying in the absence of mechanical obstruction alongside hallmark symptoms (e.g. vomiting, abdominal pain, early satiety)
- Gastric emptying scintigraphy of a solid-phase meal at four hours is the standard for diagnosis
- Most cases are idiopathic, diabetic, or post-gastric surgery

Gastroparesis is a syndrome defined by objectively delayed gastric emptying in the absence of mechanical obstruction and hallmark symptoms including early satiety, postprandial fullness, nausea, vomiting, bloating, and upper abdominal pain. Most cases in a tertiary referral setting are idiopathic (36%), post-gastric surgery (13%), or due to diabetes (29%). Gastric emptying scintigraphy of a solid-phase meal at four hours is considered the standard for diagnosis. The proportion of retained gastric material categorizes gastroparesis as mild (10%–15%), moderate (15%–35%) or severe (>35%). Scintigraphy studies of shorter duration or based on a liquid challenge have reduced diagnostic sensitivity.

Wireless capsule motility testing simultaneously measures pressure, temperature, and potential hydrogen (pH) as it traverses the GI tract with gastric emptying determined by a rapid increase in pH with capsule transit from stomach to duodenum. $^{13}$C breath testing is another alternative to scintigraphy. However, neither of these tests are widely available and both require further validation before entering routine clinical practice.

Barium follow through is superseded here by enterography and upper GI endoscopy, which both rule out mechanical obstruction.

Alternative diagnoses to consider here are functional dyspepsia, rumination syndrome, cyclical vomiting syndrome, and psychiatric disorders.

Camilleri M et al. Clinical guideline: management of gastroparesis. *Am J Gastroenterol*. 2013;108:18. Doi: 10.1038/ajg.2012.373.


## 18. A. Domperidone

- Anti-dopaminergic agents that can cross the blood–brain barrier and thereby worsen Parkinson's disease symptoms include metoclopramide, haloperidol, and prochlorperazine
- Domperidone is the anti-emetic of choice in Parkinson's disease
- The emetic centre and chemoreceptor trigger zone (CTZ) initiate nausea and vomiting

Domperidone, despite being an anti-dopaminergic agent, does not cross the blood–brain barrier, so is not able to induce the central effects that other dopamine antagonists could. It acts on dopaminergic receptors in the UGI tract as well as the CTZ, which lacks a true blood–brain barrier. Given the fact that in Parkinson's disease there is already impaired gastric emptying, domperidone's prokinetic effect makes it the most useful anti-emetic in this situation.

There are two important areas within the medulla that initiate nausea and vomiting: the emetic centre and the CTZ within the area postrema. The CTZ has five different receptors that may activate it:

1. 5-HT$_3$ receptors
2. Histamine H1 receptors
3. Muscarinic receptors
4. Dopamine D2 receptors
5. Substance P (also called 'neurokinin-1 neuropeptide')

Chemicals such as hormones, ketoacids, uraemia, opioids, and ipecac are all carried in the blood or cerebrospinal fluid (CSF) and can directly stimulate the CTZ due to the lack of a true blood–brain barrier. During pregnancy, oestrogen is thought to be the cause of morning sickness due to its direct action at the CTZ. Gastric irritation and distension, especially at the duodenum (a particularly strong stimulus), causes a massive uptake of 5HT by 5HT$_3$ receptors within the postrema. Anti-emetics that work at this site are 5HT$_3$ receptor antagonists such as ondansetron and granisetron. These are therefore safe for use in Parkinson's disease. However, they do not carry the prokinetic effect that metoclopramide or domperidone have. They could therefore be used as a second-line anti-emetic in this situation.

Dopamine antagonists such as metoclopramide and prochlorperazine are effective anti-emetics. These dopamine antagonists freely cross the blood–brain barrier and have no selectivity for dopamine receptors in the CTZ. Therefore, they can act on dopaminergic systems in other parts of the brain, worsening the symptoms of Parkinson's disease. Haloperidol has a strong anti-dopaminergic action, thereby also worsening the symptoms of Parkinson's disease.

Denholm L, Gallagher G. Physiology and pharmacology of nausea and vomiting. *Physiology*. 2018;19(9):513–516. Doi: 10.1016/j.mpaic.2018.06.010.

### 19. B. Hyoscine

- Vestibular nuclei contain muscarinic and histaminic receptors
- Anti-muscarinics (e.g. hyoscine) and anti-histaminics (e.g. cyclizine) are indicated in motion sickness
- Serotonin-receptor antagonists (ondansetron) reduce the activity of the vagus nerve, thereby suppressing the vomiting centre

Dopamine antagonists are not useful in motion sickness. Vestibular nuclei contain muscarinic and histaminic receptors, not dopaminergic receptors. Anti-muscarinic (hyoscine) and anti-histaminic (cyclizine) drugs are used in motion sickness, because both receptors are present in vestibular nuclei.

Serotonin-receptor antagonists such as ondansetron have been found to be effective in managing post-operative nausea and vomiting because of their ability to reduce activity at the vagus nerve, thereby reducing stimulation at the vomiting centre. They have also been found to be effective in managing chemotherapy-induced nausea and vomiting.

Metoclopramide is a dopamine antagonist, but in motion sickness it is not effective by itself. It is used in combination with hyoscine for its added advantage of being a prokinetic. Therefore, in practice, a combination of the two is routinely used.

Opioids cross the blood–brain barrier and stimulate the CTZ directly to induce the vomiting response. Dopamine-receptor antagonists, which also cross the blood–brain barrier, are thus recommended as the first-line treatment for opioid-induced nausea and vomiting.

Denholm L, Gallagher G. Physiology and pharmacology of nausea and vomiting. *Physiology*. 2018;19(9):513–516. Doi: 10.1016/j.mpaic.2018.06.010.

### 20. D. Lymphocytic gastritis

- Lymphocytic gastritis (LG) is associated with coeliac disease and *H. pylori* infection
- LG is a rare condition, predominantly affecting adults in the fifth to sixth decade
- *H. pylori* eradication, PPI therapy alone, or gluten-free diet lead to a reduction in intraepithelial lymphocytes (IELs)

This endoscopic image demonstrates multiple small white nodules (black asterisks), characteristic features of LG (Fig. 3.13).

LG is characterized by the accumulation of lymphocytes within the gastric epithelium. It is a rare condition with a prevalence of less than 0.3%, predominantly affecting adults in the fifth to sixth decade. Men and women are equally affected. Clinical symptoms are generally non-specific and may include dyspepsia, upper abdominal pain, heartburn, weight loss, or vomiting.

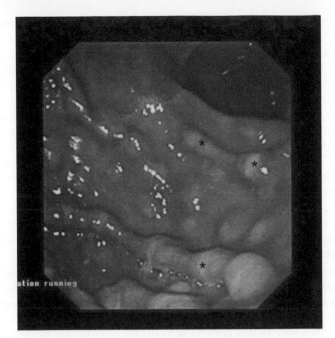

**Fig. 3.13** Endoscopic image of stomach showing lymphocytic gastritis

Image courtesy of Dr Tim Ambrose, Oxford University Hospitals NHS Foundation Trust

LG is diagnosed by characteristic endoscopic and histological findings. The most frequent endoscopic changes include erosions, nodularity, mucosal elevations, polyps, or ulcers. Local spots or mosaic structure to the mucosa may be found, most commonly (~90% of cases) in the body and antrum. Diagnosis is made histologically; the main feature is the presence of ≥25 IELs per 100 gastric surface and foveolar epithelial cells. Most of the lymphocytes present are small and may have a halo appearance. Immunohistochemistry detect CD3+ and CD8+ T lymphocytes. Foveolar epithelial hyperplasia, epithelial proliferation, and intestinal metaplasia may also be seen.

*H. pylori* infection and coeliac disease are strongly associated with the development of LG. The presence of *H. pylori* infection in LG may be up to 27%. Eradication of *H. pylori* results in fewer IELs. Spontaneous remission of LG may also be seen in PPI or H2 blocker therapy alone. In *H. pylori*-associated LG, the presence of granulocytes in the gastric mucosa is noted, which is not observed in CD-associated LG. In the context of CD, LG occurs in up to 35% of patients and is more common in women. Introduction of a gluten-free diet reduces the number of IELs. LG may also, rarely, be associated with lymphoma.

If not already excluded, a diagnosis of LG should prompt investigation for CD and *H. pylori*.

Puderecki M, Wronecki L et al. Lymphocytic gastritis. *Pol J Pathol.* 2019;70(3):155–161. Doi: 10.5114/pjp.2019.90391.

### 21. D. Ménétrier's disease

- MD is characterized by markedly thickened gastric folds in the body, and fundus with relative antral sparing
- Hypoalbuminaemia occurs secondary to protein loss in the gastric mucosa

- Foveolar hyperplasia with corkscrew morphology and preserved linear architecture are classical histopathological findings of MD

All the listed options are causes of thickened gastric folds. However, the combination of markedly thickened gastric folds and hypoalbuminaemia makes a diagnosis of MD the most likely. Correlation with histopathological findings and clinical features is important to establish the correct diagnosis.

MD is a rare, acquired, hypertrophic gastropathy. Hypertrophic gastropathies refer to conditions confined to the rugae of the body and fundus, which are associated with an excessive number of mucosal epithelial cells. MD is characterized by giant gastric folds of the body and fundus, with antral sparing endoscopically, increased gastric mucus production, decreased gastric acid secretion, malnutrition, and hypoalbuminaemia secondary to protein loss in the gastric mucosa. Men are more commonly affected and typical age of onset is between 30 and 60 years old. Importantly, MD may have an increased risk of GC.

Clinical presentation includes nausea, vomiting, abdominal pain, diarrhoea, weight loss, and peripheral oedema. The cause of MD is not fully elucidated. However, cases of MD have been reported in association with CMV, *H. pylori* infection, inflammatory bowel disease, and ankylosing spondylitis, suggesting an underlying immunopathogenesis (TGF-β mediated).

Full thickness biopsy is required. Microscopic features include massive foveolar hyperplasia, which may result in mucosal thickness of ≥1 cm and copious thick mucus production. Foveolar epithelium has a corkscrew morphology and cystically dilated deep glands. The overall linear architecture is maintained. Oxyntic glands atrophy with reduced or absent parietal cells, resulting in an increased gastric pH. The lamina propria has a predominantly chronic inflammatory cell infiltrate with scattered eosinophils.

Remission may occur spontaneously in CMV-associated MD and after *H. pylori* eradication. There is no definitive medical treatment for MD. However, trials with anti-EGFR (cetuximab) have shown some benefit. Octreotide can be used for protein loss. Total gastrectomy is reserved for patients with debilitating disease and high risk for GC.

Huh W, Coffey R et al. Ménétrier's disease: its mimickers and pathogenesis. *J Pathol Transl Med.* 2016;50:10–16. Doi:10.4132/jptm.2015.09.15

## 22. A. All the listed options

- Intraepithelial lymphocytosis is defined as IELs >20 per 100 epithelial cells
- There are multiple mimickers of coeliac disease (CD)
- CD is characterized by a predominantly neutrophilic infiltrate with few crypt abscesses

IELs are no more than 5–10 per 100 epithelial cells in healthy individuals. Intraepithelial lymphocytosis is defined as IELs >20 per 100 epithelial cells. In healthy individuals, IELs localize at the base of the surface epithelium. In the presence of intraepithelial lymphocytosis, IELs are throughout the full thickness of the epithelium.

Intraepithelial lymphocytosis in the context of preserved villous architecture can present a diagnostic challenge. Histopathological findings of CD include villous atrophy, intraepithelial lymphocytosis, increased inflammatory infiltrate in the lamina propria, and crypt hyperplasia. However, multiple differentials exist for duodenal intraepithelial lymphocytosis and villous atrophy (Table 3.2). CD is characterized by a predominantly neutrophilic infiltration. Neutrophilic crypt abscesses are less of a feature in CD. However, they are commonly seen in CD mimickers such as infection, peptic duodenitis, or autoimmune enteritis.

**Table 3.2** Differentials of duodenal intraepithelial lymphocytosis and villous atrophy

| Gluten-mediated | Infection | Immune-mediated | Drugs | Other |
|---|---|---|---|---|
| Coeliac disease | Virus (rotavirus, | Immunoglobulin | Olmesartan | Irritable bowel |
| Gluten sensitivity | enterovirus, adenovirus, | deficiencies | Non-steroidal anti- | syndrome |
| Seronegative | coronavirus, | Food allergy | inflammatory drugs | Peptic duodenitis |
| coeliac disease | cytomegalovirus) | Autoimmune enteritis | Proton pump | Post-transplant |
| Wheat allergy | Parasites (Giardia, | Vasculitides | inhibitors | lymphoproliferative |
|  | *cryptosporidum*) | Systemic autoimmune | Mycophenolate | disorders |
|  | Bacteria (*Salmonella,* | disorders (e.g. Graves' | mofetil | Lymphomas |
|  | *Shigella, Yersinia,* | disease, rheumatoid | Ipilimumab |  |
|  | *Tropheryma whipplei*— | arthritis, psoriasis, |  |  |
|  | Whipple's disease) | systemic lupus |  |  |
|  | Small intestinal bacterial | erythematosus) |  |  |
|  | overgrowth | Inflammatory bowel |  |  |
|  | *Helicobacter pylori* | disease |  |  |
|  |  | Microscopic enteritis |  |  |
|  |  | Graft vs host disease |  |  |

Data from Sergi C, Shen F, Bouma G. Intraepithelial lymphocytes, scores, mimickers and challenges in diagnosing gluten-sensitive enteropathy (celiac disease). *World J Gastroenterol.* 2017 Jan 28; 23(4): 573–589. Doi: 10.3748/wjg.v23.i4.573

Histopathological findings of intraepithelial lymphocytosis must be interpreted with clinical history, examination, and laboratory results in mind.

Sergi C, Shen F, Bouma G. Intraepithelial lymphocytes, scores, mimickers and challenges in diagnosing gluten-sensitive enteropathy (celiac disease). *World J Gastroenterol.* 2017 Jan 28;23(4):573–589. Doi: 10.3748/wjg.v23.i4.573.

### 23. D. Duodenal adenoma

- Forty per cent of duodenal adenomas (Fig. 3.14 black asterisk) are sporadic
- Between 30% and 85% of duodenal adenomas undergo malignant transformation
- ESD has a superior complete resection and recurrence rate when compared with EMR

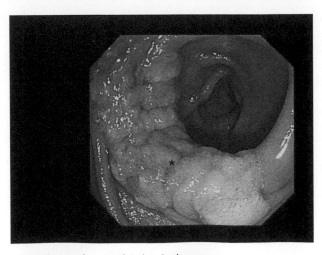

**Fig. 3.14** Endoscopic image showing duodenal adenoma

Image courtesy of Dr Tim Ambrose, Oxford University Hospitals NHS Foundation Trust

Sporadic duodenal polyps are uncommon, and can be classified according to their location and histopathological subtype. Non-ampullary duodenal adenomas are common findings in patients with FAP. Sporadic duodenal adenomas (SDA) are rare, however. Sixty per cent of duodenal adenomas are present in patients with FAP; the remaining 40% are sporadic.

Duodenal adenomas are typically multiple, sessile, and predominantly located in the distal duodenum. Between 30% and 85% of duodenal adenomas undergo malignant transformation and therefore excision, be it endoscopic or surgical, is mandatory. High-grade dysplastic lesions and large non-ampullary SDAs (≥20 mm in diameter) confer an increased risk of progression to adenocarcinoma. In patients with FAP, duodenal cancer develops from pre-existing adenomas with a cumulative risk of almost 100%.

Ampullary lesions may present clinically with obstructive jaundice or pancreatitis. Non-ampullary lesions, however, are often an incidental finding at endoscopy. Endoscopic options include snare polypectomy, EMR, ESD and argon plasma coagulation (APC). Snare polypectomy is effective with an 85% eradication rate. It may be used in combination with APC. ESD has a superior complete resection rate with no recurrence when compared with EMR. However, ESD carries higher rates of perforation (6%–50%) and bleeding when compared with EMR.

Large and/or villous adenomas are associated with a higher rate of recurrence. Post successful resection of non-ampullary SDA, initial follow-up endoscopy is recommended at three to six months to site check for recurrence. Dedicated guidance exists for upper GI endoscopic surveillance in patients with FAP.

Surgical excision is indicated in large SDAs, with severe dysplasia, suspicious for local infiltration or recurrence after complete endoscopic resection. Options include laparoscopic-assisted endoluminal surgery, laparoscopic polyp excision, duodenectomy, or pancreaticoduodenectomy. Pancreaticoduodenectomy may also be indicated in patients with FAP and severe duodenal adenomatosis.

Lim C, Cho Y. Nonampullary duodenal adenoma: current understanding of its diagnosis, pathogenesis, and clinical management. *World J Gastroenterol.* 2016;22(2):853–861. Doi:10.3748/wjg.v22.i2.853.

### 24. B. Accurate photo documentation of anatomical landmarks and abnormal findings

The European Society of Gastrointestinal Endoscopy (ESGE) have identified quality in upper GI endoscopy as a key priority. As such, key performance measures were defined in 2016 (Table 3.3).

Bisschops R et al. Performance measures for UGI endoscopy: a European Society of Gastrointestinal Endoscopy (ESGE) Quality Improvement Initiative. *Endoscopy.* 2016;48:843-864. Doi: 10.1055/s-0042-113128.

**Table 3.3** Key performance measures for upper gastrointestinal endoscopy

| Key performance measures | Minor performance measures |
|---|---|
| • Fasting instructions prior to UGI endoscopy<br>• Documentation of procedure duration<br>• Accurate photo documentation of anatomical landmarks and abnormal findings<br>• Accurate application of standardized disease-related terminology<br>• Application of Seattle protocol in Barrett's surveillance<br>• Accurate registration of complications after therapeutic UGI endoscopy | • Minimum 7-minute procedure time for first diagnostic UGI endoscopy and follow-up of gastric intestinal metaplasia<br>• Minimum 1-minute inspection time per cm circumferential Barrett's epithelium<br>• Use of Lugol chromoendoscopy in patients with a curatively treated ENT or lung cancer to exclude a second primary esophageal cancer<br>• Application of validated biopsy protocol to detect gastric intestinal metaplasia (MAPS guidelines)<br>• Prospective registration of Barrett's patients |

UGI, upper gastrointestinal; ENT, ear, nose, and throat; MAPS, management of patients with precancerous conditions and lesions of the stomach.
Reproduced with permission from Bisschops R et al., Performance measures for upper gastrointestinal endoscopy: a European Society of Gastrointestinal Endoscopy (ESGE) Quality Improvement Initiative, *Endoscopy*, 2016;48(9): 843-864. © Georg Thieme Verlag KG.

### 25. A. Decompression with large-bore nasogastric tube

- Twenty per cent of patients with pancreatic cancer develop a degree of GOO
- Stent placement or surgical bypass are treatment options in GOO
- Palliative management is the mainstay in malignant GOO

This patient has malignant GOO from pancreatic cancer. All the options are viable options. However, the appropriate immediate next step is to provide symptomatic relief with large-bore nasogastric (Ryles) tube decompression.

GOO typically develops due to progression of the pancreatic tumour resulting in extrinsic compression of the duodenum. Approximately 20% of patients with pancreatic cancer develop a degree of GOO. GOO may present with nausea, vomiting, early satiety, anorexia, or an epigastric fullness. Cross-sectional imaging confirms the diagnosis. Endoscopic assessment is key to define the degree of obstruction and a distended, fluid-filled stomach may be seen at gastroscopy. Patients often require a prolonged fast or nasogastric drainage ahead of gastroscopy. If the obstruction is incomplete, a nasojejunal feeding tube may be placed while a definitive management plan is decided.

Malignant GOO usually represents a poor prognosis. Palliative, expectant management is therefore the mainstay of treatment. Initial management includes optimal analgesia, decompression with a nasogastric tube and a plan for adequate nutrition. Endoscopic or fluoroscopic stent placement across the stricture is a readily accessible option. Stents may migrate, or become blocked or compressed, however. Surgical options include bypassing the stricture with a gastrojejunostomy. It is important, though, to determine whether surgical intervention is appropriate given the burden of disease, oncological treatment, and prognosis. In selected cases, there may be a role for short-term palliative parenteral nutrition. Such management decisions necessitate a multidisciplinary approach with input from gastroenterologists, surgeons, interventional radiologists, oncologists, and palliative care staff with the patient's wishes in mind.

McGrath C, Tsang A et al. Malignant gastric outlet obstruction from pancreatic cancer. *Case Rep Gastroenterol.* 2017;11:511–515. Doi.org/10.1159/000480070.

1.  **A 42-year-old woman presented to clinic with an incidental finding of gallstones on ultrasound performed for another indication. She had no fever, rigors, or pain. She had a moderate alcohol intake but denied any other medical problems.**

    Investigations:

    | | |
    |---|---|
    | Serum albumin | 39 g/L |
    | Serum bilirubin | 17 µmol/L |
    | Serum alanine transferase (ALT) | 42 U/L |
    | Serum alkaline phosphatase (ALP) | 104 U/L |
    | Serum C-reactive protein (CRP) | 6 mg/L |
    | Abdominal ultrasound | Three small gallstones in thin walled gallbladder with normal intra- and extrahepatic bile ducts. |

    **Which of the following most accurately reflects the patient's prognosis over the next 10 years?**

    A.  Cholecystectomy is indicated to prevent symptomatic gallstones from developing

    B.  Fifty per cent chance of developing Mirizzi syndrome

    C.  Less than 1% chance of developing pancreatitis, cholecystitis, or biliary obstruction

    D.  More than 90% chance of remaining asymptomatic

    E.  Twenty per cent chance of developing biliary colic

*Best of Five MCQs for the European Specialty Examination in Gastroenterology and Hepatology.* Thomas Marjot, Colleen G C McGregor, Tim Ambrose, Aminda N De Silva, Jeremy Cobbold, and Simon Travis, Oxford University Press (2021). © Oxford University Press. DOI: 10.1093/oso/9780198834373.003.0004

2. **A 64-year-old man underwent a cholecystectomy for right upper-quadrant pain.**

Investigations:

| | |
|---|---|
| Cholecystectomy specimen | The muscle wall is thickened with multiple prolapsed glands in the subserosal tissue (Rokitansky–Ashoff sinuses). The glands are variably dilated. |

### What is the most likely diagnosis?

A. Acute cholecystitis

B. Adenomyomatosis (ADM)

C. Gallbladder adenocarcinoma

D. Gallbladder empyema

E. Porcelain gallbladder

3. **A 55-year-old woman was found incidentally to have gallbladder calcification on a computed tomography pulmonary angiogram (CTPA) performed to investigate a shortness of breath on the acute medical take. She did not have a pulmonary embolism and was discharged with an outpatient computed tomography (CT) abdomen. She was asymptomatic with no other comorbidities.**

Investigations:

| | |
|---|---|
| Serum bilirubin | 12 µmol/L |
| Serum alkaline phosphatase (ALP) | 120 U/L |
| Serum alanine transferase (ALT) | 18 U/L |
| Serum albumin | 35 g/L |
| CT abdomen | Gallbladder contains several calculi with intramural spotty calcification of the gallbladder wall. |

### What is the most appropriate next step for this patient?

A. Cholecystectomy

B. Endoscopic retrograde cholangiopancreatography (ERCP)

C. Endoscopic ultrasound (EUS)

D. Magnetic resonance cholangiopancreatography (MRCP)

E. Observation

4.  A 39-year-old man had a laparoscopic cholecystectomy for acute cholecystitis. Twelve hours after the operation, he developed abdominal pain although it was not peritonitic. Bile was also found in the surgical drain. CT abdomen showed no collections and ERCP demonstrated a low-grade bile leak from the duct of Luschka with no filling defects in the biliary tree.

    What would be the next best management approach?

    A. Conservative management with prophylactic antibiotics
    B. ERCP and plastic biliary stent insertion
    C. ERCP and sphincterotomy
    D. Nasobiliary drainage
    E. Repeat laparoscopy and surgical repair

5.  A 75-year-old man presented with right upper-quadrant pain, jaundice, and fever. He had a myocardial infarction six months ago and received a drug-eluting coronary artery stent. He takes daily aspirin 75 mg, clopidogrel 75 mg, bisoprolol 5 mg and atorvastatin 80 mg. He still drives and enjoys playing golf. He remains septic despite 48 hours of intravenous co-amoxiclav and gentamicin.

    Investigations:

    | | |
    |---|---|
    | Serum bilirubin | 71 μmol/L |
    | Serum alkaline phosphatase (ALP) | 317 U/L |
    | Serum alanine transferase (ALT) | 43 U/L |
    | Serum albumin | 35 g/L |
    | International normalized ratio (INR) | 1.4 |
    | Haemoglobin | 120 g/L |
    | White cell count | 12 × 10⁹/L |
    | Platelet count | 150 × 10⁹/L |
    | Serum C-reactive protein (CRP) | 70 mg/L |
    | Blood cultures | *Escherichia coli* |
    | Ultrasound abdomen | Common bile duct (CBD) dilatation with probable calculi. Sludge and gallstones in non-inflamed gallbladder. |
    | MRCP | (Fig. 4.1) |

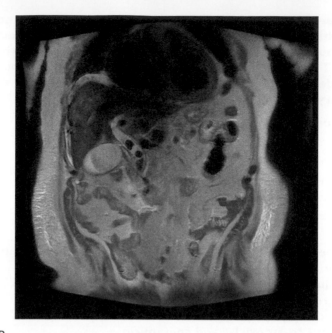

**Fig. 4.1** MRCP

### What is the best treatment option for sepsis source control?

A.  Broaden antimicrobial cover

B.  ERCP with sphincterotomy and stone extraction

C.  ERCP and plastic stent

D.  Extracorporeal shock wave lithotripsy

E.  Percutaneous transhepatic cholangiogram and internal–external biliary drain

6. **A 30-year-old woman who was 34 weeks' pregnant presented with right upper-quadrant pain. She had a temperature of 38.2°C, heart rate 128 beats per minute and blood pressure 85/60 mmHg.**

   Investigations:

   | | |
   |---|---|
   | Abdominal ultrasound | Dilated CBD (15 mm) with no obvious filling defect and dilated intrahepatic ducts. Multiple small stones within a thin walled gallbladder. |
   | Haemoglobin | 110 g/L |
   | White cell count | 18.3 × 10⁹/L |
   | Platelet count | 162 × 10⁹/L |
   | Prothrombin time | 12.5 seconds |
   | Serum bilirubin | 73 μmol/L |
   | Serum alkaline phosphatase (ALP) | 556 U/L |
   | Serum alanine transferase (ALT) | 67 U/L |
   | Serum C-reactive protein (CRP) | 187 mg/L |

   **What is the most appropriate next step in the management of this patient?**

   A. CT abdomen

   B. ERCP

   C. Expectant management

   D. Induce delivery

   E. MRCP

7. **A 40-year-old woman presented with recurrent episodes of nocturnal right upper-quadrant pain radiating to the back, and vomiting over the past one month.**

   Investigations:

   | | |
   |---|---|
   | Serum bilirubin | 45 μmol/L |
   | Serum alkaline phosphatase (ALP) | 258 U/L |
   | Serum alanine transferase (ALT) | 65 U/L |
   | Serum amylase | 39 U/L |
   | Abdominal ultrasound | Several gallbladder calculi. Normal bile duct calibre. |
   | MRCP | (Fig. 4.2) |
   | EUS | (Fig. 4.3) |

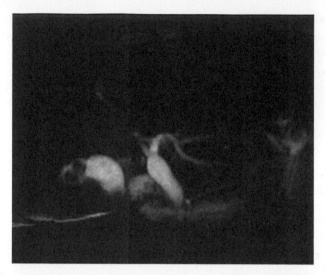

**Fig. 4.2** MRCP

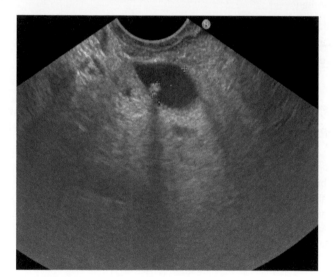

**Fig. 4.3** Endoscopic ultrasound image

## What is the diagnosis?

A. Biliary microlithiasis

B. Cholecystitis

C. Choledochal cyst

D. Cholelithiasis

E. Gallbladder polyp

8.  **A 36-year-old man, who had recently moved to the UK from Kashmir, presented to the emergency department with episodic severe right upper-quadrant pain.**

    Investigations:
    Ultrasound abdomen                     The distal CBD contains several hypoechoic
                                           tubular structures with well-defined echogenic
                                           walls seen making curling movements.

    **Which of the following is the most likely cause?**

    A.  *Ascaris lumbricoides*
    B.  *Clonorchis sinensis*
    C.  *Entamoeba histolytica*
    D.  *Fasciola hepatica*
    E.  *Opisthorchis viverrini*

9.  **A 28-year-old-man was seen in clinic with a five-year history of recurrent episodic right upper-quadrant pain and two previous episodes of cholangitis requiring ERCP and clearance of CBD calculi. His pain had persisted despite cholecystectomy two years before.**

    Investigations:

    | | |
    |---|---|
    | Serum bilirubin | 25 µmol/L |
    | Serum alanine transferase (ALT) | 75 U/L |
    | Serum alkaline phosphatase (ALP) | 230 U/L |
    | Haemoglobin | 125 g/L |
    | Platelet count | 245 × 10⁹/L |
    | Liver stiffness | 4.5 kPa |
    | Abdominal ultrasound | Multiple foci of intrahepatic microlithiasis in both lobes of the liver. No CBD calculi or duct dilatation. |
    | Genetic analysis | Homozygous mutation (c.139C>T) in ABCB4 gene |

    **What is the best next management strategy?**

    A.  Cholangioscopy and electrohydraulic lithotripsy (EHL)
    B.  Ezetimibe
    C.  High dose vitamin C
    D.  Liver transplantation (LT)
    E.  Ursodeoxycholic acid

10. **Question focused on knowledge of the procedure rather than diagnostics/patient management.**

    **Which of the following statements about cholangioscopy is most correct?**

    A. Air embolism is a recognized complication of dual-operator cholangioscopy (DOC)

    B. Biliary sphincterotomy is usually not required

    C. It is associated with a low rate of clearance of extrahepatic bile duct stones unable to be removed with conventional ERCP

    D. It is associated with higher rates of cholangitis compared with conventional ERCP

    E. Single-operator cholangioscopy has superior image quality compared with the dual-operator technique

11. **A 35-year-old man with large-duct primary sclerosing cholangitis (PSC) developed jaundice, worsening liver biochemistry, and fevers.**

    Investigations:
    MRCP                         (Fig. 4.4)

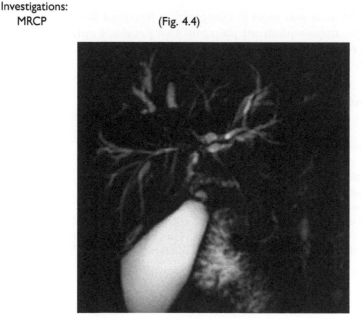

**Fig. 4.4** MRCP

    **Which of the following statements is true with regard to the MRCP finding?**

    A. It is associated with specific genetic polymorphisms affecting bile acid transport

    B. It occurs in 50% of patients with PSC over the course of their disease

    C. Management with biliary stenting is associated with fewer short-term complications than balloon dilatation at ERCP

    D. Prophylactic antibiotics are not required prior to investigation with ERCP

    E. Serum carbohydrate antigen CA 19-9 is a good surveillance strategy for development of cholangiocarcinoma (CCA)

12. **A 75-year-old man presented with a two-month history of progressive jaundice and weight loss. An MRCP showed a suspicious stricture in the mid CBD.**

    **Which of the following is an established risk factor for CCA?**
    A. Caucasian ethnicity
    B. Cirrhosis
    C. *Fasciola hepatica*
    D. Hepatitis E
    E. Primary biliary cholangitis

13. **A 55-year-old man with a history of recurrent pancreatitis presented with a one-week history of painless jaundice. Ultrasound and MRCP revealed dilated common hepatic and intrahepatic ducts with suspicion of a distal CBD stricture. Staging CT revealed no mass lesion, vessel, or nodal involvement. Cholangiogram at ERCP confirmed a short distal CBD stricture. Brush cytology was obtained and the stricture was stented (Fig. 4.5).**

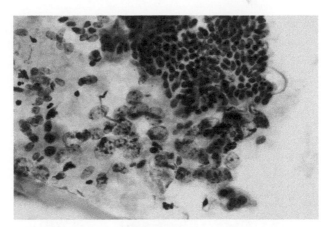

**Fig. 4.5** Brush cytology specimen from biliary stricture. See also Plate 10

    **What is the next step in management?**
    A. EUS tissue sampling
    B. Refer for chemotherapy
    C. Refer for cholangioscopy
    D. Refer for surgery
    E. Repeat ERCP and brushing

14. **A 68-year-old woman presented with a one-week history of painless jaundice, dark urine, and pale stools. There was pruritus and weight loss. She had no other medical history and World Health Organisation (WHO) performance status 0. She was referred to the hepatopancreatobiliary multidisciplinary team (MDT) meeting.**

Investigations:

| | |
|---|---|
| Serum bilirubin | 222 µmol/L |
| Serum alanine transferase (ALT) | 262 U/L |
| Serum alkaline phosphatase (ALP) | 290 U/L |
| Serum gamma-GT | 386 U/L |
| Serum albumin | 34 g/L |
| INR | 1.0 |
| Haemoglobin | 140 g/L |
| White cell count | 7.7 × 10⁹/L |
| Platelet count | 319 × 10⁹/L |
| Serum CA 19-9 | 1,033 U/ml |
| Serum CEA | 2.8 µg/ml |
| Serum CA 125 | 15 U/ml |
| CT abdomen and pelvis with contrast | (Fig. 4.6) |

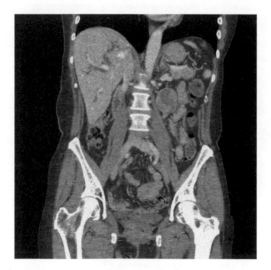

**Fig. 4.6** CT abdomen and pelvis

What is the most likely outcome of the multidisciplinary team meeting with regard to the next step in her management?

A. Chemotherapy

B. ERCP, brushings, and metal stent

C. ERCP, brushings, and plastic stent

D. PET-CT

E. Surgery

15. **A 66-year-old man presented with five months' history of weight loss and two months' history of jaundice. He had no other past medical history.**

    Investigations:
    | | |
    |---|---|
    | Serum bilirubin | 91 µmol/L |
    | Serum alkaline phosphatase (ALP) | 425 U/L |
    | Serum alanine transferase (ALT) | 77 U/L |
    | MRCP | (Fig. 4.7) |

    ### Which of the following is most likely to support a benign diagnosis?

    A. Absence of arterial or portal venous invasion

    B. Bulky pancreas and hypodense wedge-shaped renal lesions

    C. Elevated serum immunoglobulin G subclass 4 (IgG4)

    D. Enhancing thickened bile duct wall

    E. Hilar mass lesion

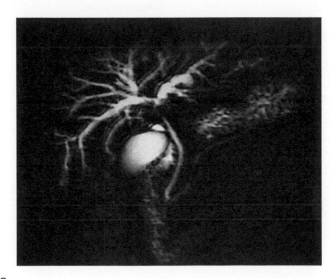

**Fig. 4.7** MRCP

**16.** **A 55-year-old man with hepatitis C cirrhosis and HCC had a liver transplant three months ago. He presented with a history of progressive jaundice.**

Investigations:

| | |
|---|---|
| Serum bilirubin | 88 μmol/L |
| Serum alkaline phosphatase (ALP) | 104 U/L |
| Serum alanine transferase (ALT) | 442 U/L |
| Serum albumin | 34 g/L |
| Serum C-reactive protein (CRP) | 7 mg/L |
| Serum tacrolimus level | 8 ng/mL |
| Blood cultures | Negative |
| MRCP | (Fig. 4.8) |
| transplant operation note | Modified piggyback common hepatic artery to common hepatic artery at gastroduodenal artery. Duct-to-duct anastomosis. DCD (donation after circulatory death) donor. CMV positive-positive. |

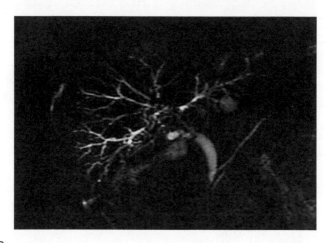

**Fig. 4.8** MRCP

### What is the next best investigation?

A. CMV DNA titre

B. CT liver triple phase

C. ERCP

D. Liver biopsy

E. Ultrasound abdomen

17. **A 30-year-old woman was reviewed in clinic after a recent inpatient stay with cholangitis. During her admission, an ultrasound scan showed a dilated CBD. Subsequent ERCP did not reveal choledocholithiasis but it did show a fusiform dilatation of the CBD. An MRCP was arranged as an outpatient, which confirmed spindle-like dilatation along the length of the CBD. A diagnosis of choledochal cyst type I was made. The patient was currently asymptomatic.**

    **What is the most appropriate management?**

    A.  Cholecystoenterostomy

    B.  Expectant management and ERCP as required for episodes of cholangitis

    C.  MRCP every two years and surgical excision if progressive duct dilatation occurs

    D.  Surgical excision

    E.  Surgical excision only if the patient becomes symptomatic

18. **A 25-year-old man was referred with abnormal liver function tests.**

    Investigations:

    | | |
    |---|---|
    | Serum bilirubin | 19 µmol/L |
    | Serum alkaline phosphatase (ALP) | 340 U/L |
    | Serum alanine transferase (ALT) | 48 U/L |
    | MRCP | Fusiform extrahepatic duct dilatation with distal tapering. |

    **Use of which recreational drug is most likely to be responsible?**

    A.  3,4-Methylenedioxymethamphetamine (MDMA)

    B.  Amphetamine

    C.  Ketamine

    D.  Methadone

    E.  Nitrous oxide

**19. A 54-year-old Nigerian man who had recently moved to the United Kingdom presented to the emergency department with severe pneumococcal pneumonia.**

Investigations:

| | |
|---|---|
| Haemoglobin | 110 g/dl |
| White cell count | $6 \times 10^9$/L |
| Platelet count | $106 \times 10^9$/l |
| HIV antibody | Positive |
| CD4+ count | 9 cells/µL |
| HIV viral load | $1.7 \times 10^7$/mL |
| Serum bilirubin | 95 µmol/L |
| Serum alanine transferase (ALT) | 79 U/L |
| Serum alkaline phosphatase (ALP) | 390 U/L |
| MRCP | CBD dilatation with smooth margins and terminal tapering. Multiple alternating stenosis and saccular dilatations of the intrahepatic biliary tree of both liver lobes. No gallstones visualized. |

**Which opportunistic infection is most associated with this condition?**

A. *Cryptosporidium parvum*

B. *Cytomegalovirus* (CMV)

C. *Giardia intestinalis*

D. Microsporidia

E. *Pneumocystis jirovecii*

**20. What is the 10-year incidence of recurrent PSC after liver transplantation?**

A. 5%

B. 10%

C. 20%

D. 50%

E. 75%

chapter

4

# BILIARY DISORDERS

ANSWERS

## 1. E. Twenty per cent chance of developing biliary colic

- Asymptomatic gallstones have a 20% chance of becoming symptomatic with biliary colic over the next 10 years
- Asymptomatic gallstones have a low (2%–3%) risk of being complicated by pancreatitis, cholecystitis, or biliary obstruction, and therefore cholecystectomy is not routinely recommended

Asymptomatic gallstones are found in 10%–20% of the global adult population and generally do not require therapy. Patients with asymptomatic gallstones have a 20% chance of becoming symptomatic with biliary colic over the next 10 years. The onset of gallstone-associated pain indicates a higher chance of developing complications (cholecystitis, choledocholithiasis) and provides a rational for cholecystectomy in symptomatic patients unless surgical risk is prohibitive. Patients with asymptomatic gallstones only have a 2%–3% chance of developing pancreatitis, cholecystitis, and biliary obstruction, and cholecystectomy is therefore not recommended for patients with asymptomatic stones. Mirizzi's syndrome is a rare complication of gallstones. It refers to biliary obstruction with jaundice either as a direct consequence of stone impaction or from inflammation when a large stone resides in Hartmann's pouch of the gallbladder. This causes obstructive jaundice via pressure on the CBD and is treated with cholecystectomy.

Lammert F, Gurusamy K, Ko CW et al. Gallstones. *Nat Rev Dis Primers.* 2016 Apr 28;2:16024. Doi: 10.1038/nrdp.2016.24.

## 2. B. Adenomyomatosis

- ADM is a benign cause of gallbladder thickening that is commonly asymptomatic
- Histologically, it is characterized by outpouchings of the mucosa into thickened muscle wall (Rokitansky–Aschoff sinuses)
- Care must be taken to differentiate ADM from gallbladder carcinoma, which may be aided by use of MRCP

Gallbladder ADM is a relatively common, asymptomatic, and benign cause of diffuse or focal gallbladder wall thickening, which is commonly identified incidentally during investigation for other pathologies. Histologically, it is characterized by epithelial proliferation and hypertrophy of the muscles of the gallbladder wall with outpouchings of the mucosa into thickened muscular layer, known as 'Rokitansky–Aschoff sinuses'. ADM is identified in 1%–9% of cholecystectomy specimens and is associated with gallstones in >50% of cases. While ADM is a benign condition, it must be differentiated from gallbladder carcinoma, which carries a very poor prognosis. Ultrasound is often the first-line diagnostic test with MRCP reserved for cases when an experienced radiologist cannot make a definitive diagnosis of ADM using ultrasound alone. ADM theoretically requires no specific treatment, except when symptomatic, with or without gallstones.

Golse N, Lewin M, Rode A et al. Gallbladder adenomyomatosis: diagnosis and management. *J Visc Surg.* 2017 Oct;154(5):345–353. Doi: 10.1016/j.jviscsurg.2017.06.004.

### 3. A. Cholecystectomy

- Porcelain gallbladder is associated with gallbladder carcinoma
- Spotty mural calcification has much higher risk of malignancy than homogenous complete calcification
- Current guidelines recommend cholecystectomy for porcelain gallbladder although evidence is weak

This woman has porcelain gallbladder. Porcelain gallbladder is rare and is detected in less than 0.1% of cholecystectomy specimens. It is associated with the presence of gallstones in 95% of patients, which are thought to contribute to chronic gallbladder inflammation scarring, hyalinization and calcification. Porcelain gallbladder is associated with an increased risk of gallbladder malignancy but a poor causal relationship has been established. Patients are usually asymptomatic and the condition is often discovered incidentally on abdominal imaging. CT can confirm the condition with a high degree of accuracy.

While early studies described an incidence of carcinoma in calcified gallbladders as high as 20%, more recent series suggest a far lower rate of ~3%. Spotty mucosal calcification as seen in this case is associated with a much higher carcinoma rate compared to homogenous wall calcification.

The management of porcelain gallbladder is controversial. European Association for Study of the Liver (EASL) recommend that asymptomatic patients with porcelain gallbladder may undergo cholecystectomy although the quality of evidence is very low. However, given that the risk of carcinoma appears to be lower than previously observed, some experts suggest observation particularly in those with homogenous wall calcification.

EASL Clinical Practice Guidelines on the prevention, diagnosis and treatment of gallstones. *J Hepatol.* 2016 Jul;65(1):146–181. Doi: 10.1016/j.jhep.2016.03.005.

### 4. B. ERCP and plastic biliary stent insertion

- Bile leak occurs in <1% post-laparoscopic cholecystectomy
- It commonly presents as abdominal pain and leak of bilious fluid from wound sites or surgical drains
- In the absence of peritonism and intrabdominal collections, endoscopic management with ERCP and plastic biliary stenting is the preferred treatment modality

Bile leak is a well-recognized and serious complication after cholecystectomy, occurring more commonly after a laparoscopicy (~0.9%) compared with an open approach. The cystic duct stump is the most common site of leak, followed by the duct of Luschka, CBD, common hepatic duct, and gallbladder bed. Bile leaks are also reported in the setting of LT with both duct-to-duct anastomosis and hepatojejunostomy. The most common clinical feature of bile leaks is abdominal pain and percutaneous leakage of bilious fluid either from wound sites or from surgical drains. The management of bile leaks (not caused by complete CBD transection) usually involves an endoscopic approach aiming to create a low-pressure flow direction for the bile to drain away from the leak, which allows it to epithelialize and seal. This is most commonly achieved by endoscopic biliary sphincterotomy and/or endoscopic biliary stenting, which leads to bile leak resolution in >90%.

Choice of treatment at ERCP should be guided on a case-by-case basis. Biliary stenting provides faster leak resolution than sphincterotomy alone, and it is equally effective whether sphincterotomy is performed or not. Therefore, in the absence of obstructing biliary lesions (e.g. retained stones), current European guidelines recommend insertion of a plastic biliary stent without performance of sphincterotomy, and removal of the stent four to eight weeks later.

Dumonceau JM, Tringali A, Papanikolaou IS. Biliary stenting: indications, choice of stents and results: European Society of Gastrointestinal Endoscopy (ESGE) clinical guideline. *Endoscopy*. 2018 Sep;50(9):910–930. Doi: 10.1055/a-0659-9864.

### 5.  C. ERCP and plastic stent

- ERCP and plastic stent placement without sphincterotomy can be safely performed for biliary decompression without interruption to antiplatelet therapy

MRCP shows stacked stones in the CBD (Fig. 4.9). While it is safe to continue low-dose aspirin for all endoscopic therapies (apart from endoscopic submucosal dissection, colonic endoscopic mucosal resection [EMR] (>2 cm), upper gastrointestinal EMR, and ampullectomy), the management strategy here is complicated by the patient's clopidogrel. P2Y12 receptor antagonists (clopidogrel, prasugrel, ticagrelor) increase the risk of bleeding with interventional procedures but need to be balanced against the risk of coronary stent thrombosis. ERCP for biliary stenting without sphincterotomy is classified as at low risk of peri-procedural bleeding and represents the best option in this case, given no improvement on medical therapy and the need for urgent source control of the sepsis. Percutaneous options are best avoided to reduce the risk of complications from bleeding. Extracorporeal shock wave lithotripsy can be used for problematic, large CBD stones as an alternative to surgery but usually requires subsequent ERCP and sphincterotomy to extract stone fragments. Definitive CBD stone management and a cholecystectomy should be

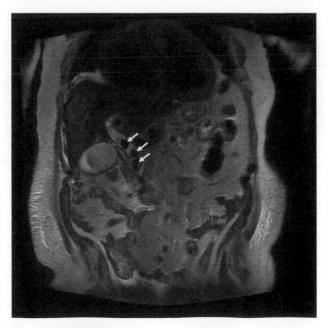

**Fig. 4.9** MRCP showing multiple CBD calculi

planned in this case following discussion with cardiology regarding when it is safe to discontinue the P2Y12 receptor antagonist.

Veitch AM, Vanbiervliet G, Gershlick AH et al. Endoscopy in patients on antiplatelet or anticoagulant therapy, including direct oral anticoagulants: BSG and ESGE guidelines. *Gut.* 2016 Mar;65(3):374–389. Doi: 10.1136/gutjnl-2015-311110.

## 6. B. ERCP

- Pregnancy should not deter ERCP when it is indicated for cholangitis and systemic inflammatory response syndrome (SIRS)
- Temporary decompression with biliary stenting followed by a completion ERCP after delivery is often the most appropriate strategy

In this case, there is a high probability of ascending cholangitis requiring either ERCP-directed stenting or stone extraction. Ultrasound is useful for looking at dilated ducts, but does not always visualize obstructing stones within the CBD. Patients with ascending cholangitis should undergo ERCP to relieve the obstruction as soon as possible, particularly those with severe sepsis and SIRS, as in this case. Pregnancy should not deter one from performing ERCP when it is indicated because, despite the radiation exposure, in the context of ascending cholangitis, it is life-saving. Positioning of the patient may be more challenging during ERCP, but is not impossible. Radiation exposure should be kept to a minimum, and a shield worn to protect the unborn baby. Because of the technical difficulties of performing an ERCP during pregnancy, the definitive aim of duct clearance in CBD stone disease is often compromised. Temporary decompression with biliary stenting followed by a completion ERCP after delivery is an appropriate strategy. This also reduces the risk of pancreatitis at the index ERCP, which may compromise the pregnancy.

Cappell MS. Risks versus benefits of gastrointestinal endoscopy during pregnancy. *Nat Rev Gastroenterol Hepatol.* 2011 Oct 4;8(11):610–634. Doi: 10.1038/nrgastro.2011.

## 7. A. Biliary microlithiasis

- EUS should be performed to exclude microlithasis in patients with recurrent biliary-type pain when ultrasound and MRCP have proven non-diagnostic
- MRCP has slightly inferior diagnostic value for microlithiasis than EUS but is more cost effective

In patients with recurrent biliary-type pain, when ultrasound and MRCP have proven non-diagnostic, an EUS should be considered to exclude microlithiasis before labelling them with a functional biliary sphincter disorder (formally sphincter of Oddi dysfunction). The MRCP shows gallbladder calculi (cholelithiasis) but no evidence of CBD stones (choledocholithiasis) (Fig. 4.10). Cholelithiasis alone does not explain the raised bilirubin. The EUS image shows a 2.7 mm CBD calculi (microlithiasis) (Fig. 4.11). This patient should be referred for ERCP and sphincterotomy followed by a cholecystectomy.

While EUS has a slightly higher diagnostic odds ratio compared with MRCP, the latter has proven more cost-effective. Therefore, MRCP is often favoured following non-diagnostic ultrasound, with EUS performed as a third-line investigation when clinical suspicion remains after a non-diagnostic MRCP.

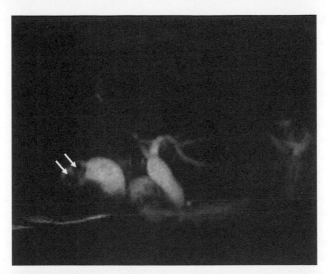

**Fig. 4.10** MRCP showing gallbladder calculi

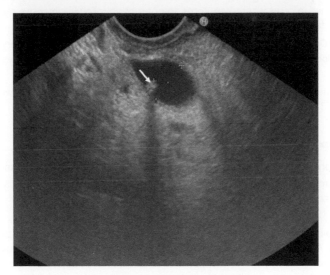

**Fig. 4.11** Endoscopic ultrasound image showing CBD microlithiasis

Meeralam Y, Al-Shammari K, Yaghoobi M et al. Diagnostic accuracy of EUS compared with MRCP in detecting choledocholithiasis: a meta-analysis of diagnostic test accuracy in head-to-head studies. *Gastrointest Endosc.* 2017 Dec;86(6):986–993. Doi: 10.1016/j.gie.2017.06.009.

## 8. A. Ascaris lumbricoides

- Ascariasis affects 25% of the global population and is common in India, China, Africa, and Latin America
- Hepatobiliary and pancreatic infestation leads to ampullary obstruction, biliary colic, cholangitis, and acute pancreatitis
- Treatment is with antihelminthic agents +/− removal of nematodes via ERCP

Ascariasis describes human colonization acts with the nematode, *Ascaris lumbricoides*. It affects 25% of the global population and is ubiquitous in the Indian subcontinent, China, Africa, and Latin America, although it can rarely be found in Europe and then typically in rural areas. Most infections are asymptomatic with clinical disease restricted to individuals with heavy worm load, whereby multiple organ systems can become involved with associated clinical presentations including the gastrointestinal tract (obstruction, peritonitis, appendicitis), lungs (pneumonia, asthma) and hepatobiliary and pancreatic ducts (cholangitis, cholecystitis, hepatic abscesses, hepatolithiasis, or acute pancreatitis). Hepaticobiliary and pancreatic ascariasis (HPA) is caused by proximal movement of the organisms from the jejunum (its natural habitat) into the duodenum and ampulla of Vater, causing biliary obstruction and associated complications. In addition, the writhing movements of live worms induce sphincter spasm causing severe biliary colic. Ultrasound has an excellent sensitivity for hepatobiliary ascariasis but is less reliable in pancreatic duct disease where MRCP or ERCP may be required. Antihelmintic drugs (e.g. mebendazole) are the mainstay of therapy with endotherapy for HPA performed in cases where symptoms do not subside following intensive medical treatment and/or ascrides fail to move out of the ductal lumen.

The liver flukes *Opisthorchis viverrini*, *Clonorchis sinensis*, and *Fasciola hepatica* are very thin, tend to reside in peripheral small and medium-sized bile ducts, and beyond the spatial resolution of ultrasound.

Khuroo MS, Rather AA, Khuroo NS et al. Hepatobiliary and pancreatic ascariasis. *World J Gastroenterol.* 2016 Sep 7;22(33):7507–7517. Doi: 10.3748/wjg.v22.i33.7507.

## 9. E. Ursodeoxycholic acid

- Low-phospholipid associated cholelithiasis (LPAC) is caused by mutations in the ABCB4 gene
- It is characterized by gallstone disease <40 years, intrahepatic lithiasis, and biliary colic post cholecystectomy
- Treatment is with urosodeoxycholic acid

Low-phospholipid associated cholelithiasis (LPAC) is a rare genetic disease associated with mutations in the ABCB4 gene encoding for the biliary carrier protein MDR3. Because of low biliary phospholipid concentrations, cholesterol gallstone disease develops before the age of 40 years with intrahepatic bile duct and gallbladder cholesterol stones and recurrent biliary symptoms after cholecystectomy. Further diagnostic clues are provided by a family history of cholelithiasis in first-degree relatives and recurrent bile duct stones. While ABCB4 gene sequencing may provide additional information, it is not necessary to make the diagnosis of LPAC. Treatment revolves around ursodeoxycholic acid (15 mg/kg body weight per day), which yields dissolution of biliary calculi. Rarely, intrahepatic lithiasis can lead to secondary biliary cirrhosis requiring LT.

EASL Clinical Practice Guidelines on the prevention, diagnosis and treatment of gallstones. *J Hepatol.* 2016 Jul;65(1):146–181. Doi: 10.1016/j.jhep.2016.03.005.

## 10.  D. It is associated with higher rates of cholangitis compared with conventional ERCP

- Chalangiopancreatoscopy allows direct visualization of the biliary and pancreatic ducts, and can help with diagnosis of ductal lesions and removal of difficult stones
- The technique carries a higher risk of cholangitis compared with conventional ERCP

Per-oral cholangiopancreatoscopy enables direct endoscopic visualization of the biliary and pancreatic ductal systems during ERCP and usually requires sphincterotomy. Traditional DOC, the so-called 'mother–daughter' techinique, requires one endoscopist to control the cholangioscope and a second to control the duodenoscope. Adding cholangioscopic appearance of bile duct lesions to biopsy/brush sampling has been shown to improve diagnostic yield. EHL of ductal calculi is the most common therapeutic application of DOC, and manages to achieve duct clearance in 77%–96% of cases where standard ERCP has been unsuccessful. Cholangiopancreatoscopy is associated with increased risk of cholangitis compared with standard ERCP because of intraductal irrigation, and therefore prophylactic antibiotics are always required. A more recent innovation is the single-operator fibre-optic cholangioscope system (SpyGlassTM), which has removed many of the logistical difficulties inherent in requiring two endoscopists, although it is limited by reduced image quality and the small diameter of the working channel. Direct cholangioscopy refers to the use of ultraslim endoscopes designed to directly enter the CBD. This technique is technically demanding and the high intrabiliary pressures from air insufflation has been associated with paradoxical embolism of hepatic venous air and cerebrovascular accidents.

Tringali A, Lemmers A, Meves V et al. Intraductal biliopancreatic imaging: European Society of Gastrointestinal Endoscopy (ESGE) technology review. *Endoscopy*. 2015 Aug;47(8):739–753. Doi: 10.1055/s-0034-1392584.

## 11.  B. It occurs in 50% of patients with PSC over the course of their disease

- Dominant strictures (DS) in PSC are associated with increased risk of CCA and mortality
- CA 19-9 has poor sensitivity for the detection of CCA
- Balloon dilatation should be the initial treatment of choice for DS in PSC

The MRCP image (Fig. 4.12) shows a long DS involving the CBD and common hepatic duct (CHD) (arrow), hilar stricture, and proximal dilatation of intrahepatic ducts (arrowheads).

DS occur in 50% of PSC patients and are defined as an extrahepatic stenosis ≤1.5 mm diameter in the CBD or ≤1 mm in the main hepatic ducts within 2 cm of the hilum. DS are associated with an increased risk of CCA and mortality. Development of DS have been associated with polymorphisms in CD14, a key mediator of the innate immune system. ERCP and ductal sampling should be considered in PSC in the case of (i) worsening symptoms (jaundice, cholangitis, pruritus); (ii) rapid increase of cholestatic enzyme levels; or (iii) new DS or progression of existing stricture(s) identified at MRCP. Antibiotics should be given routinely before ERCP in PSC patients because they are at high risk for incomplete biliary drainage and cholangitis. For symptomatic DS, dilatation or stenting at ERCP has been shown to improve survival and may alter the natural history of the disease. Data are lacking in asymptomatic DS. In a recent randomized trial, both balloon dilatation and short-term stenting were shown to have equal clinical benefit, but there were significantly more side effects in the stenting group (pancreatitis and cholangitis). CA 19-9 in isolation has a low sensitivity (14%) for detection of CCA in PSC. Currently, there is no proven beneficial surveillance strategy for CCA in DS.

Aabakken L, Karlsen TH, Albert J, Role of endoscopy in primary sclerosing cholangitis: ESGE and EASL Clinical Guideline. *Endoscopy*. 2017 Jun;49(6):588–608. Doi: 10.1055/s-0043-107029.

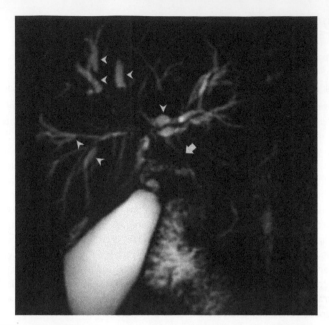

**Fig. 4.12** MRCP showing CBD stricture (arrow) and proximal biliary dilatation (arrowheads)

## 12. B. Cirrhosis

- The hepatobiliary flukes *Opisthorchis viverrini* and *Clonorchis sinensis* are important risk factors for CCA in Southeast Asia
- PSC is the most common risk factor for CCA in Western populations
- Other risk factors for CCA include hepatolithiasis, cirrhosis, hepatitis B virus (HBV), hepatitis C virus (HCV) infection, and choledochal cysts

CCAs are biliary epithelial tumours involving the intrahepatic, perihilar, and distal biliary tree, and they are the second most common hepatic malignancy after HCC. Although most CCAs are sporadic, there are several established risk factors. Age-adjusted incidence rates are highest in Hispanic and Asian populations, and lowest in non-Hispanic white and black populations. Some of the geographical variation may be accounted for by exposure to environmental risk factors. For example, in Southeast Asia, there is a high prevalence of infection with the hepatobiliary flukes *Opisthorchis viverrini* and *Clonorchis sinensis*, which contribute to chronic biliary inflammation and development of CCA. *Fasciola hepatica* is another common liver fluke in Asia and Africa but, although it can cause biliary pain and obstruction, it is not an established risk factor for CCA. Hepatolithiasis is another risk factor for intrahepatic CCA in Asia, and can occur alongside or independently of fluke infection. Meta-analysis has confirmed cirrhosis, HBV and HCV infection as major independent risk factors for CCA with odds ratios of 23, 5, and 5 respectively. In the West, PSC is the most common predisposing condition for CCA with an annual risk of development of CCA between 0.5% and 1.5%, with a lifetime prevalence of 5%–10%. Primary biliary cholangitis is not an established risk factor for CCA. Other risk factors for CCA include choledochal cystic diseases, including Caroli's disease, which is characterized by multiple segmental dilatations of intrahepatic bile ducts and congenital hepatic fibrosis.

Rizvi S, Gores GJ. Pathogenesis, diagnosis, and management of cholangiocarcinoma. *Gastroenterology.* 2013 Dec;145(6):1215–1229. Doi: 10.1053/j.gastro.2013.10.013.

### 13. D. Refer for surgery

- Brush cytology of biliary strictures has a typically low sensitivity but high specificity for the detection of malignancy

The history of recurrent pancreatitis suggests the possibility of pancreatitis-related benign distal CBD stricture in the absence of any mass lesion on imaging. However, the brush cytology clearly shows malignant changes throughout with increased nuclear-cytoplasmic ratio, nuclear crowding, and overlapping with three-dimensional cell clusters. While sensitivities have been reported to be variable (6%–64%) and typically low (41.6% in a meta-analysis), the specificity reaches 98%–99%. EUS tissue sampling, or cholangioscopy, is a reasonable next step if the brush cytology was negative or equivocal. This patient had a localized distal CBD malignant stricture likely to be CCA and should be referred for a Whipple's operation.

Burnett AS, Calvert TJ, Chokshi RJ et al. Sensitivity of endoscopic retrograde cholangiopancreatography standard cytology: 10-y review of the literature. *J Surg Res.* 2013 Sep;184(1):304–311. Doi: 10.1016/j.jss.2013.06.028.

### 14. B. ERCP, brushings, and metal stent

- Biliary decompression in pancreatobiliary cancers should be performed after MDT discussion on resectability whenever possible
- An uncovered metal stent should be avoided if there is uncertainty in the diagnosis of cancer because it is difficult to remove endoscopically and makes surgery technically challenging

A CT scan shows intrahepatic bile duct dilation and a large malignant-appearing left para-aortic lymph node (Fig. 4.13). Given the patient's presentation, a hepatopancreatobiliary cancer should be suspected. The para-aortic lymph node suggests metastatic disease and precludes surgery. A PET-CT does not alter management in this case, and is reserved to investigate for locoregional lymph node involvement and distant metastasis when considering resectability. Biliary decompression is required before initiating chemotherapy. Therefore, an ERCP allows biliary sampling and decompression at the same time. The advantage of a metal stent over a plastic stent is its durability and patency, which reduces the need for repeat ERCP and stent change, particularly in patients who are expected to survive over three months. The patency rates of metal stents are significantly greater than those of plastic stents (12 months vs 3 months). Initial stent insertion for biliary obstruction should be a plastic or covered metal stent if the diagnosis and resectability are undecided. EUS and fine needle aspiration biopsy may improve the diagnosis of CCA if brush cytology is negative. The ERCP image for this patient is shown in Fig. 4.14. It demonstrates a common hepatic duct stricture (arrowheads) suggestive of a CCA. This patient has started chemotherapy after successful biliary decompression.

Khan SA, Davidson BR, Goldin RD et al. BSG Guidelines for the diagnosis and treatment of cholangiocarcinoma: an update. *Gut.* 2012 Dec;61(12):1657–1669. Doi: 10.1136/gutjnl-2011-301748.

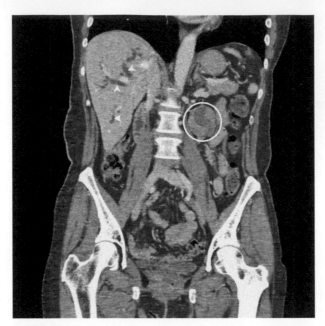

**Fig. 4.13** CT abdomen and pelvis showing intrahepatic biliary dilatation (arrowheads) and large para-aortic lymph node (circled)

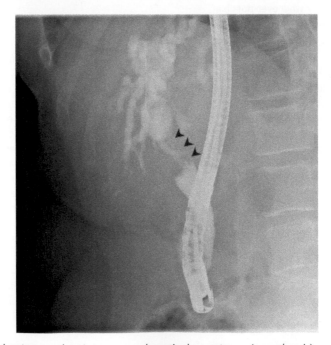

**Fig. 4.14** Cholangiogram showing common hepatic duct stricture (arrowheads)

## 15. B. Bulky pancreas and hypodense wedge-shaped renal lesions

- IgG4-related sclerosing cholangitis (IgG4-SC) can mimic CCA and/or PSC
- Diagnosis of IgG4-SC relies on careful interpretation of histopathological appearances, radiological features, and serological abnormalities in an appropriate clinical scenario (HiSORT criteria)

This patient has a hilar stricture (Fig. 4.15; arrow head) with intrahepatic duct dilatation (Fig. 4.15; arrows) on the MRCP image. The main differential diagnosis is IgG4-related sclerosing cholangitis (IgG4-SC) and hilar CCA. IgG4-SC has a male preponderance with typical age of 50–60 at presentation. It is the most common extrapancreatic manifestation in patients with autoimmune pancreatitis (AIP type 1). Four main cholangiographic subtypes of IgG4-SC have been reported but are not specific to discriminate from CCA, particularly in localized malignant disease.

Serum IgG4 levels are elevated in 65%–80% of patients at diagnosis of IgG4-SC. However, they are also raised in 5%–25% of inflammatory, autoimmune, and malignant conditions. Serum CA 19-9 can also be raised in up to 63% of IgG4-SC patients. Cross-sectional imaging is important because it can show thickened bile duct walls, a mass lesion, evidence of other organ involvement, and any vascular invasion. Brush cytology and FNA have poor sensitivity for the diagnosis of IgG4-SC but are useful to exclude malignancy. Intraductal biopsies can show characteristic histological features. This patient had pancreatic and renal involvement on cross-sectional imaging characteristic of IgG4-related disease.

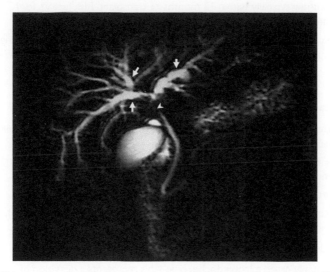

**Fig. 4.15** MRCP image showing hilar stricture (arrowhead) and intrahepatic duct dilatation (arrows)

Culver EL, Barnes E. IgG4-related sclerosing cholangitis. *Clin Liver Dis (Hoboken)*. 2017 Jul 28;10(1):9–16. Doi: 10.1002/cld.642.

## 16. B. CT liver triple phase

- Biliary strictures post-LT can be anastomotic (AS) or non-anastomotic (NAS)
- In NAS, vascular imaging with triple phase CT or ultrasound doppler is essential to exclude hepatic artery thrombosis or stenosis
- Diffuse NAS in the context of a patent hepatic artery is called ischaemic cholangiopathy (IC)

This patient presented with jaundice three months after LT. MRCP shows diffuse irregularity and mild dilatation of the intrahepatic bile ducts. There is an anastomosis between the non-dilated donor common hepatic duct and the dilated native CBD.

Post-transplant biliary strictures can be AS strictures at the site of bile duct anastomosis (choledochocholedochostomy or choledochojejunostomy) or NAS biliary strictures.

AS strictures occur in 5%–10% usually within the first year post-transplantation and are attributable to intraoperative technical issues (e.g. small calibre of the bile ducts, donor-recipient bile duct size mismatch, AS tension and excessive use of electrocauterization for control of bleeding). Management of AS is mainly with stenting or dilatation at ERCP.

NAS strictures occur as a result of hepatic artery thrombosis (HAT), hepatic artery stenosis (HAS) or IC. The blood supply to the biliary tree is derived nearly exclusively from the hepatic artery and therefore CT triple phase liver or ultrasound with dopplers is the essential first investigation to exclude hepatic artery thrombus or stenosis. Diffuse NAS in the presence of a patent hepatic artery is termed 'IC'. IC can be asymptomatic with progressive cholestasis or manifest as recurrent biliary sepsis occurring typically within 12 months of transplant. Risk factors for IC include prolonged ischaemia time, DCD and cytomegalovirus (CMV) infection.

Mourad MM, Algarni A, Liossis C et al. Aetiology and risk factors of ischaemic cholangiopathy after liver transplantation. *World J Gastroenterol*. 2014 May 28;20(20):6159–6169. Doi: 10.3748/wjg.v20.i20.6159.

## 17. D. Surgical excision

- Choledochal cysts are congenital dilatations of the CBD and 20% of cases only become symptomatic in adulthood
- They have a high rate of malignant transformation to CCA and therefore surgical excision is recommended

In 1977, Todani described five types of choledochal cyst:[1]

*Type I*: This consists of dilatation of the CBD, which may be cystic (A), focal (B), or fusiform (C), and does not include the intrahepatic ducts

*Type II*: This describes a diverticulum of the CBD

*Type III*: Commonly called a 'choledochocoele', this represents a dilatation of the distal CBD, which some believe is actually a duodenal diverticulum

*Type IV*: This consists of multiple dilatations of the intra- and extra-hepatic biliary tree (A), or just the extrahepatic ducts (B)

*Type V*: This is also known as 'Caroli's disease' and involves multiple intrahepatic dilatations.

Choledochal cysts are congenital dilatations of the CBD, which most commonly present in infancy before the age of 10 years with jaundice and biliary colic. Approximately 20% of cases only become

1 Reprinted from *The American Journal of Surgery*, 134, 2, Todani et al., 'Congenital bile duct cysts: Classification, operative procedures, and review of thirty-seven cases including cancer arising from choledochal cyst', pp. 263–269. Copyright 1977, with permission from Elsevier.

symptomatic in adulthood. Choledochal cysts occur in a female to male ratio of 4:1 and predispose to stone disease, duct structuring, pancreatitis, and malignant transformation to CCA in 10%–30%. Surgical excision is therefore the treatment of choice.

Yoon JH. Magnetic resonance cholangiopancreatography diagnosis of choledochal cyst involving the cystic duct: report of three cases. *Br J Radiol.* 2011;84: e18–22.

## 18. C. Ketamine

- Diffuse, fusiform extrahepatic duct dilatation and intrahepatic duct dilatation and beading are recognized biliary complications of ketamine abuse
- Liver function tests and cholangiographic appearances can improve with drug cessation

Ketamine abuse has emerged as a risk factor for biliary cholangiopathy. Over time, chronic stimulation of N-methyl-D-aspartic acid receptor in bile duct smooth muscle induces inflammation and fibrosis, ultimately resulting in biliary strictures and dilatation. Affected patients are usually asymptomatic initially and only manifest abnormal liver function tests after one to two years, indicating that chronicity and repeated exposure are important in disease pathogenesis. Several cholangiographic patterns of biliary tract abnormalities are recognized including diffuse extrahepatic duct dilatation (46%), fusiform extrahepatic duct dilatation with distal tapering (40%), and intrahepatic duct dilatation or beading with normal extrahepatic ducts (14%). Cessation of ketamine use correlates with improvement in LFTs and improved MRCP findings in ~20%. Chronic methadone use induces sphincter of Oddi dysfunction and is associated with CBD and pancreatic duct dilatation, but not with the fusiform dilatation and stricturing observed in this case.

Seto WK, Mak SK, Chiu K. Magnetic resonance cholangiogram patterns and clinical profiles of ketamine-related cholangiopathy in drug users. *J Hepatol.* 2018 Jul;69(1):121–128. Doi: 10.1016/j.jhep.2018.03.006.

## 19. A. *Cryptosporidium parvum*

- Patients with advanced HIV can develop cholangiopathy commonly due to biliary colonization with *cryptosporidium parvum*
- This typically causes papillary stenosis with associated CBD dilatation
- Management is with antiretroviral therapy and ERCP with spincterotomy

Hepatobiliary disease in HIV can be classified into three categories: i) diseases associated with immunosuppression including AIDS cholangiopathy, acalculous cholecystitis, AIDS-related neoplasms (non-Hodgkin lymphoma and Kaposi sarcoma), and vanishing bile duct syndrome, ii) drug-induced hepatotoxicity secondary to highly active antiretroviral therapy (HAART), and iii) worsening co-infection with hepatitis B and C viruses associated with accelerated progression of fibrosis. In addition, patients with HIV are at increased risk of non-alcoholic fatty liver disease and nodular regenerative hyperplasia.

This patient has AIDS cholangiopathy, which is a syndrome of biliary obstruction and liver damage secondary to infection-related bile duct strictures. It is associated with advanced immunosuppression in AIDS patients and is now primarily seen only in instances of poor access to HAART and medication non-compliance. *Cryptosporidium parvum* is the most common pathogen associated with AIDS cholangiopathy being isolated in 20%–57% of patients. CMV is the next most common, being found in 10%–20% with lesser associations documented for Microsporidium, *Giardia, Histoplasma* and *Mycobacterium avium* complex. No infectious pathogen is identified in 20%–40% of cases. The most common cholangiographic finding is a smoothly tapered stricture in the distal CBD consistent with papillary stenosis with or without multifocal intrahepatic duct dilatation and strictures. Treatment includes optimization of immune function using HAART alongside ERCP and sphincteromy to relieve papillary stenosis. Targeted antimicrobial therapy of culprit opportunistic infections is often ineffective (e.g. gancyclovir and CMV-related cholangitis) and currently there is no effective eradication therapy for *Cryptosporidium parvum*.

Naseer M, Dailey FE, Juboori AA et al. Epidemiology, determinants, and management of AIDS cholangiopathy: a review. *World J Gastroenterol.* 2018 Feb 21;24(7):767–774. Doi: 10.3748/wjg.v24. i7.767.

## 20. C. 20%

- Recurrent PSC (rPSC) after LT occurs in 20% of patients over 10 years
- rPSC results in graft failure in approximately half of patients
- Risk factors for rPSC include male gender, CMV mismatch, living-related donation, and the presence of active inflammatory bowel disease

PSC is currently the fifth most frequent indication for LT, most commonly in in the context of decompensated cirrhosis or HCC. Additional PSC-specific indications for transplantation include recurrent bacterial cholangitis and hilar CCA in selected LT centres. rPSC after LT is estimated to occur in 20%–25% over a 10-year period with a mean time to diagnosis of approximately five years.

A diagnosis of rPSC should only be made in the context of typical cholangiographic and histological findings after excluding other causes of post-LT biliary disease including HAT/HAS, ductopenic rejection, and CMV infection. Risk factors of rPSC include male gender of recipient, gender mismatch, CMV mismatch, living-related donation, the presence and activity of inflammatory bowel disease, early post-LT cholestasis, and certain human leukocyte antigen genotypes. While Roux-en-Y biliary reconstruction has traditionally been employed during LT for PSC, recent meta-analysis has shown comparable rates of bile leaks, rPSC, and graft survival when using duct-to-duct anastomosis. Unlike recurrence of other autoimmune liver diseases (primary biliary cholangitis and autoimmune hepatitis), rPSC is associated with decreased graft survival in nearly half of cases and fourfold overall increased risk of death. Pharmacologic agents, including ursodeoxycholic acid, have no proven benefit in reducing rates of rPSC. While colectomy before or at the time of LT has been shown to confer protection against the development of rPSC, the evidence is conflicting. Furthermore, colectomy in patients with end-stage liver disease is associated with increased mortality and morbidity, and therefore this practice has not been adopted by most LT centers.

Montano-Loza AJ, Bhanji RA, Wasilenko S et al. Systematic review: recurrent autoimmune liver diseases after liver transplantation. *Aliment Pharmacol Ther.* 2017 Feb;45(4):485–500. Doi: 10.1111/apt.13894.

# chapter 5

# PANCREATIC DISORDERS

## QUESTIONS

1. **A 37-year-old woman with type 1 diabetes mellitus presented to the emergency department with a four-hour history of severe epigastric pain radiating through to the back.**

   Investigations:

   | | |
   |---|---|
   | Serum bilirubin | 36 µmol/L |
   | Serum alanine aminotransferase (ALT) | 152 U/L |
   | Serum alkaline phosphatase (ALP) | 168 U/L |
   | Serum albumin | 30 g/L |
   | Serum amylase | 1,200 U/L |
   | HbA1c | 72 mmol/mol |
   | Serum triglycerides | 9 mmol/L |

   **What is the most likely aetiology of this patient's acute pancreatitis?**

   A. Alcohol

   B. Drug induced

   C. Gallstone related

   D. Hypertriglyceridemia

   E. Tumour at the ampulla

2. **A 38-year-old man with ileocaecal Crohn's disease presented to the emergency department with severe abdominal pain and a serum amylase of 2,134 U/L. He was recently started on azathioprine 250 mg once a day.**

   **Which of the following statements is correct about azathioprine-induced pancreatitis in inflammatory bowel disease?**

   A. It affects <1% of patients

   B. It is a dose-independent complication

   C. It usually manifests as severe acute pancreatitis

   D. It usually occurs after more than three months of treatment

   E. There is a low rate of repeat pancreatitis on re-exposure

*Best of Five MCQs for the European Specialty Examination in Gastroenterology and Hepatology.* Thomas Marjot, Colleen G C McGregor, Tim Ambrose, Aminda N De Silva, Jeremy Cobbold, and Simon Travis, Oxford University Press (2021). © Oxford University Press. DOI: 10.1093/oso/9780198834373.003.0005

3.  **A 68-year-old woman was admitted to hospital with an episode of gallstone-related cholangitis. On resolution of her acute infection, endoscopic retrograde cholangiopancreatography (ERCP) was planned to clear residual gallstones from her common bile duct.**

    **Which of the following should be administered peri-procedurally to reduce the risk of post-ERCP pancreatitis (PEP)?**

    A.  Antioxidants

    B.  Diclofenac

    C.  Glyceryl trinitrate

    D.  Pentoxifylline

    E.  Somatostatin

4.  **A 57-year-old male is admitted to hospital with severe acute epigastric pain that radiates through to the back.**

    Investigations:

    | | |
    |---|---|
    | Haemoglobin | 122 g/L |
    | White cell count | $14.6 \times 10^9$/L |
    | Platelet count | $198 \times 10^9$/L |
    | Serum sodium | 135 mmol/L |
    | Serum potassium | 4.3 mmol/L |
    | Serum urea | 5.5 mmol/L |
    | Serum creatinine | 83 µmol/L |
    | Serum C-reactive protein (CRP) | 180 mg/L |
    | Serum bilirubin | 20 µmol/L |
    | Serum alanine transferase (ALT) | 66 U/L |
    | Serum alkaline phosphatase (ALP) | 179 U/L |
    | Serum albumin | 21 g/L |
    | Serum amylase | 1,011 U/L |

    **Which radiological investigation is most appropriate in the acute setting?**

    A.  Abdominal ultrasound

    B.  Computed tomography (CT) abdomen and pelvis with contrast

    C.  ERCP

    D.  Magnetic resonance cholangiopancreatography (MRCP)

    E.  Non-contrast CT abdomen and pelvis

5.  **A 50-year-old man with a history of excessive alcohol consumption is admitted to hospital with acute abdominal pain.**

Observations and investigations:

| | |
|---|---|
| Temperature | 38.2°C |
| Heart rate | 119 beats per minute |
| Blood pressure | 90/52 mmHg |
| Respiratory rate | 24 breaths per min |
| Patient weight | 75 kg |
| Oxygen saturations (FiO$_2$ 28%) | 94% |
| Haemoglobin | 138 g/L |
| White cell count | 14 × 10$^9$/L |
| Platelet count | 390 × 10$^9$/L |
| Serum amylase | 1,209 U/L |

**What would be the best initial resuscitation strategy?**

A. 1.5L Ringer's lactate over one hour

B. 1L hydroxyethyl starch (HES) over one hour

C. 750 ml Ringer's lactate over one hour

D. Prophylactic antibiotics and 1.5L normal saline over one hour

E. Prophylactic antibiotics and 750 ml Ringer's lactate over one hour

6.  **A 32-year-old woman with a history of excessive alcohol consumption is admitted to hospital with acute abdominal pain.**

Observations and investigations:

| | |
|---|---|
| Temperature | 38.2°C |
| Heart rate | 104 beats per minute |
| Blood pressure | 113/76 mmHg |
| Respiratory rate | 21 breaths per minute |
| Patient weight | 75 kg |
| Oxygen saturations (FiO$_2$ 28%) | 94% |
| Haemoglobin | 138 g/L |
| White cell count | 11.8 × 10$^9$/L |
| Platelet count | 388 × 10$^9$/L |
| Serum amylase | 980 U/L |

**What is the most appropriate nutritional strategy?**

A. Bowel rest for 48 hours

B. Enteral feeding via nasogastric tube

C. Enteral feeding via nasogastric tube when abdominal pain and inflammatory markers begin to improve

D. Oral diet when abdominal pain and inflammatory markers begin to improve

E. Parenteral nutrition

7.  **A 53-year-old woman presented to the emergency department with upper abdominal pain radiating through to the back. She had a heart rate of 105 beats per minute, blood pressure 110/60 mmHg, temperature 38°C, oxygen saturations 97% on air. She had no comorbidities, took no medications, and did not drink alcohol.**

Investigations:

| | |
|---|---|
| Haemoglobin | 130 g/L |
| White cell count | 17 × 10⁹/L |
| Neutrophil count | 14 × 10⁹/L |
| Serum amylase | 3,014 U/L |
| C-reactive protein | 206 mg/L |
| Serum bilirubin | 95 umol/L |
| Serum alanine transferase (ALT) | 76 U/L |
| Serum alkaline phosphatase (ALP) | 205 U/L |
| Abdominal ultrasound | Increased pancreatic volume with marked parenchymal heterogeneity consistent with acute pancreatitis. One 5 mm gallstone in the distal common bile duct with proximal dilation to 9 mm. |

### What would be the most appropriate timing of ERCP?

A. As an elective procedure once pancreatitis episode has resolved

B. There is no need for ERCP if amylase, Liver function tests (LFTs), and abdominal pain improve with conservative measures alone

C. Within 24 hours

D. Within 72 hours

E. Within one week

8.  **A 45-year-old man presented with persisting abdominal pain three months after an episode of acute gallstone pancreatitis.**

    Investigations:
       MRCP                                        Fig. 5.1

    **Which of the following would be the best management option?**

    A.  Conservative management

    B.  Conventional endoscopic transmural drainage

    C.  Endoscopic ultrasound (EUS)-guided transmural drainage

    D.  Percutaneous drainage

    E.  Surgical cystogastrostomy

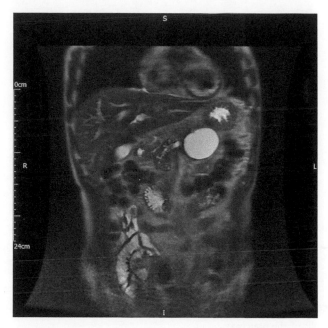

**Fig. 5.1** MRCP

Image courtesy of Dr Andrew Slater, Consultant Radiologist, OUH NHS Trust andrew.slater@ouh.nhs.uk

9. **A 52-year-old man presented with a history of intermittent abdominal pain over the last six-months.**

   **What is the diagnosis shown in the MRCP (Fig. 5.2)?**

   A. Annular pancreas

   B. Chronic pancreatitis (CP)

   C. IgG4 disease

   D. Pancreas divisum

   E. Primary sclerosing cholangitis

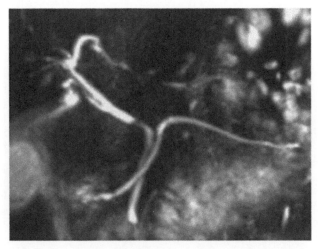

**Fig. 5.2** MRCP

Image courtesy of Dr Helen Bungay, Consultant Radiologist, Oxford University Hospitals NHS Foundation Trust

10. **Which cells are responsible for the secretion of secretin?**

   A. Acinar cells of the pancreas

   B. Alpha cells of the pancreas

   C. Delta cells of the pancreas

   D. Enteroendocrine cells in the duodenum

   E. S-cells in the duodenum

**11.** A 66-year-old man was referred with a three-month history of weight loss and malodourous pale stool. He was a long-term heavy smoker and drank 28 units of alcohol per week. Blood tests including inflammatory markers and amylase were normal. Faecal elastase (FE) was less than 50 ng/ml.

Which of the following options regarding CP is true?

A. CT has a specificity of 75% for CP

B. Hereditary CP carries a low risk of pancreatic cancer

C. Pancreatic enzyme supplements should be administered once a day at the lowest dose to avoid side effects

D. Patients with an additional risk factor for osteoporosis should have a baseline DEXA scan at diagnosis

E. Progression to CP after a single attack of acute pancreatitis occurs in 10% of patients

**12.** A 65-year-old-man with a long history of heavy smoking described 9-months of worsening offensive loose stool and weight loss.

Which of the following statements regarding pancreatic exocrine insufficiency (PEI) is correct?

A. Co-efficient of fat absorption is the gold standard for detection of mild PEI

B. FE >200 microgram/g has a high negative predictive value for mild–moderate PEI

C. MRCP with secretin has highest sensitivity for diagnosis

D. Severe PEI usually occurs within five years of the onset of CP

E. Vitamin deficiencies can occur in the absence of steatorrhoea

**13.** Which of the following is most correct regarding pain in CP?

A. Less than 10% of patients who achieve pain relief with EUS-guided coeliac plexus block will have ongoing pain relief after two years

B. Pain improves with pancreatic enzyme supplementation

C. Pain usually 'burns out' after more than 10 years from diagnosis

D. Pain usually presents after the development of steatorrhoea

E. Treatment with morphine is preferred over tramadol

**14.** A 58-year-old man presented with a four-week history of jaundice, pruritus, and weight loss. He had a history of eczema and allergic rhinitis. A CT scan revealed a bulky head of the pancreas, an irregular main pancreatic duct, distal common bile duct obstruction, localized lymphadenopathy and bilateral enlarged kidneys.

Which of the following is the best treatment option?

A. Biliary stent

B. Prednisolone

C. Rituximab

D. Supportive management

E. Surgical resection

15. **A 45-year-old male publican presented to the emergency department with one month of worsening episodic, sudden onset, severe upper abdominal pain, post-prandial vomiting, and weight loss.**

Investigations:

| | |
|---|---|
| Haemoglobin | 13 g/L |
| White cell count | $15.1 \times 10^9$/L |
| Serum C-reactive protein (CRP) | 120 mg/L |
| Serum bilirubin | 25 µmol/L |
| Serum alanine transferase (ALT) | 50 U/L |
| Serum alkaline phosphatase (ALP) | 120 U/L |
| Serum amylase | 180 U/L |
| CT abdomen with contrast | Focal thickening and abnormal enhancement of the second portion of the duodenum with an enlarged pancreatic head |
| Gastroscopy | Duodenal wall oedema and stenosis from D1 to D2. |
| Duodenal histology | Brunner's gland hyperplasia with multiple spindle cells |

### Which of the following statements regarding this condition is correct?

A. Endoscopic stenting of the minor papilla is the mainstay of treatment

B. High-dose prednisolone is the optimal first-line therapy

C. Pancreatoduodenectomy is often required

D. Serum levels of CA 19-9 are often elevated

E. Serum levels of IgG4 are often elevated

16. **A 70-year-old man presented with abdominal pain and weight loss. On clinical examination, he was jaundiced. Observations including temperature, heart rate, and blood pressure were all unremarkable. He had no comorbidities and his performance status was 0.**

Investigations:

| | |
|---|---|
| CT triple phase pancreas | 3 cm solid mass in the head of the pancreas, highly suspicious for pancreatic carcinoma. No locoregional lymph nodes or metastatic disease. Mild common bile duct dilatation (8 mm) but no intrahepatic biliary dilatation. |
| CT chest | Normal |
| Haemoglobin | 120 g/L |
| White cell count | 4 × 10⁹/L |
| Platelet count | 252 × 10⁹/L |
| International normalized ratio (INR) | 1.0 |
| Serum bilirubin | 75 µmol/L |
| Serum alanine transferase (ALT) | 35 U/L |
| Serum alkaline phosphatase (ALP) | 150 U/L |
| Serum C-reactive protein (CRP) | 3 mg/L |

**What is the next best intervention for this patient?**

A. EUS

B. ERCP

C. Percutaneous biopsy of pancreatic mass

D. Staging laparoscopy

E. Whipple procedure

17. **Which of the following statements about CA 19-9 is correct?**

A. A level ≥500 U/ml is diagnostic of pancreatic adenocarcinoma

B. Is unable to be produced by 1% of the population

C. Level is elevated in 50% of patients with advanced pancreatic adenocarcinoma

D. Level is not elevated in hepatocellular carcinoma

E. Level positively correlates with serum bilirubin

18. **Which syndrome is most associated with the development of pancreatic neuroendocrine tumours (p-NETs)?**

A. Familial adenomatous polyposis

B. Lynch syndrome

C. Multiple endocrine neoplasia type 1

D. Multiple endocrine neoplasia type 2A

E. Multiple endocrine neoplasia type 2B

19. **Which of the following pancreatic cystic neoplasms has the lowest malignant potential?**
    A. Branch duct intraductal papillary neoplasm
    B. Cystic pancreatic endocrine neoplasm
    C. Main duct intraductal papillary neoplasm
    D. Mucinous cystic neoplasms
    E. Serous cystadenoma

20. **A 50-year-old man was incidentally noted to have a pancreatic cystic lesion on a CT abdomen performed to investigate diverticulitis. A subsequent MRCP was performed.**

    Investigations:

    MRCP        20 mm cystic lesion in the head of the pancreas with connection to the pancreatic duct consistent with branch duct intraductal papillary mucinous neoplasm (IPMN). The main pancreatic duct is dilated to 11 mm

    **What is the next best management strategy?**
    A. Discharge with no follow-up required
    B. Surgical resection
    C. Surveillance at six months, one year, and then annually with magnetic resonance imaging (MRI)
    D. Surveillance with MRI after one year
    E. Symptom-based follow-up

## 1. C. Gallstone related

- Gallstones are responsible for 40% of acute pancreatitis
- A >3-fold elevation of ALT in the presence of acute pancreatitis has a positive predictive value of 95% in diagnosing acute gallstone pancreatitis
- Hypertriglyceridemia is not thought to be a risk for acute pancreatitis at levels below 11 mmol/L

Although alcohol is thought to account for >30% of cases of acute pancreatitis, there is nothing in the question stem to suggest a history of excessive alcohol consumption. There is also no history of recent new medication that makes drug-related pancreatitis unlikely. Although an ampullary tumour is possible, the young age of the patient and no family history of pancreatic malignancy make this a less likely diagnosis. The patient has hypertriglyceridemia. However, the serum triglyceride level is insufficiently elevated to cause acute pancreatitis. Even in the context of a normal calibre common bile duct, the presence of gallstones within the gallbladder of a patient with acute pancreatitis and no other more likely aetiology should prompt further investigation of gallstone-related disease. Furthermore, an elevated ALT ≥3-fold—the upper limit of normal in the presence of acute pancreatitis—has a positive predictive value of 95% in diagnosing acute gallstone pancreatitis.

Sleisenger and Fordtran's *Gastrointestinal and Liver Disease*. 10th ed. 2 vols, 2016. Chapter 58: Acute Pancreatitis.

## 2. B. It is a dose-independent complication

- Two to three per cent of patients with inflammatory bowel disease (IBD) treated with azathioprine will develop azathioprine-induced pancreatitis
- It usually manifests as mild disease within one month of treatment initiation and rapidly improves on treatment withdrawal

Azathioprine-induced pancreatitis is an idiosyncratic, dose-independent drug reaction affecting 2%–7% of treated patients with IBD. Risk factors associated with its onset include female gender, cigarette smoking, glucocorticoid exposure, and certain human leukocyte antigen polymorphisms. There is no association with polymorphisms in the thiopurine methyltransferase enzyme. The temporal relationship between initiation of azathioprine and symptom onset usually helps clarify the diagnosis, with most cases occurring within one month of commencing treatment. Other potential causes of acute pancreatitis in IBD must also be considered, however, including drug-related pancreatitis (e.g. 5-aminosalicylates, metronidazole), choledocholithiasis (with increased prevalence of gallstones in Crohn's disease), and from related autoimmune conditions (primary sclerosing cholangitis and autoimmune pancreatitis). In most cases, the pancreatitis is mild and

*Best of Five MCQs for the European Specialty Examination in Gastroenterology and Hepatology.* Thomas Marjot, Colleen G C McGregor, Tim Ambrose, Aminda N De Silva, Jeremy Cobbold, and Simon Travis, Oxford University Press (2021). © Oxford University Press. DOI: 10.1093/oso/9780198834373.003.0005

rapidly responds to azathioprine withdrawal. There is a high rate of recurrence with azathioprine re-introduction.

Ledder O, Lemberg DA, Day AS. Thiopurine-induced pancreatitis in inflammatory bowel diseases. *Expert Rev Gastroenterol Hepatol.* 2015 Apr;9(4):399–403. Doi: 10.1586/17474124.2015.992879.

### 3. B. Diclofenac

- The risk of PEP is 3.5% in unselected cases
- The European Society of Gastrointestinal Endoscopy (ESGE) recommends 100 mg rectal diclofenac or indomethacin for all patients undergoing ERCP unless contraindicated

PEP is the most common complication of ERCP occurring in 3.5% of patients. Most cases are mild–moderate but death occurs in 3%. Patient risk factors for PEP include functional biliary sphincter disorder (formerly Sphincter of Oddi dysfunction, female gender, and previous pancreatitis. Procedural risk factors include prolonged cannulation attempts, pancreatic guidewire passage, and pancreatic injection. ESGE 2014 guidelines recommend the routine administration of diclofenac or indomethacin either pre- or post-procedure. The estimated number needed to treat to prevent one episode of pancreatitis is 15. Both glyceryl trinitrate and somatostatin have conflicting evidence to support their use with heterogeneity of dosages or routes of administration used in different trials. The other medications listed are ineffective in reducing PEP.

Dumonceau JM, Andriulli A, Elmunzer BJ et al. Prophylaxis of post-ERCP pancreatitis: European Society of Gastrointestinal Endoscopy Guideline. *Endoscopy.* 2014 Sep;46(9):799–815. Doi: 10.1055/s-0034-1377875.

### 4. A. Abdominal ultrasound

- All patients with acute pancreatitis should have an abdominal ultrasound at presentation to look for gallstones as the underlying aetiology
- Early CT imaging does not help prognosticate or improve outcomes but can be useful after 72 hours in deteriorating patients to exclude pancreatic necrosis and/or collections

International Association of Pancreatology (IAP)/American Pancreatic Association (APA) guidelines recommend the use of ultrasound abdomen for all patients presenting with acute pancreatitis to establish the possibility of a gallstone aetiology, although an ALT level >150 U/L within 48 hours after symptoms onset discriminates biliary pancreatitis with a positive predictive value of >95%.

Contrast CT in acute pancreatitis is indicated in cases of diagnostic uncertainty to help confirm disease severity based on clinical predictors, and in the setting of clinical deterioration where pancreatic necrosis and peripancreatic fluid collections amenable to surgical/radiological intervention may be identified. These complications take several days to manifest and therefore optimal timing for initial CT assessment is at least 72–96 hours after onset of symptoms. Early CT does not add to prognostic scoring systems or improve clinical outcome.

IAP/APA Evidence-based guidelines for the management of acute pancreatitis. *Pancreatology.* 2013 Jul–Aug;13(4 Suppl 2):e1–15. Doi: 10.1016/j.pan.2013.07.063.

### 5. C. 750 ml Ringer's lactate over one hour

- In acute pancreatitis, Ringer's lactate decreases the incidence of systemic inflammatory response syndrome (SIRS) compared with resuscitation with normal saline

- Meta-analysis has demonstrated no evidence to support the routine use of antibiotic prophylaxis in patients with severe acute pancreatitis

There have been few head-to-head trials on the effects of different fluid regimes on outcomes in acute pancreatitis. However, there is randomized control data suggesting that resuscitation with Ringer's lactate decreases the incidence of SIRS compared with resuscitation with normal saline. The use of HES is discouraged because it has been found to increase the rates of renal failure and mortality, as compared with Ringer's lactate in patients with severe sepsis. Note that Ringer's lactate is very similar but not identical to Hartmann's solution. Although fluid resuscitation is important, particularly in severe acute pancreatitis, there is randomized control evidence that overly aggressive resuscitation can increase morbidity and mortality. Patients resuscitated with fluid infusion rate of 5–10 ml/kg/h experienced less need for mechanic ventilation, abdominal compartment syndrome, sepsis, and mortality as compared with patients assigned to receive infusion rates of 10–15 ml/kg/h. Meta-analysis has demonstrated no evidence to support the routine use of antibiotic prophylaxis in patients with severe acute pancreatitis.

IAP/APA Evidence-based guidelines for the management of acute pancreatitis. *Pancreatology*. 2013 Jul–Aug;13(4 Suppl 2):e1–15. Doi: 10.1016/j.pan.2013.07.063.

## 6. B. Enteral feeding via nasogastric tube

- The presence of SIRS at baseline and 48 hours helps grade severity of pancreatitis, predict outcome, and guide approach to nutritional management
- In severe pancreatitis, defined by the presence of SIRS, enteral feeding reduces systemic infections, multi-organ failure, and mortality

Determining the optimal nutritional strategy in acute pancreatitis requires an assessment of severity. Despite a range of validated predictive scoring systems, the joint international guidelines recommend using the presence of SIRS to define severe pancreatitis because of its widespread familiarity and simplicity. SIRS is defined by the presence of two or more of the following criteria: (1) temperature <36°C or >38°C (2) heart rate >90/min, (3) respiratory rate >20/min, and (4) white blood cells >12 or >10% bands. Persistent SIRS (>48 hours) carries a 25% mortality compared with 8% mortality for transient SIRS.

In mild–moderate pancreatitis, oral feeding with a full solid diet can start as soon as clinically tolerated. In those intolerant to oral feeding, enteral tube feeding (using standard polymeric formulae) should be commenced within 24–48 hours of admission. In severe pancreatitis, defined by the presence of SIRS, enteral tube feeding (via either a nasojejunal or nasogastric tube) is the preferred route and has been proven to reduce systemic infections, multi-organ failure, need for surgical intervention, and mortality. While placement of a nasogastric feeding tube is more straightforward, a number of patients will not tolerate nasogastric feeding because of delayed gastric emptying and may require nasojejunal tube placement. Parenteral nutrition is reserved for patients who do not meet nutritional requirements via the oral or enteral route. Where parenteral is indicated, parenteral L-glutamine should also be supplemented because it may reduce infection rates and mortality.

Arvanitakis M, Ockenga J, Bezmarevic M et al. ESPEN guideline on clinical nutrition in acute and chronic pancreatitis. *Clin Nutr*. 2020 Jan 22. pii: S0261-5614(20)30009-1. Doi: 10.1016/j.clnu.2020.01.004.

## 7. C. Within 24 hours

- In patients with gallstone pancreatitis and coexisting cholangitis, an ERCP should be performed urgently (<24 hours)
- In patients with gallstone pancreatitis without cholangitis, the need and timing of ERCP remain unclear

The role and timing of ERCP in acute gallstone pancreatitis is controversial and was subject to Cochrane systematic review and meta-analysis in 2012. This demonstrated that routine ERCP (<72 hours) did not significantly affect mortality or local/systemic complications, regardless of pancreatitis severity compared with conservative treatment alone. Furthermore, no statistically significant effect of the timing of ERCP (<24 hours vs <72 hours) on mortality was demonstrated. Therefore, in uncomplicated gallstone pancreatitis, it is reasonable to treat conservatively for at least the first 48 hours.

However, meta-analysis did clearly demonstrate that early ERCP (<24 hours) improved mortality and local and systemic complications in patients with acute gallstone pancreatitis and co-existing cholangitis, which is evident in this case (jaundice, fever, choledocholithiasis, and common bile duct dilatation).

IAP/APA Evidence-based guidelines for the management of acute pancreatitis. *Pancreatology*. 2013 Jul–Aug;13(4 Suppl 2):e1–15. Doi: 10.1016/j.pan.2013.07.063.

## 8. C. EUS-guided transmural drainage

- Most pancreatic pseudocysts can be managed conservatively with drainage only required for cases with symptoms, obstructive complications, or pseudocyst infection
- EUS-guided transmural stenting represents the best and safest method of achieving pseudocyst drainage

The MRCP image shows a large pancreatic pseudocyst (Fig. 5.3; arrow). Pancreatic pseudocysts complicate 10%–20% and 20%–40% of cases of acute and chronic pancreatitis respectively. In CP, the risk of pseudocysts is particularly high with underlying alcohol aetiology. Up to 70% of pseudocysts will resolve spontaneously, particularly following an episode of acute pancreatitis, and, even without resolution, most pseudocysts rarely lead to significant symptoms or complications. Most pseudocysts can therefore be managed conservatively with intervention reserved for patients with symptoms (usually abdominal pain) or complications including biliary and/or gastric outlet obstruction, pseudocyst bleeding, or infection. In these problematic cases, a range of treatment modalities are available. Traditionally, a surgical cystogastrostomy was performed, which involved an open or laparoscopic procedure to create an anastomosis between the lumen of the cyst cavity and the stomach. However, endoscopic approaches are now preferred, yielding similar technical success rates with lower rates of complications. Conventional endoscopic drainage involves visualizing the pseudocyst bulge in the gastric wall, advancing a guidewire into the pseudocyst cavity, and deploying one or more plastic stents. While this can safely be used for visibly bulging pseudocysts, most pseudocysts are now drained under EUS guidance to allow safer access and a decrease in complications. Trials comparing percutaneous versus endoscopic drainage have demonstrated equivalent technical success rates but a decreased re-intervention rate and shorter hospital stays among patients drained endoscopically.

Tyberg A, Karia K, Gabr M et al. Management of pancreatic fluid collections: a comprehensive review of the literature. *World J Gastroenterol*. 2016 Feb 21;22(7):2256–2270. Doi: 10.3748/wjg.v22.i7.2256.

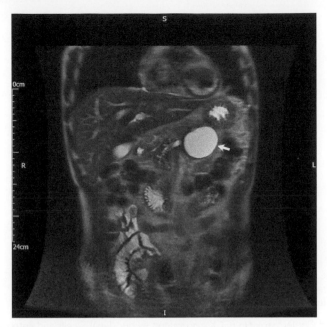

**Fig. 5.3** MRCP image showing pancreatic pseudocyst (arrow)

### 9. D. Pancreas divisum

- Pancreas divisum results from failure of ventral and dorsal pancreatic ducts to fuse, and occurs in 4%–14% of the population
- Poor pancreatic drainage through the minor papilla can result in recurrent pancreatitis
- Annular pancreas is characterized by pancreatic tissue wrapping around the descending duodenum, and can rarely cause duodenal obstruction and ulceration

Pancreas divisum is the most common congenital pancreatic ductal abnormality occurring in 4%–14% of the population. It is characterized by a failure of the dorsal and ventral pancreatic anlage to fuse during gestation resulting in two separate duct systems: the dorsal pancreatic duct (Santorini duct) directly entering the minor papilla, and the ventral duct (Wirsung) entering the major papilla. In most cases, there is no communication between the two ducts with most of the pancreas drained via the dorsal duct and minor papilla (Fig. 5.2). Most patients are asymptomatic. However, it can be associated with recurrent pancreatitis due to inadequate pancreatic drainage. Up to 26% of patients with idiopathic recurrent pancreatitis have pancreas divisum. Annular pancreas is a much rarer anomaly (1/20,000 people) in which a band of pancreatic tissue surrounds the descending duodenum, either completely or incompletely, and is in continuity with the head of the pancreas. The anomaly is often discovered incidentally in asymptomatic patients although it can be associated with duodenal stenosis and ulceration, acute pancreatitis, and biliary obstruction.

Yu J1, Turner MA, Fulcher AS et al. Congenital anomalies and normal variants of the pancreaticobiliary tract and the pancreas in adults: Part 2, Pancreatic duct and pancreas. *AJR Am J Roentgenol*. 2006 Dec;187(6):1544-1553.

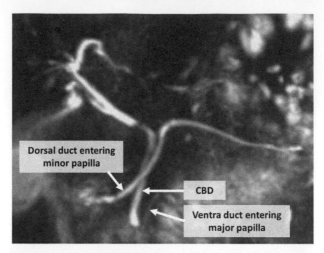

**Fig. 5.4** MRCP image showing pancreas divisum

### 10. E. S-cells in the duodenum

- Secretin and Cholecystokinin (CCK), produced by duodenal S-cells and enteroendocrine cells respectively, promote secretion of bicarbonate-rich fluid and digestive enzymes from the pancreas
- Secretin-stimulated MRCP improves pancreatic duct distension and signaling, and can be used to help characterize anatomical abnormalities

The acinar cells of the exocrine pancreas are radially orientated around a central lumen into which >2L of bicarbonate-rich fluid containing digestive enzymes and proenzymes are secreted each day. This secretion is upregulated both by neural stimulation from the vagus nerve and from humoral factors, principally secretin and CCK. Secretin is produced by duodenal S-cells in response to low luminal pH derived from the transit of acidic gastric secretions. Secretin stimulates the pancreatic acinar cells and duodenal Brunner's glands to secrete neutralizing water and bicarbonate, as well as to directly downregulate acid production by gastric parietal cells. The exogenous administration of intravenous secretin during MRCP image acquisition can improve pancreatic duct visualization by increasing duct calibre and signal intensity. Secretin-stimulated MRCP therefore has a role in the detection and characterization of pancreatic duct abnormalities, communications with fistulae or pseudocysts, and in Sphincter of Oddi dysfunction.

CCK is produced by duodenal enteroendocrine cells in response to a meal, and promotes the production and secretion of digestive enzymes from the exocrine pancreas. CCK also increases hepatic bile production, stimulates the contraction of the gallbladder, and induces Sphincter of Oddi relaxation. CCK-stimulated cholescintigraphy, which involves assessment of gallbladder contractility and emptying after injection of CCK, and a radiolabelled tracer can be used in carefully selected cases to investigate functional gallbladder disorders.

The endocrine pancreas is comprised of alpha, beta, delta, and epsilon cells that produce glucagon, insulin, somatostatin, and ghrelin respectively.

Kumar V, Abbas A, Aster J. *Robbins & Cotran Pathologic Basis of Disease*. 10th ed. June 2020.

## 11. E. Progression to CP after a single attack of acute pancreatitis occurs in 10% of patients.

- Alcohol consumption is the most common cause of CP
- Pancreatic insufficiency is best managed with pancreatic enzyme replacement with dose uptitrated to control maldigestion-related symptoms (e.g. steatorrhoea, weight loss)
- All patients with CP should be screened for osteoporosis at baseline with dual-energy X-ray absorptiometry (DEXA)

CP is accompanied by the progressive destruction of both islet cells and acinar tissue. Malabsorption only becomes evident once >90% of pancreatic acinar tissue has been destroyed. Progression to CP following a single attack of acute pancreatitis occurs in 10%. The most common aetiology for CP is alcohol excess with smoking and genetic mutations also significant risk factors. Hereditary pancreatitis should be considered in young patients with otherwise unexplained CP and carries a significantly elevated risk of secondary pancreatic cancer. Pancreatic calcification occur in >90% of patients with CP and are pathognomonic in the appropriate clinical context. Contrast-enhanced CT is reported to have moderate sensitivity and very high specificity (close to 100%).

Malabsorption (exocrine insufficiency), including of fat-soluble vitamins (A, D, E, and K), should be managed with adequate pancreatic enzyme replacement therapy starting at a minimum lipase dose of 40,000–50,000 PhU with main meals and half that dose with snacks. This should be uptitrated as necessary, aiming for the relief of maldigestion-related symptoms (e.g. steatorrhoea, weight loss, flatulence) and normalization of nutritional status. Monitoring for osteoporosis should be done by DEXA scan at baseline and repeated every two years in those with osteopenia.

Löhr JM, Dominguez-Munoz E, Rosendahl J et al. United European gastroenterology evidence-based guidelines for the diagnosis and therapy of chronic pancreatitis (HaPanEU). *United European Gastroenterol J*. 2017 Mar;5(2):153–199. Doi: 10.1177/2050640616684695.

## 12. E. Vitamin deficiencies can occur in the absence of steatorrhoea

- Vitamin deficiencies can occur with mild–moderate pancreatic endocrine insufficiency well before the onset of steatorrhoea
- FE is not capable of excluding mild–moderate PEI
- Direct tests involving the collection of duodenal juice in response to a hormonal stimulus are the accepted reference standard for PEI

Mild–moderate exocrine insufficiency can be compensated and asymptomatic, with severe disease (manifesting as steatorrhoea) only developing once pancreatic lipase falls <10% of normal. Patients with 'compensated' PEI do, however, have an increased risk of nutritional deficiencies, particularly of fat-soluble vitamins (A, D, E, K). The most common causes of PEI include CP and cystic fibrosis. Additional causes include pancreatic neoplasms, post-pancreatic resection and acute necrotizing pancreatitis. Coeliac disease can also lead to PEI, secondary to villous atrophy and impaired CCK production. Severe PEI and steatorrhea tend to manifest over a decade from initial diagnosis of CP. FE is a simple test for the indirect and non-invasive evaluation of pancreatic secretion. It is not capable of excluding mild–moderate PEI and there is no consensus regarding the threshold levels for diagnosis. However, very low FE values are most probably associated with PEI, whereas high values (>500 microg/g) allow its exclusion. The coefficient of fat absorption is the accepted, but rarely used, gold standard for the diagnosis of steatorrhoea. It involves measuring total faeces over three days while consuming a fat-controlled diet. Alternative indirect tests include a $^{13}$C-labelled mixed triglyceride breath test and estimation of pancreatic secretion volume with secretin-MRCP. Both are limited by sensitivity and availability for use in routine clinical practice. Direct tests involve the collection of duodenal juices in response to a hormonal stimulus (secretin or CCK) and are the accepted reference standard allowing the quantification of pancreatic exocrine secretion.

Löhr JM, Dominguez-Munoz E, Rosendahl J et al. United European gastroenterology evidence-based guidelines for the diagnosis and therapy of chronic pancreatitis (HaPanEU). *United European Gastroenterol J*. 2017 Mar;5(2):153–199. Doi: 10.1177/2050640616684695.

## 13. A. Less than 10% of patients who achieve pain relief with EUS-guided coeliac plexus block will have ongoing pain relief after two years

- Pain is the predominant symptom in CP, occurring in 94% of cases
- Management includes alcohol cessation, oral analgesia, and targeted endoscopic/surgical therapy for structural lesions (e.g. pseudocysts, ductal calculi)
- The pain relief of EUS-guided coeliac plexus block is often short-lived

Pain is the first presentation of CP in most patients and is usually the most disabling symptom of the condition. Only about 6% of patients with CP report being pain free. There is no good evidence to suggest that ongoing inflammation and parenchymal destruction will ultimately lead to reduction in pain over time. The mechanisms underlying pain in CP are complex and include structural pathology (e.g. pseudocysts, common bile duct, and duodenal obstruction) and ductal lesions (e.g. strictures, calculi) that may respond to targeted radiological or endoscopic therapy. However, a large group of patients will have neurogenic pain when no clear alternative source of pain can be identified. In these cases, cessation of alcohol, and possibly smoking, can improve pain. Pharmacological analgesia should follow the principles of the 'pain relief ladder' provided by the World Health Organization. Many patients will require opiates, in which case tramadol is preferred over morphine because of its association with fewer gastrointestinal side effects for the same degree of analgesia. Adjuvant analgesics may include antidepressants, anticonvulsants (e.g. gabapentin), and anxiolytics. EUS-guided coeliac plexus blocks can improve pain in half of patients, but the effect is often short with <10% experiencing pain relief for >24 weeks.

Löhr JM, Dominguez-Munoz E, Rosendahl J et al. United European gastroenterology evidence-based guidelines for the diagnosis and therapy of chronic pancreatitis (HaPanEU). *United European Gastroenterol J*. 2017 Mar;5(2):153–199. Doi: 10.1177/2050640616684695.

## 14. B. Prednisolone

- Autoimmune pancreatitis type 1 (AIP) is the pancreatic manifestation of IgG4-related disease (IgG4-RD), and often presents with a pancreatic mass and jaundice mimicking pancreatic cancer
- Associated features include multi-organ involvement, history of atopy, and elevated serum IgG4 and IgE

AIP is the pancreatic manifestation of IgG4-RD: an immune-mediated condition associated with fibro-inflammatory mass-forming lesions that can occur at nearly any anatomic site. It often presents as a multi-organ disease, and may be confused with malignancy, infection, or other inflammatory conditions. There is a male preponderance and often a clinical history of atopy. Serum IgG4 levels are raised in most (65%–80%) patients. However, they are non-specific and can be elevated in other malignant and inflammatory conditions, and 5% of healthy individuals. While the classical imaging description of AIP is with a diffuse sausage-shaped pancreas, half of patients have a discrete pancreatic head mass mimicking cancer. Localized lymphadenopathy is common and does not distinguish it from malignancy. Evidence of extra-pancreatic organ involvement supports the diagnosis. IgG4-RD is corticosteroid-responsive and prednisolone therapy would be the optimal first-line therapy. Biliary stenting has a role if there is evidence of biliary sepsis or corticosteroid treatment will be delayed because of a suspicion of malignancy. Rituximab is currently reserved as third-line therapy for patients who have relapsed or developed side effects on steroids, usually after a trial of an immunomodulator (e.g. Azathioprine).

Culver EL, Chapman RW. IgG4-related hepatobiliary disease: an overview. Nat Rev Gastroenterol Hepatol. 2016 Oct;13(10):601–612. Doi: 10.1038/nrgastro.2016.

### 15. C. Pancreatoduodenectomy is often required

- Para-duodenal 'groove' pancreatitis occurs in the tissue between the duodenal wall and the pancreatic head
- It can be differentiated from peri-pancreatic cancer and autoimmune pancreatitis by classical histopathology and imaging characteristics
- Pancreatoduodenectomy leads to complete pain relief in 75% of patients

Para-duodenal pancreatitis (groove pancreatitis) is an uncommon segmental CP affecting the 'groove' area between the pancreatic head, duodenum, and common bile duct. It often surrounds the minor ampulla and accessory duct. It predominantly affects males aged 40–50 years with a history of alcohol abuse, and can cause severe intermittent upper abdominal pain, nausea, and vomiting (due to disordered gastric emptying and duodenal stenosis). Weight loss can be severe, mimicking pancreatic cancer.

Serum pancreatic and hepatic enzymes are often slightly elevated whereas serum carbohydrate antigen (CA 19-9) and IgG4 levels are usually normal. The duodenum is usually oedematous, nodular, or cobblestone in appearance with stenosis on endoscopic evaluation. Histology from duodenal biopsies show duodenal wall cysts, Brunner gland hyperplasia, dilation of Santorini's duct, and protein plaques in the pancreatic duct. Imaging with EUS, CT, or magnetic resonance (MR) may demonstrate focal thickening and abnormal enhancement of the second portion of the duodenum, and cystic change in the duodenal wall.

Conservative treatment options include analgesia and smoking/alcohol cessation. Endoscopic stenting of the minor papilla has been reported, but long-term outcomes remain unclear. Pancreatoduodenectomy is the treatment of choice when the condition remains difficult to distinguish from pancreatic carcinoma or with persisting symptoms when resection leads to complete pain relief in >75%.

Jani B, Rzouq F, Saligram S et al. Groove pancreatitis: a rare form of chronic pancreatitis. N Am J Med Sci. 2015 Nov;7(11):529–532. Doi: 10.4103/1947-2714.170624.

#### 16. A. EUS

- In potentially resectable pancreatic tumours, EUS is required prior to surgery to help identify lymph node involvement and vascular invasion
- Pre-operative biliary drainage in patients with biliary obstruction, without cholangitis secondary to resectable pancreatic tumours, is associated with a higher rate of post-operative complications

This patient has a potentially resectable pancreatic mass with mild biliary obstruction but no evidence of cholangitis or metastatic disease on cross-sectional imaging. In this setting, the European Society for Medical Oncology recommend further assessment with EUS, which is now widely used in the staging of pancreatic cancer prior to surgery. EUS can detect metastatic lymph nodes and vascular invasion not seen on imaging, and helps to predict overall resectability. It can also acquire tissue via fine needle aspiration, which can confirm the primary diagnosis and help stage disease by sampling atypical portocaval lymph nodes or incidental hepatic metastases. Percutaneous biopsy of a liver metastasis can be used in metastatic disease, but percutaneous biopsy of the pancreas is contra-indicated in potentially resectable cases because of the risk of peritoneal seeding. In uncomplicated biliary obstruction secondary to resectable pancreatic cancer, as in this case, pre-operative drainage should be avoided because it is associated with higher rates of post-operative complications. In cases of cholangitis where biliary decompression is necessary, further studies are needed to determine the best treatment modality (e.g. ERCP vs percutaneous transhepatic cholangiogram; plastic vs metal stenting). Staging laparoscopy in addition to imaging and EUS has been suggested by some groups in order to exclude peritoneal metastases but it is not widely practised.

Ducreux M, Cuhna AS, Caramella C et al. Cancer of the pancreas: ESMO clinical practical guidelines. *Ann Oncol.* 2015 Sep;(26 Suppl 5):v56–68. Doi: 10.1093/annonc/mdv295.

#### 17. E. Level positively correlates with serum bilirubin

- CA 19-9 does not have the necessary sensitivity or specificity to facilitate its use in the diagnosis of pancreatic adenocarcinoma
- Cholestasis from any cause can cause an elevation in CA 19-9

The carbohydrate antigen sialyl Lewis A is more commonly referred to as 'CA 19-9', the name of the monoclonal antibody currently used for its detection. Elevated CA 19-9 is best studied in the context of pancreatic adenocarcinoma being elevated in >80% patients with advanced disease. However, it can also be elevated in a range of other benign and malignant conditions, and therefore does not carry the necessary sensitivity or specificity to be utilized in the diagnosis of pancreatic cancer. CA 19-9 is related to the Lewis blood group antigens and only patients belonging to the Le ($\alpha$-$\beta$+) or Le ($\alpha$+$\beta$-) blood groups will express the CA 19-9 antigen. Approximately 6% of the caucasian population and 22% of the black population are Le($\alpha$-$\beta$-) and do not generate the specific sialyl antigen. Conversely, CA 19-9 strongly correlates with the level of bilirubin and can be elevated with any cause of cholestasis. CA 19-9 does have significant prognostic value and a failure of CA 19-9 level to normalize after pancreatic cancer resection is associated with a poor prognosis and suggests residual disease. CA 19-9 can also be used as a surrogate marker of response to chemotherapy with a ≥20%–50% decrease in CA 19-9 associated with a positive tumour response and increased survival. A pre-operative serum CA 19-9 level ≥500 U/ml predicts worse prognosis after surgery.

Ducreux M, Cuhna AS, Caramella C et al. Cancer of the pancreas: ESMO clinical practical guidelines. *Ann Oncol.* 2015 Sep;26 (Suppl 5):v56–68. Doi: 10.1093/annonc/mdv295.

## 18. C. Multiple endocrine neoplasm type 1

- Multiple endocrine neoplasia type 1 is the main inherited cause of p-NETs
- Other rare inherited causes are Von Hippel–Lindau disease, neurofibromatosis type 1 (von Recklinghausen's syndrome) and tuberous sclerosis

P-NETs are a heterogeneous group of tumours derived from the endocrine pancreatic cells (e.g. $\alpha$-, $\beta$-, $\delta$-, and $\gamma$-cells) and represent just <2% of all pancreatic neoplasms. They express at least two of the following markers: chromogranin A, synaptophysin and/or neuron-specific enolase, and can secrete a variety of neuropeptides leading to a range of clinical symptoms (e.g. carcinoid syndrome). Most p-NETs occur as sporadic tumours although a proportion occur as part of an inherited syndrome. Multiple endocrine neoplasia type 1 remains the most important inherited condition, responsible for 20%–30% of gastrinomas and 5% of insulinomas. Other inherited conditions predisposing to p-NETS are Von Hippel–Lindau disease, neurofibromatosis type 1 (von Recklinghausen's syndrome), and tuberous sclerosis.

Falconi M, Eriksson B, Kaltsas G, et al. Consensus guidelines update for the management of functional p-NETs (F-p-NETs) and non-functional p-NETs (NF-p-NETs). *Neuroendocrinology*. 2016;103(2):153–171. Doi: 10.1159/000443171.

## 19. E. Serous cystadenoma

- Secondary cystic changes can occur in frankly malignant pancreatic adenocarcinomas
- Cystic lesions with malignant potential include IPMNs, mucinous cystic neoplasms, and solid pseudopapillary neoplasms
- Serous cystadenomas and simple cysts are benign

Three to fourteen per cent of patients undergoing routine imaging are now incidentally found to have pancreatic cysts. Multiple types are recognized with varying natural histories and malignant potential. The most aggressive cystic lesions are typically cystic changes in frankly malignant, otherwise solid lesions, such as ductal adenocarcinoma or neuroendocrine tumours. Lesions with malignant potential include IPMN and mucinous cystic neoplasm. Solid pseudopapillary neoplasm has a known, but low, risk for malignancy. The other end of the spectrum comprises benign neoplasms (such as serous cystadenoma) and non-neoplastic lesions (such as simple cysts, lymphoepithelial cysts). Serous cystadenomas can be macrocystic, which appear similar to mucinous lesions on imaging, or microcystic, which have a typical honeycomb appearance and central scar.

Stark A, Donahue TR, Reber HA et al. Pancreatic cyst disease: a review. *JAMA*. 2016 May 3;315(17):1882–1893. Doi: 10.1001/jama.2016.4690.

## 20. B. Surgical resection

- Absolute indications for surgical resection of IPMN include jaundice, pancreatic duct dilatation >10 mm, and solid mass
- Patients not meeting criteria for surgery should have six-month follow-up in the first year, and then yearly follow-up with MRI or EUS

IPMN can be classified according to their association with the pancreatic ducts. Main-duct IPMNs are characterized by dilation of the main pancreatic duct (MPD) of >5 mm, for which other causes of ductal obstruction have been ruled out, are mostly located in the pancreatic head and carry the highest risk of malignancy. Branch duct IPMNs are grape-like cysts (>5 mm) that communicate with the main duct. They have a preference for the uncinate process, can be multifocal, and have lower risk of malignancy. Absolute indications for surgical resection in patients with suspected IPMN include jaundice, an enhancing mural nodule ≥5 mm, a solid mass, a positive malignant cytology, or a dilated MPD diameter measuring ≥10 mm. Patients outside these criteria require six-month follow-up in the first year, and then yearly follow-up with MRI/EUS if no indications for surgery arise.

*European evidence-based guidelines on pancreatic cystic neoplasms. The European Study Group on Cystic Tumours of the Pancreas. Gut.* 2018 May;67(5):789–804. Doi: 10.1136/gutjnl-2018-316027.

1.  **A 32-year-old man was reviewed in the emergency department with diarrhoea secondary to enteropathogenic *Escherichia coli* infection. Oral rehydration therapy (ORT) was suggested to improve hydration status.**

    **Through which ion transporter does ORT act?**

    A.  Cystic fibrosis transmembrane conductance regulator (CFTR)

    B.  Epithelial sodium channel (ENaC)

    C.  Glucose transporter 1 (GLUT1)

    D.  Sodium/glucose cotransporter 1 (SGLT1)

    E.  Sodium/potassium/chloride cotransporter 1 (NKCC1)

2.  **A 46-year-old woman presented with a 5-month history of profuse diarrhoea despite fasting, and associated abdominal bloating. She complained of increasing fatigue and flushing, and appeared dehydrated.**

    Investigations:

    | | |
    |---|---|
    | Haemoglobin | 125 g/L |
    | Serum sodium | 144 mmol/L |
    | Serum potassium | 1.9 mmol/L |
    | Serum urea | 7.3 mmol/L |
    | Serum creatinine | 136 µmol/L |
    | Plasma viscosity | 1.76 mPa/s |

    **Which of the following is the most likely diagnosis?**

    A.  Bile acid diarrhoea

    B.  Carcinoid syndrome

    C.  Coeliac disease

    D.  Vasoactive intestinal polypeptide (VIP)oma

    E.  *Vibrio cholera* infection

*Best of Five MCQs for the European Specialty Examination in Gastroenterology and Hepatology.* Thomas Marjot, Colleen G C McGregor, Tim Ambrose, Aminda N De Silva, Jeremy Cobbold, and Simon Travis, Oxford University Press (2021). © Oxford University Press.
DOI: 10.1093/oso/9780198834373.003.0006

3.  **A 37-year-old with diarrhoea was reviewed in outpatients and was interested to understand more about gut hormones.**

    **Regarding gut hormones, which of the following statements is true?**

    A.  Cholecystokinin is produced by I cells of the small intestine in response to ingested carbohydrate

    B.  Gastrin is produced by G cells of the duodenum in response to raised gastric pH

    C.  Glucagon-like peptide 1 stimulates glucose-dependent glucagon release from the pancreatic islets

    D.  Glucagon-like peptide 2 (GLP-2) inhibits gastric emptying and gastric acid production, induces small bowel mucosal growth, and stimulates mesenteric blood flow

    E.  Somatostatin increases gut motility and stimulates pancreatico-biliary secretions

4.  **You reviewed a 47-year-old patient in clinic with a body mass index (BMI) of 34 kg/m². They asked for your opinion on the role of leptin in obesity.**

    **Which of these statements is true?**

    A.  Ethnicity exerts a significant effect on leptin concentrations

    B.  Leptin is a product of the *lep* gene primarily expressed in adipocytes

    C.  Most patients with obesity have low serum leptin

    D.  Overeating reduces circulating leptin levels

    E.  Supraphysiological doses of leptin may reduce food intake in patients of normal weight

5.  **A 43-year-old woman with a BMI of 37 kg/m² was referred for gastric bypass surgery. She was consented for a research study investigating satiety hormones in those undergoing bariatric surgery.**

    **Which of the following statements best describes the behaviour of ghrelin?**

    A.  Levels fall before meal ingestion but gradually rise in the subsequent two hours

    B.  Levels remain unchanged before and after meal ingestion

    C.  Levels rise sharply before and fall shortly after meal ingestion

    D.  Levels rise sharply before meal ingestion and remain high afterwards for several hours

    E.  Levels are unchanged before meal ingestion but fall rapidly afterwards

6.  **A 47-year-old man presented with intermittent, watery diarrhoea. He had a 25-year history of type I diabetes with retinopathy and peripheral neuropathy requiring an insulin pump. Investigations were unremarkable and autonomic enteropathy was suspected.**

    **Which of the following neurotransmitters is most responsible for activating sensory neurones following stimulation of stretch receptors in the bowel?**

    A.  Acetylcholine

    B.  Nitric oxide

    C.  Serotonin

    D.  Substance P

    E.  Vasoactive intestinal peptide (VIP)

7.  **A 25-year-old scientist was referred for a second opinion due to persistent abdominal pain, nausea, abdominal distension, and weight loss. All investigations had been normal and enteric dysmotility was suspected. She enquired about measuring small bowel contractility.**

    **Which of the following would you recommend as best for measuring small intestinal contractile patterns?**

    A.  Barium follow through

    B.  Catheter-based manometry

    C.  Lactulose hydrogen breath test

    D.  Scintigraphy

    E.  Wireless motility capsule

8.  **A 38-year-old man presented with recurrent abdominal pain, every other day, for the previous three months.**

    **Which of the following most favours a diagnosis of irritable bowel syndrome (IBS)?**

    A.  Bloating

    B.  Early satiety

    C.  Mucus discharge per rectum

    D.  Nausea

    E.  Worsening pain with defecation

9. **A 37-year-old woman with a history of functional abdominal pain was referred for a second opinion and was keen to know about options for managing her ongoing pain. She had had no response to antispasmodics, amitriptyline, duloxetine, or hypnotherapy.**

    **Which of the following should you recommend next?**

    A. Fentanyl patch

    B. Gabapentin

    C. Oxycodone immediate release

    D. Sacral nerve stimulator

    E. Sertraline

10. **You have been invited to present to the local coeliac disease patient support group about the practicalities of a gluten-free diet.**

    **Which one of the following foods and drinks could be included in a gluten-free diet?**

    A. Barley squash

    B. Champagne

    C. Couscous

    D. Porridge oats

    E. Scotch eggs

11. **A 29-year-old white British nursery worker attended clinic with a two-year history of abdominal bloating, discomfort, and an alternating bowel habit. She had not lost weight, had no rectal bleeding or skin rashes, but was frequently tired. She had a sister with type 1 diabetes.**

Investigations:

| | |
|---|---|
| Haemoglobin | 121 g/L |
| White cell count | 5.4 × 10⁹/L |
| Platelet count | 174 × 10⁹/L |
| Mean corpuscular volume (MCV) | 87 fL |
| Serum ferritin | 12 µg/L |
| Serum C-reactive protein (CRP) | 0.2 mg/L |
| Serum vitamin B12 | 358 ng/L |
| Serum folate | 1.9 µg/L |
| Serum vitamin D | 51 nmol/L |
| immunoglobin A tissue transglutaminase antibody (IgA TTG) | <0.2 U/ml |
| Total IgA | 0.05 g/L |
| human leukocyte antigen (HLA) status | DQ 2.5 heterozygote |
| Gastroscopy | Macroscopically normal |
| Duodenal histology | Marsh 3C villous atrophy and crypt hyperplasia with intraepithelial lymphocytosis |

**What is the most appropriate test to establish a diagnosis?**

A. Faecal calprotectin

B. *Helicobacter pylori* serology

C. HIV serology

D. Periodic-acid Schiff (PAS) staining of duodenal biopsies

E. Serum IgG TTG antibody

12. **A 27-year-old man presented to clinic with persistent abdominal discomfort, bloating, and alternating bowel habit. He had been diagnosed with coeliac disease 12 months ago.**

Investigations:

|  | At diagnosis | At present |
|---|---|---|
| Haemoglobin | 116 g/L | 134 g/L |
| MCV | 87 fL | 93 fL |
| Serum ferritin | 8 µg/L | 42 µg/L |
| Serum vitamin B12 | 246 ng/L | 283 ng/L |
| Serum folate | 2.2 µg/L | 4.9 µg/L |
| IgA TTG | 1800 U/ml | 7 U/ml |
| Duodenal histology | Marsh 3C villous atrophy and crypt hyperplasia with intra-epithelial lymphocytosis | Fig. 6.1 |

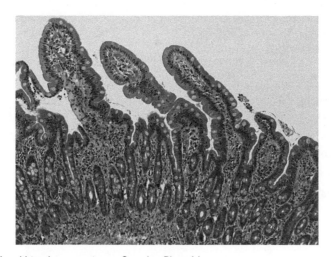

**Fig. 6.1** Duodenal histology specimen. See also Plate 11

Image courtesy of Dept of Histopathology, Oxford University Hospitals NHS Foundation Trust

### How would you classify the histological features?

A. Enteropathy-associated T-cell lymphoma (EATL)

B. Marsh I

C. Marsh 3A

D. Marsh 3C

E. Normal

13. **A 23-year-old patient with coeliac disease was worried about their bone health.**

    **Which of the following statements is true?**

    A. A bone density scan does not need to be performed until the age of 50

    B. Bone density will not increase during the first year of a gluten-free diet

    C. Calcium intake should be at least 1,000 mg per day

    D. Patients with ongoing villous atrophy require annual bone density scans

    E. The risk of osteoporosis and bone fracture is not increased in patients with coeliac disease

14. **A 25-year-old man presented as an emergency with abdominal pain, distension, vomiting and weight loss of 6 kg in two months. Over the past few days he had occasionally opened his bowels and had noted some blood on the paper when wiping. He had a past history of coeliac disease and insisted he was compliant with a gluten-free diet. Axillary and inguinal lymphadenopathy was present.**

    Investigations:

    | | |
    |---|---|
    | Haemoglobin | 113 g/L |
    | MCV | 79.4 fL |
    | Serum ferritin | 13 µg/L |
    | IgA TTG | 359 U/ml |
    | Faecal occult blood | Positive |

    **Which of the following is the most likely diagnosis?**

    A. Coeliac disease exacerbation

    B. Colorectal cancer

    C. EATL

    D. Graves' disease

    E. Lactose intolerance

15. **A 51-year-old woman was referred for assessment of diarrhoea. She complained of episodes of abdominal pain, bloating, and vomiting. She was troubled by facial flushing although wondered if this was the menopause. She had a recent diagnosis of asthma, and a history of previous parathyroidectomy and resection of a pituitary microadenoma.**

    Investigations:

    | | |
    |---|---|
    | Gastroscopy | Normal |
    | Ileocolonoscopy | Normal |
    | CT enterography | There is no small bowel inflammation but there is a suggestion of a mid-ileal small bowel mass. Several poorly characterized liver lesions are seen. MRI liver recommended. |
    | Thyroid-stimulating hormone (TSH) | 0.38 mU/L |
    | 24-hour urinary 5-hydroxyindolacetic acid (5-HIAA) | 523 µmol |

    **What is the most likely diagnosis?**

    A. Multiple endocrine neoplasia (MEN) I

    B. MEN2A

    C. MEN2B

    D. Thyrotoxicosis

    E. Zollinger-Ellison syndrome

16. **A 48-year old homeless man was admitted with a one week history of confusion and diarrhoea, passing loose, watery stool several times a day with urgency. He drank approximately 140 units of alcohol a week. He was confused with disorientation to place and time. An Abbreviated Mental Test Score was 2/10. There was no evidence of confabulation. On examination he was alert, but confused, with normal neurological examination and no nystagmus or ophthalmoplegia. He had poor dentition. He had a non-itchy, erythematous, symmetrical rash, predominantly on his face, neck, hands and forearms, with some blebs and blisters.**

    **Which nutritional deficiency would best explain the presentation?**

    A. Cobalamin (B12)

    B. Folate (B9)

    C. Niacin (B3)

    D. Pyridoxine (B6)

    E. Thiamine (B1)

17. **A 37-year-old Caucasian woman was referred with fatigue, bloating, and looser stools. She had a history of alcohol excess and ankylosing spondylitis, and was prone to urinary tract infections for which she took long-term prophylactic dose trimethoprim.**

    Investigations:

    | | |
    |---|---|
    | Haemoglobin | 95 g/L |
    | MCV | 105 fL |
    | Serum ferritin | 276 µg/L |
    | Serum folate | 1.4 µg/L |
    | Serum vitamin B12 | 358 ng/L |
    | Serum CRP | 4.3 mg/L |

    **What is the most likely cause of her folate deficiency?**

    A. Coeliac disease

    B. Crohn's disease

    C. Dietary deficiency in the context of alcohol excess

    D. Small intestinal bacterial overgrowth

    E. Trimethoprim

18. **A 76-year-old man was referred to clinic with abnormal blood tests. There was no history of loose stools, abdominal pain, or weight loss. He had a past medical history of type 2 diabetes. His only medications were metformin, aspirin, and ranitidine when required.**

    Investigations:

    | | |
    |---|---|
    | Haemoglobin | 98 g/L |
    | MCV | 113 fL |
    | Serum ferritin | 276 µg/L |
    | Serum folate | 2.4 µg/L |
    | Serum vitamin B12 | 123 ng/L |
    | Intrinsic factor antibodies | Negative |

    **Which is the most likely underlying cause of his presentation?**

    A. Gastric cancer

    B. Metformin

    C. Pancreatic insufficiency

    D. Pernicious anaemia

    E. Ranitidine

19. **An 80-year-old man presented with a three-week history of progressive discolouration and oligo-arthralgia of his lower limbs. He denied any history of trauma. He lived alone but had no past medical history and was not on any regular medications. On examination, he appeared frail and unkempt. Widespread ecchymosis of the lower limbs with perifollicular haemorrhage and corkscrew hair was noticed.**

Investigations:

| | |
|---|---|
| Haemoglobin | 111 g/L |
| MCV | 77 fL |
| White cell count | $6.0 \times 10^9$/L |
| Platelet count | $300 \times 10^9$/L |
| Serum CRP | 4 mg/L |
| Serum ferritin | 13 µg/L |
| Serum folate | 8 µg/L |
| Serum vitamin B12 | 250 ng/L |
| Coagulation screen | Normal |
| Urinalysis | Normal |

**Which micronutrient deficiency is the most likely cause for his presentation?**

A. Copper

B. Nicotinamide

C. Vitamin C

D. Vitamin D

E. Vitamin K

20. **A 35-year-old woman presented with increasing orthopnoea and breathlessness on minimal exertion. On examination, her jugular venous pressure (JVP) was raised, she had pitting oedema to her thighs, and her breath sounds were reduced bibasally. She had recently arrived in the UK from rural China to visit her cousin. She felt generally weak and her cousin said that her mood was different from usual.**

Investigations:

| | |
|---|---|
| Full blood count | Normal |
| TSH | 5.9 mU/L |
| Free T4 | 9.8 pmol/L |
| Free T3 | 2.1 pmol/L |
| Chest radiograph | Blunted costophrenic angles and cardiomegaly |
| Echocardiogram | Dilated left ventricle, globally reduced systolic function |

**Which micronutrient deficiency is the most likely cause for her presentation?**

A. Magnesium

B. Niacin

C. Selenium

D. Vitamin B12

E. Zinc

21. **A 19-year-old woman was reviewed in outpatients for abdominal pain, diarrhoea, and excessive flatulence. Her symptoms were worsened when drinking milk and lactose intolerance was suspected.**

    **Which of the following statements is true?**

    A. Lactase persistence in Caucasians is due to a loss-of-function mutation in the lactase gene

    B. Lactose malabsorption in adults is most commonly caused by lactase non-persistence

    C. SGLT1 and GLUT2 transport the monosaccharides into enterocytes via passive diffusion

    D. The brush border enzyme, lactase, cleaves lactose into two glucose monosaccharides

    E. The diagnosis should be suspected in the presence of a positive lactulose-hydrogen breath test

22. **A 66-year-old man presented with an eight-week history of non-bloody diarrhoea, flatulence, and fatigue. He had a past history of systemic sclerosis.**

    Investigations:

    | | |
    |---|---|
    | Haemoglobin | 105 g/L |
    | MCV | 100 fL |
    | Serum folate | 18.2 µg/L |
    | Gastroscopy | Normal |
    | Colonoscopy | Normal |
    | Duodenal histology | Villi of normal height and shape. Focal intraepithelial lymphocytosis, no increase in chronic inflammatory cells in the lamina propria |

    **What is the most appropriate management?**

    A. Budesonide

    B. Co-amoxiclav

    C. Creon

    D. Gluten-free diet

    E. Prednisolone

23. **A 56-year-old man with a history of Crohn's disease and previous ileocaecal resection presented with non-bloody diarrhoea with urgency. He denied abdominal pain, fever, nausea, vomiting, or weight loss. Examination was unremarkable. He had no extra-intestinal manifestations of inflammatory bowel disease. He was 178 cm tall and weighed 75 kg.**

    Investigations:

    | | |
    |---|---|
    | Haemoglobin | 130 g/L |
    | Haematocrit | 45% |
    | White cell count | $6.5 \times 10^9$/L |
    | Platelet count | $278 \times 10^9$/L |
    | Erythrocyte sedimentation rate | 12 mm/1$^{st}$ hr |
    | Serum vitamin B12 | 350 ng/L |
    | Red cell folate | 410 µg/L |
    | C-reactive protein (CRP) | 9 mg/L |

    **Which medication is most likely to be effective for treating the diarrhoea?**

    A. Budesonide

    B. Ciprofloxacin

    C. Colestyramine

    D. Mesalazine

    E. Prednisolone

24. **A 43-year-old builder was reviewed for abdominal pain and iron deficiency anaemia. He also complained of joint aches and ankle swelling. He took omeprazole for heartburn but vehemently denied any other medications.**

    Investigations:

    | | |
    |---|---|
    | Gastroscopy | Gastritis and multiple duodenal ulcers |
    | Ileocolonoscopy | Normal |
    | Magnetic resonance enterography | Widespread ileal ulceration with diaphragm-like structures |
    | Serum gastrin | 104 pmol/L (non-fasting) |
    | Haemoglobin | 79 g/L |
    | MCV | 73.8 fL |
    | Serum albumin | 29 g/L |

    **What is the diagnostic test?**

    A. Echocardiogram

    B. Fasting serum gastrin level

    C. NSAID metabolites

    D. Renal biopsy

    E. Vasculitis screen

25. **A 37-year-old man presented with a two-week history of chills, abdominal pain, and constipation. There were faint pink macules on his trunk. He had recently returned from a trekking holiday in Nepal. He received the oral typhoid vaccine one year ago.**

    Investigations:

    | | |
    |---|---|
    | Haemoglobin | 120 g/L |
    | White cell count | $3.0 \times 10^9$/L |
    | Platelet count | $175 \times 10^9$/L |
    | Serum C-reactive protein (CRP) | 120 mg/L |
    | Serum alanine transferase (ALT) | 200 U/L |
    | Blood cultures (×2) | Negative after 48 hours |
    | HIV | Negative |
    | Hepatitis A, B, C, E virus serology | Negative |
    | Dengue virus serology | Negative |
    | Thick and thin film | Negative |

    ## Which is the most sensitive diagnostic test for this disease?

    A. Blood culture incubation for >72 hours

    B. Bone marrow culture

    C. Stool cultures

    D. Urine culture

    E. Widal test

## 1. D. SGLT1

- SGLT1 enables absorption of sodium (and water) when coupled with glucose
- Some infections (e.g. enteropathogenic *E. coli*) inhibit the activity of SGLT1, rendering oral rehydration therapies less effective
- Targeting ion transporters may provide novel drug therapies for managing infectious diarrhoea

Transporters are transmembrane proteins that mediate transport of ions and other solutes. Intestinal epithelial cells control the absorption and secretion of electrolytes through various ion transporters to maintain fluid balance. Infectious causes of diarrhoea may affect both secretory and/or absorptive transporters. Oral rehydration therapies typically comprise combinations of glucose, salt, and water, and take advantage of the preservation of SGLT1 function in infectious diarrhoea. Therefore, sodium and fluid absorption can be achieved if glucose is provided while the (usually self-limiting) infection resolves. Novel forms of oral rehydration therapies include starch (to drive sodium absorption in the colon by providing short chain fatty acids) and zinc (which may work through altering chloride homeostasis). Enteropathogenic *E. coli* can inhibit the activity of SGLT1, and patients with this infection are less responsive to oral rehydration therapies.

Other ion transporters include the EnaC, which functions in the distal colon to mediate sodium absorption. This is decreased in murine *Salmonella* infections. (NKCC1 is located on the basolateral membrane and supplies chloride for secretion. Expression of this transporter may be increased in *Salmonella* and some *E. coli* infections. CFTR mediates chloride efflux from the apical surface of intestinal epithelial cells and is an attractive target for novel drug therapies. GLUT1 is a glucose transporter alone and has no role in the function of oral rehydration therapies.

Das S, Jayaratne R, Barrett KE. The role of ion transporters in the pathophysiology of infectious diarrhea. *Cell Mol Gastroenterol Hepatol.* 2018;6(1):33–45. Doi:10.1016/j.jcmgh.2018.02.009.

## 2. D. Vasoactive intestinal polypeptide (VIP)oma

- Typical features of VIPoma include secretory diarrhoea, hypokalaemia, and dehydration
- It is a rare type of functioning neuroendocrine tumour, typically pancreatic
- Somatostatin analogues and surgery form part of management

Patients with VIPoma, or Verner–Morrison syndrome, complain of high-volume diarrhoea despite fasting and are found to have hypochlorhydria, hypokalaemia (serum potassium <3 mmol/L), hyperglycaemia, and hypercalcaemia with signs of dehydration. Flushing occurs in 20% of patients and abdominal pain, fatigue, and bloating may also be present.

VIP stimulates fluid and electrolyte secretion from intestinal epithelium and bile duct cholangiocytes. VIPoma is a rare form of functioning neuroendocrine tumour that affects an estimated 1 in

*Best of Five MCQs for the European Specialty Examination in Gastroenterology and Hepatology.* Thomas Marjot, Colleen G C McGregor, Tim Ambrose, Aminda N De Silva, Jeremy Cobbold, and Simon Travis, Oxford University Press (2021). © Oxford University Press. DOI: 10.1093/oso/9780198834373.003.0006

10 million people per year. They are typically pancreatic (over 90%) and are usually diagnosed in adults, age 30–50 years, and more commonly in women. VIPoma should be suspected in patients with >700 mL/day secretory diarrhoea and confirmed with serum VIP greater than 75 pg/mL.

Cross-sectional imaging may reveal the primary tumour but an octreotide scan or endoscopic ultrasound may be needed. Management involves fluid rehydration with potassium and the use of a somatostatin analogue (e.g. octreotide) to decrease secretion of VIP. Surgical resection may be needed but over 50% may be metastatic at the point of diagnosis. Median survival is 96 months from diagnosis.

Flushing and diarrhoea can be associated with carcinoid syndrome but it is unusual to develop profound hypokalaemia. The history is too long for *Vibrio cholera* infection. Bile acid diarrhoea and coeliac disease are unlikely in this case.

Farina DA, Krogh KM, Boike JR. Chronic diarrhoea secondary to newly diagnosed VIPoma. *Case Rep Gastroenterol.* 2019;13:225–229. Doi:10.1159/000494554.

### 3. D. Glucagon-like peptide 2 (GLP-2) inhibits gastric emptying and gastric acid production, induces small bowel mucosal growth, and stimulates mesenteric blood flow

- GLP-2 is intestinotrophic and released in response to luminal nutrients
- GLP-2 analogues (e.g. teduglutide) are used for the management of short bowel syndrome. See Table 6.1 for details on gastrointestinal hormones

**Table 6.1** Gastrointestinal hormones

| Hormone | Site of production | Release pattern | Action |
|---|---|---|---|
| Cholecystokinin | I cells, small intestine | Stimulated by ingested fat and protein | Delays gastric emptying, stimulates gallbladder contraction |
| Gastrin | G cells, stomach | Stimulated by high pH, high-grade gastric distension, amino acids, histamine, acetylcholine; inhibited by somatostatin, carbohydrate and fat | Stimulates gastric acid production, gastric hypertrophy |
| Glucagon-like peptide 1 | L cells, small intestine | Stimulated by carbohydrate ingestion | Inhibits gastric emptying, glucagon release, and appetite; stimulates glucose-dependent insulin release |
| Glucagon-like peptide 2 | L cells, small intestine | Stimulated by carbohydrate ingestion | Inhibits gastric emptying and gastric acid production; stimulates small bowel mucosal growth, increases mesenteric blood flow |
| Somatostatin | D cells, stomach, small intestine, pancreas | Stimulated by gastrin, gastric acid, vasoactive intestinal polypeptide, low-grade gastric distension, acetylcholine; inhibited by catecholamines | Inhibits production of most gut hormones including gastrin production, reduces pancreatico-biliary secretions, reduces gastrointestinal motility and gallbladder contraction |

Ahmed M, Ahmed S. Functional, diagnostic and therapeutic aspects of gastrointestinal hormones. *Gastroenterology Res.* 2019;12(5):233–244. Doi: 10.14740/gr1219.

## 4. E. Supraphysiological doses of leptin may reduce food intake in patients of normal weight

- Leptin is the 'satiety' hormone and levels increase in response to eating
- Levels reflect overall fat mass and obese patients have high levels
- Obese patients are poorly responsive to supraphysiological doses

Leptin is a product of the *ob* gene and acts on leptin receptors to reduce food intake. It is predominantly produced in fat cells but is also found in the placenta and breast milk. Leptin acts to signal to the brain the quantity of stored fat. Most patients with obesity therefore have high serum levels reflecting their increased fat mass. Abnormalities in the leptin gene resulting in complete leptin deficiency are rare but are associated with obesity and hyperphagia. Unlike their normal or lean counterparts, obese patients are resistant or tolerant to supraphysiological doses of leptin. Overeating increases serum leptin concentrations before any changes are seen in fat mass.

The mode of action of leptin to reduce food intake is through decreased expression of neuropeptide Y in the hypothalamus, increased transcription of pro-opiomelanocortin and alpha-melanocyte-stimulating hormone. Leptin also has direct effects on bone health and immune function.

Serum leptin is higher in women than men, and in pregnancy. Ethnicity has no effect on leptin concentrations.

Farr OM, Gavrieli L, Mantzoros CS. Leptin applications in 2015: what have we learned about leptin and obesity? *Curr Opin Endocrinol Diabetes Obes*. 2015;22(5):353–359. Doi:10.1097/MED.0000000000000184.

## 5. C. Levels rise sharply before and fall shortly after meal ingestion

- Ghrelin levels increase during fasting and fall in response to ingested nutrients
- Bariatric surgery alters the pattern of ghrelin secretion, reducing the pre-meal surge

Ghrelin is predominantly produced from oxyntic glands in the stomach (predominantly fundus) with lower amounts found in the duodenum, pancreas, pituitary gland, and kidney. Levels increase during fasting with a surge shortly before meals, driven by a cephalic response to meals. Ghrelin levels then fall after eating, largely driven by carbohydrate ingestion and less so by protein and fat. The fall is not dependent upon gastric distension. Ghrelin further acts to increase gastric emptying and secretion of growth hormone, and so may affect bone metabolism.

Basal levels of ghrelin are inversely related to BMI. Furthermore, in obesity, the normal postprandial suppression of ghrelin is impaired. Following bypass surgery and sleeve gastrectomy, ghrelin levels are lower and the pre-meal surge is lacking, which may be one reason why energy balance is improved following this surgery. Ghrelin levels are increased in the Prader-Willi syndrome and may contribute to hyperphagia.

Makris MC, Alexandrou A, Papatsoutsos EG et al. Ghrelin and obesity: identifying gaps and dispelling myths. A reappraisal. *In Vivo*. 2017;31(6):1047–1050.

## 6. C. Serotonin

- The enteric nervous system (ENS) controls intestinal motility through a network of neurons and neurotransmitters
- Serotonin is released in response to intestinal stretch

ENS is one division of the autonomic nervous system in addition to the sympathetic and parasympathetic divisions. It comprises the myenteric plexus (located between longitudinal and circular smooth muscle layers) and the submucosal plexus (located in the submucosa) of neurons. The ENS can operate independently of the brain and spinal cord through a network of interneurons, intrinsic primary afferent neurons (IPANs), motor neurons, and mechano/chemoreceptors. However, mostly there is communication between the ENS and the central nervous system through parasympathetic (cholinergic: increases intestinal smooth muscle activity) and sympathetic (noradrenergic: decreases intestinal smooth muscle activity) connections.

Luminal distension activates IPANs either directly (through mechanoreceptors) or indirectly (through release of serotonin from enterochromaffin cells in the epithelium). IPANs then activate interneurons that, in turn, activate either proximal excitatory or distal inhibitory motor neurons. Excitatory motor neurons release acetylcholine and substance P, while inhibitory motor neurons release nitric oxide, vasoactive intestinal polypeptide, and β-nicotinamide adenine dinucleotide. This results in luminal propulsion of contents from the mouth to the anus.

The basic electrical rhythm (BER) is a pacemaker-like activity triggered by the interstitial cells of Cajal that coordinates peristaltic activity: it cannot cause a contraction but it can increase muscle tension. Contractions only occur as the BER wave is depolarizing. Diabetic autonomic enteropathy may result from a combination of damage to neurons, impaired pacemaker function, or altered neurotransmitter release.

Rao M, Gershon MD. The bowel and beyond: the enteric nervous system in neurological disorders. *Nat Rev Gastroenterol I Iepatol.* 2016;13(9):517–528. Doi:10.1038/nrgastro.2016.107.

## 7. B. Catheter-based manometry

- Small bowel physiology testing is rarely available outside specialist centres and can usually only be recommended if the results would alter clinical management
- Catheter-based manometry is preferred over wireless motility capsules for measuring contractile patterns
- Transit tests are limited by significant variability

Catheter-based manometry using multiple pressure sensors is the most accurate means of measuring small bowel contractility patterns both for amplitude and propagation. Sensors are usually placed in the duodenum and proximal jejunum for practical reasons, and physiology of the remaining small bowel is inferred. The pattern of motility can provide information on neuropathic versus myopathic conditions. Wireless motility capsules can provide information on amplitude of contractions at given points through the small bowel but not on propagation of contractions.

Small bowel scintigraphy may be used to accurately measure transit time although the technique lacks standardization and is not widely available. An alternative modality is the wireless motility capsule that uses pH monitoring to determine passage through the pylorus and the ileocaecal valve from which small bowel transit time can be calculated. However, passage through the ileocaecal valve using pH alone is only accurate in about 90% of patients and the technique has yet to be fully validated. Lactulose hydrogen breath tests can infer small bowel transit from the hydrogen surge resulting from lactulose arriving in the caecum, but the tests are troubled by false negative/positive results. Barium follow-through studies can give anatomical information but are not useful for measuring transit time or contractility patterns.

Keller J, Bassotti G, Clarke J et al. Expert consensus document: advances in the diagnosis and classification of gastric and intestinal motility disorders. *Nat Rev Gastroenterol Hepatol.* 2018;15(5):291–308. Doi:10.1038/nrgastro.2018.7.

## 8. E. Worsening pain with defecation

- IBS can be suspected in patients with abdominal pain associated with defecation or change in stool frequency or form
- The Rome IV are the current diagnostic criteria
- Exclusion of other conditions is essential in patients with alarm symptoms such as weight loss or rectal bleeding

The Rome IV criteria for the diagnosis of IBS were released in 2016. Notable changes from the previous criteria include the removal of the word 'discomfort' and the recognition that pain may either be relieved or worsened by defecation. Symptoms such as nausea, rectal mucus, early satiety, and bloating may be present in patients with IBS but do not form part of the diagnostic criteria. Exclusion of other pathologies should be considered in, for example, patients over 50 years of age, persistent weight loss, rectal bleeding, predominant diarrhoea, abdominal masses, or raised inflammatory markers.

### Diagnostic criteria (Rome IV) for irritable bowel syndrome

Recurrent abdominal pain at least one day per week in the past three months on average, associated with at least two of the following criteria, and with symptom onset at least six months previously:

1. Related to defecation (either increasing or improving pain)
2. Associated with change in stool frequency
3. Associated with change in stool form (appearance)

Four subtypes of IBS are recognized based on the predominant stool consistency: constipation, diarrhoea, mixed, or unclassified.

Lacy BE, Mearin F, Chang L et al. Bowel disorders. *Gastroenterology.* 2016;150:1393–1407. Doi:10.1053/j.gastro.2016.02.031.

## 9. B. Gabapentin

- Initial pharmacological management includes tricyclic antidepressants and serotonin noradrenergic reuptake inhibitors
- Step-up therapy should include gabapentin or pregabalin
- Opiates should not be used in this condition

General measures for managing functional abdominal pain include validation of symptoms, education about the underlying condition, and setting of achievable goals. Drugs may be used to modulate pain pathways. Dysfunction of the brain-gut pain axis may arise at a number of levels including peripheral sensitization (such as that seen in post-infectious IBS), central sensitization at the spinal dorsal horn, and descending modulation from the brain of pain pathways.

Low-dose amitriptyline at night can be considered first line although somnolence and cholinergic side effects can limit use. Serotonin-noradrenergic reuptake inhibitors (e.g. duloxetine or venlafaxine) are promising agents for managing chronic pain conditions and can be used second line. Psychological therapies such as cognitive behavioural therapy, relaxation therapy, hypnotherapy, and stress management can be considered particularly for patients with clear symptom association to psychological triggers. Gabapentin and pregabalin act on the pain-signalling areas. Of the central nervous system and are used in a number of chronic pain syndromes. These should be considered in refractory cases.

Opiates should be avoided because of the risk of hyperalgesia, narcotic bowel syndrome, and psychological dependence. There is no role for sacral nerve stimulation in the management of functional abdominal pain.

Farmer AD, Aziz Q. Mechanisms and management of functional abdominal pain. *J R Soc Med.* 2014;107(9):347–354. Doi:10.1177/0141076814540880.

## 10. B. Champagne

Any foods made of barley, wheat, or rye are not gluten free. Most porridge oats are not strictly gluten free due to contamination, but patients with coeliac disease can eat oats if specifically labelled as gluten-free. Barley waters/squash, malted milk drinks, ales, beers, lagers, and stouts are not gluten free. However, wine, spirits, sherry, port, cider, and other soft drinks are. Breaded and battered foods are not gluten free unless specified as such on the packaging. Many grains have to be avoided including couscous, bulgar wheat, semolina, and spelt. However, buckwheat, polenta, quinoa, and rice can be eaten.

Levels of susceptibility to gluten vary between patients with coeliac disease. Foods labelled as gluten-free have 20 parts per million, or fewer, of gluten, and this is the case both in Europe and the United States. Given the complexities of a gluten-free diet, all patients should be referred to a specialist dietitian at diagnosis. This will also ensure that patients do not become deplete in micronutrients. Adherence to a gluten-free diet is improved when the patient is well educated.

Ludvigsson JF et al. Diagnosis and management of adult coeliac disease: guidelines from the British Society of Gastroenterology. *Gut.* 2014;63:1210–1228. Doi:10.1136/gutjnl-2013-306578.

## 11. E. Serum IgG TTG antibody

- Seronegative villous atrophy, where coeliac serology is negative in the presence of duodenal villous atrophy, has a wide differential, with coeliac disease and *Helicobacter pylori* infection the most common causes
- Selective IgA deficiency is a common primary immunodeficiency that confers an increased risk of coeliac disease
- In selective IgA deficiency, IgG coeliac antibodies should be performed to confirm the diagnosis

Seronegative villous atrophy (SNVA) has a wide differential, with coeliac disease and chronic infections the most common causes. Crohn's disease, drugs (non-steroidal anti-inflammatory agents, angiotensin 2 receptor blockers, mycophenolate mofetil, among others), autoimmune enteropathy, and common variable immunodeficiency (CVID) are rarer causes. Seronegative coeliac disease is more common in individuals of European descent, and those with a family history of autoimmunity. Iron and folate deficiency are common, B12 deficiency less so. HLA haplotype status can be useful for its negative predictive value.

Selective IgA deficiency (prevalence 1/400), as in this case, is associated with an increased risk of coeliac disease. IgA coeliac serology is frequently negative. An IgG coeliac antibody can be performed that would confirm the diagnosis. The other options are less likely in this case.

Aziz I, Peerally MF, Barnes JH et al. The clinical and phenotypical assessment of seronegative villous atrophy; a prospective UK centre experience evaluating 200 adult cases over a 15-year period (2000–2015). *Gut.* 2017;66(9):1563–1572. Doi:10.1136/gutjnl-2016-312271.

## 12. B. Marsh I

- The Marsh-Oberhuber classification is the most common system for assessing the severity of histological changes in coeliac disease (Table 6.2)
- Duodenal histology will improve in most patients after 6–12 months on a gluten-free diet, although mild changes, such as intraepithelial lymphocytosis, commonly persist
- Patients with coeliac disease are more likely to have IBS, which can lead to persistent abdominal symptoms despite resolution of villous atrophy

**Table 6.2** Modified Marsh-Oberhuber classification of coeliac disease duodenal histology

| Classification | Description | Intraepithelial lymphocytosis | Crypt hyperplasia | Villous atrophy |
| --- | --- | --- | --- | --- |
| Marsh 0 | Normal | No | No | No |
| Marsh I | Intraepithelial lymphocytosis | Yes | No | No |
| Marsh 2 | Intraepithelial lymphocytosis and crypt hyperplasia | Yes | Yes | No |
| Marsh 3A | Partial villous atrophy | Yes | Yes | Yes (partial) |
| Marsh 3B | Subtotal villous atrophy | Yes | Yes | Yes (subtotal) |
| Marsh 3C | Total villous atrophy | Yes | Yes | Yes (total) |

Fig. 6.2 shows Marsh I changes, with preserved villous height. While many patients with coeliac disease will have an improvement in their degree of villous atrophy on a gluten-free diet, it is common for intraepithelial lymphocytosis to persist, even with good dietary adherence. Some villous atrophy may persist, most commonly in older patients, but it raises the possibility of ongoing

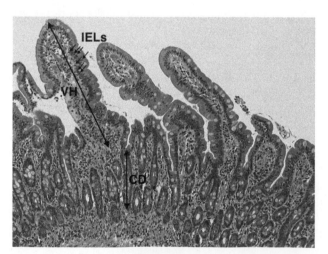

**Fig. 6.2** (VH—large double-headed arrow) and crypt depth (CD—small double-headed arrow), but an increased number of intraepithelial lymphocytes (IELs—small arrows).

Image courtesy of Dept of Histopathology, Oxford University Hospitals NHS Foundation Trust

gluten exposure, particularly if serum tissue transglutaminase IgA antibody levels are persistently raised and symptoms continue.

Persistent symptoms of bloating and alternating bowel habit in the context of a resolution of villous atrophy and nutritional deficiency may indicate coexisting IBS. IBS is more common in patients with coeliac disease and should be treated with similar strategies to IBS seen in isolation.

Ludvigsson JF, Bai JC, Biagi F et al. Diagnosis and management of adult coeliac disease: guidelines from the British Society of Gastroenterology. *Gut.* 2014;63:1210–1228. Doi:10.1136/gutjnl-2013-306578.

## 13. C. Calcium intake should be at least 1,000 mg per day

- Management of bone health is a critical component of long-term care of patients with coeliac disease
- Bone density scans should be considered for all patients at baseline but particularly those at higher risk of osteoporosis
- Bone density has been shown to increase within the first year of a gluten-free diet

Both osteoporosis and bone fracture rates are increased with coeliac disease but this risk is reduced by good adherence to a gluten-free diet and improvement in villous atrophy. After one year of a gluten-free diet, bone density can be expected to improve.

Calcium, alkaline phosphatase, and vitamin D should be measured at baseline and supplemented as needed. Daily calcium intake should be at least 1,000 mg. Baseline dual energy X-ray absorptiometry (DEXA) scanning should be considered for all patients but particularly those with other risk factors for poor bone health. Those with osteopenia and osteoporosis require repeat DEXA every two to three years. Loss of bone density at a faster rate than expected should prompt a review of diet, measurement of Vitamin D levels, and consideration of alternative causes (e.g. hypogonadism). Those with normal bone density should be reassessed every five years.

For those with osteoporosis, if there are concerns about absorption of oral bisphosphonates, intravenous preparations can be considered. Involvement of metabolic bone specialists may be needed for complex cases.

Al-Toma A, Volta U, Auricchio R et al. European Society for the Study of Coeliac Disease (EssCD) guideline for coeliac disease and other gluten-related disorders. *United European Gastroenterol J.* 2019;7(5):583–613. Doi:10.1177/2050640619844125.

## 14. C. EATL

- Coeliac disease is associated with EATL; B symptoms are uncommon
- EATL often presents with subacute obstructive symptoms, weight loss, gastrointestinal bleeding, or perforation

It is likely that this patient has been non-compliant with a gluten-free diet, despite his insistence to the contrary, or has refractory coeliac disease. The constellation of symptoms is concerning for small bowel obstruction and the iron deficiency anaemia with positive coeliac serology suggests poorly managed disease. The lymphadenopathy is concerning. Coeliac disease is associated with the T cell lymphoma, EATL. Typical symptoms of lymphomas (e.g. fevers and night sweats) are usually absent. EATL often presents with subacute obstructive symptoms, weight loss, gastrointestinal bleeding, or perforation.

While it was previously suggested that other forms of cancer (e.g. colorectal) might be associated with coeliac disease, the evidence now suggests that this is not the case. Colorectal cancer in this age group is extremely rare. There is a higher incidence of lactose intolerance in people with coeliac disease compared with the general population. However, this would not cause intermittent constipation. Similarly, Graves' disease is more common in people with coeliac disease compared with the general population. However, this would cause diarrhoea, not constipation.

Al-Toma A, Volta U, Auricchio R et al. European Society for the Study of Coeliac Disease (EssCD) guideline for coeliac disease and other gluten-related disorders. *United European Gastroenterol J.* 2019;7(5):583–613. Doi:10.1177/2050640619844125.

### 15. A. Multiple endocrine neoplasia (MEN) 1

- Symptoms of carcinoid syndrome (diarrhoea, flushing, wheezing) result from the secretion of serotonin into the systemic circulation
- Elevated 24 h urinary 5-HIAA can suggest the diagnosis
- Carcinoid tumours can be seen in MEN1

MEN1 is an autosomal dominant condition and typically comprises tumours of the parathyroid, anterior pituitary, and pancreas (the 3 'P's) but some patients will develop carcinoid tumours. The symptoms of carcinoid tumours are usually only apparent after the disease has metastasized and the tumour products are no longer inactivated by the liver. Typical symptoms include diarrhoea, wheezing, and flushing. However, cardiac fibrosis can also occur. Flushing episodes may be provoked by eating, drinking alcohol, and heightened emotions. Carcinoid crisis with severe hypotension may result in the context of anaesthesia. Patients may develop symptoms of intermittent small bowel obstruction, as in this case, depending on the size of the primary tumour.

Measurement of 24-hour urinary excretion of 5-HIAA is a useful diagnostic test and measures the end product of serotonin metabolism. Importantly, patients should avoid serotonin/tryptophan rich foods for 72 hours prior to the collection to reduce the risk of a false positive. These include pineapple, kiwi fruit, aubergine, and walnuts. Chromogranin A, B, and C are non-specific markers of neuroendocrine tumours.

Niederle B, Pape UF, Costa F et al. ENETS consensus guidelines update for neuroendocrine neoplasms of the jejunum and ileum. *Neuroendocrinology.* 2016;103(2):125–138. Doi:10.1159/000443170.

### 16. C. Niacin (B3)

- Niacin deficiency can lead to pellagra, characterized by photosensitive dermatitis, neuropsychiatric complications including delirium and dementia, and diarrhoea
- Poor nutrition and alcohol abuse are risk factors, and other water-soluble vitamin deficiencies may coexist
- A high index of suspicion of vitamin deficiency is appropriate in patients with malnutrition, homelessness, or alcoholism, because such deficiencies can mimic alcohol intoxication, withdrawal, or mental illness

Pellagra is caused by severe niacin deficiency, and is characterized by the '4 Ds' of dermatitis, delirium/dementia, and diarrhoea, with the fourth D, death, if treatment is not instigated. The skin manifestation of pellagra is a photosensitive erythematous rash, sometimes with blistering, affecting sun-exposed areas such as the hands, forearms, face, and neck. Diarrhoea can be severe. The confusion of pellagra is described as a delirium (with disorientation) in the early stages.

Endemic niacin deficiency is rare in developed countries, with meat, fish, mushrooms, peanuts, yeast products, and fortified cereals all good dietary sources. It may be under-recognized in those with significant malnutrition and/or alcohol abuse. Deficiencies in other water-soluble vitamins, such as thiamine, may coexist with niacin deficiency. Therefore, intravenous B vitamin supplementation, such as Pabrinex®, is indicated because it contains thiamine, riboflavin, pyridoxine, and ascorbic acid in addition to nicotinamide (niacin).

Powell-Tuck J et al. Vitamins and trace elements. In: Warrell DA, Cox TM, Firth JD, editors. *The Oxford Textbook of Medicine* (5th ed.). Oxford: Oxford University Press; 2011.

## 17. E. Trimethoprim

- Folate is required for DNA synthesis and haematopoeisis
- Green leafy vegetables and liver are good sources of folate
- Dihydrofolate reductase is required for a key step of folate metabolism and may be inhibited by certain medications

Folate (or vitamin B9) is a water-soluble member of the vitamin B family that is not biologically active (folic acid is the chemically synthesized version of the vitamin). It is found in animal products and leafy green vegetables in the polyglutamate form, and is cleaved to the monoglutamate form in the jejunum, where it is absorbed. Uptake occurs via passive and carrier-mediated routes. It is reduced to dihydrofolate, then tetrohydrofolate, through the actions of dihydrofolate reductase. Folate is required for DNA and RNA synthesis and haematopoesis, but not neuronal function (unlike vitamin B12). Excess folate is excreted in the urine because it is water-soluble. Body stores are 0.5–20 mg and last weeks to months.

Causes of folate deficiency include dietary deficiency (e.g. in the context of alcohol excess), increased utilization of folate (pregnancy, lactation, chronic haemolytic anaemia), intestinal malabsorption (coeliac disease, small bowel Crohn's disease), or medications that inhibit dihydrofolate reductase (methotrexate, trimethoprim).

Small bowel bacterial overgrowth usually results in elevated folate due to production by bacteria. Isolated folate deficiency in the presence of normal ferritin and B12 makes coeliac disease or a dietary deficiency unlikely. The presence of a normal CRP and ferritin makes Crohn's disease less likely.

Zheng Y, Cantley LC. Toward a better understanding of folate metabolism in health and disease. *J Exp Med.* 2019;216(2):253–266. Doi:10.1084/jem.20181965.

## 18. B. Metformin

- B12 metabolism is complex and deficiency can occur due to problems at any step
- Metformin and proton pump inhibitors can result in deficiency
- Dietary sources of B12 include liver, dairy products, and eggs

Cobalamin (vitamin B12) is a water-soluble vitamin that is not synthesized by humans but is found in high levels in meat, dairy products, eggs, and liver. Total body stores are 2–5 mg, and 50% is stored in the liver. Deficiency can take up to three to five years to become apparent but may manifest with megaloblastic anaemia, peripheral neuropathy, or subacute combined degeneration of the spinal cord. Hypersegmented neutrophils and cytopenias may be seen on blood film as a result of DNA synthesis inhibition.

B12 metabolism is complex. Ingested B12 is bound to proteins that are dissociated by gastric acid. Free B12 then binds to R-proteins in the stomach and travels with intrinsic factor, produced by gastric parietal cells, to the duodenum. Here, pancreatic proteases cleave the R-protein, allowing B12 to bind to intrinsic factor. This complex then travels to the terminal ileum where it is absorbed—this final process requires calcium.

Deficiency may be caused through dietary insufficiency, gastric acid hyposecretion (autoimmune atrophic gastritis, chronic *Helicobacter pylori* infection, proton pump inhibitor use (rarely with H2 receptor antagonist use), surgical gastrectomy), pernicious anaemia, pancreatic exocrine insufficiency, terminal ileal disease/resection, metformin (secondary to altered calcium homeostasis), and nitrous oxide (inhibits B12 function).

Gastric cancer is unlikely in the absence of iron deficiency or weight loss. Pancreatic insufficiency is not suggested in the absence of loose stool or weight loss. Pernicious anaemia is less likely given the negative intrinsic factor antibodies.

Hunt A, Harrington D, Robinson D. Vitamin B12 deficiency. *BMJ.* 2014;349:g5226. Doi:10.1136/bmj.g5226.

### 19. C. Vitamin C

- Vitamin C (ascorbic acid) deficiency presents with the clinical syndrome scurvy, which results in defective collagen synthesis
- The typical presenting signs are follicular hyperkeratosis and perifollicular haemorrhage
- Scurvy is treated with ascorbic acid replacement at 250 mg daily in divided doses

Vitamin C has a number of important actions including promotion of iron absorption and formation of cross-linking in connective tissues. It is mainly absorbed in the jejunum and terminal ileum. Almost complete absorption occurs if <100 mg per dose is administered orally but absorption reduces at doses higher than this with the excess unmetabolized ascorbic acid excreted in urine. Good dietary sources of vitamin C are citrus fruits, green vegetables, tomatoes, and potatoes.

The clinical syndrome associated with vitamin C deficiency is scurvy. Although now rare, scurvy may be seen among the poor, elderly, or in those consuming excess alcohol. Symptoms of scurvy reflect impaired connective tissue formation, resulting in haemorrhagic manifestations such as petechiae, ecchymoses, perifollicular haemorrhage, and haemorrhagic gums and joints. Plasma and leucocyte vitamin C levels are the mainstay of laboratory-based diagnosis. The condition is treated by administration of ascorbic acid supplements at 250 mg daily in divided doses. Symptoms can improve in a matter of days with supplementation.

Granger M, Eck P. Dietary vitamin C in human health. *Adv Food Nutr Res.* 2018;83:281–310. Doi:10.1016/bs.afnr.2017.11.006.

### 20. C. Selenium

- Keshan disease is a cardiomyopathy secondary to dietary selenium deficiency affecting women of childbearing age in areas of China
- Selenium deficiency can affect the production of thyroid hormones, and cause skeletal muscle weakness and mood changes

Selenium is found in seafood, kidney, liver, and some grains/seeds, and it has high bioavailability. It is absorbed in the small intestine and patients with extensive small bowel resections may be at risk of selenium deficiency. However, selenium supplementation is now a core component of parenteral nutrition so deficiency is now rare in this cohort.

Within the body, it is a component of selenoproteins including glutathione peroxidase and iodo-thyronine deiodinase 2. Cytosolic glutathione peroxidase-1 protects cardiomyocytes against oxidative damage but requires selenoproteins to maximize antioxidant capacity and reduce production of pro-inflammatory cytokines. Selenium deficiency may result in dilated cardiomyopathy, which may be reversible with supplementation. Iodo-thyronine deiodinases convert thyroxine (T4) to its more active form triiodothyronine (T3). Therefore, a deficiency in selenium may result in reduced production of thyroid hormones. Selenium also has roles in immune cell function including natural killer cells and cell-mediated immunity. Severe deficiency may result in skeletal muscle dysfunction and mood changes.

A differential diagnosis for this presentation would include wet beri-beri although this would not be expected to cause the abnormal thyroid parameters seen here.

Avery JC, Hoffman PR. Selenium, selenoproteins, and immunity. *Nutrients*. 2018;10(9):E1203. Doi:10.3390/nu10091203.

## 21. B. Lactose malabsorption in adults is most commonly caused by lactase non-persistence

- Lactose intolerance defines the occurrence of typical intestinal symptoms of abdominal pain, bloating, and diarrhoea in patients with lactose malabsorption
- Lactase persistence is due to a dominant gain-of-function mutation in the lactase gene
- The lactose-hydrogen (not lactulose-hydrogen) breath test may suggest the diagnosis although there is a risk of false negative or false positive results

Lactose malabsorption is common worldwide with lowest rates in Scandinavian countries and higher rates in areas of the Far East. Lactase activity is highest at the time of birth and decreases in most populations through childhood. Most cases of lactose malabsorption in adults are due to lactase non-persistence (i.e. primary, genetic disease). In Caucasians, persistence of lactase activity is due to a dominant, gain-of-function mutation within the lactase gene on chromosome 2 and only patients with two wild type genes should be considered to have lactase non-persistence.

Lactase breaks down the disaccharide lactose into glucose and galactose monosaccharides, which are then readily absorbed by active transport (SGLT1 and GLUT2) into the enterocyte. Symptoms result from the action of intestinal microbes on undigested lactose, which results in the production of short chain fatty acids, methane, hydrogen, and carbon dioxide.

The lactose-hydrogen breath test measures expired breath hydrogen in response to an oral lactose load. However, some patients are hydrogen non-producers (resulting in false negatives) or have altered bowel anatomy, small intestinal bacterial overgrowth, or rapid GI transit (resulting in false positives). Alternative diagnostic modalities include measuring duodenal lactase activity, genetic testing in Caucasians, and the serum gaxilose test.

Misselwitz B, Butter M, Verbeke K et al. Update on lactose malabsorption and intolerance: pathogenesis, diagnosis and clinical management. *Gut*. 2019;68(11):2080–2091. Doi: 10.1136/gutjnl-2019-318404.

## 22. B. Co-amoxiclav

- Treatment for small intestinal bacterial overgrowth (SIBO) should comprise management of reversible causes and antibiotic therapy, which may be empirical, long-term, or cyclical
- Low B12 and elevated folate are characteristic of SIBO but are not always seen
- Hydrogen breath testing with glucose or lactulose is the most accessible method of diagnosing SIBO because small intestinal aspiration and culture is invasive and cumbersome

The most likely diagnosis is SIBO in the context of impaired gut motility secondary to systemic sclerosis. The formal definition of SIBO is an increase in the number of bacteria to more than

$10^5$ CFU/ml or the presence of atypical flora on small intestinal aspirates. Treatment includes addressing any primary cause and using antibiotics such as metronidazole, co-amoxiclav, co-trimoxazole, ciprofloxacin, norfloxacin, and rifaximin. Some patients may require cyclical antibiotics on rotation. Drugs such as anticholinergics and opioids should be avoided because they slow gut transit and may exacerbate symptoms.

Intraepithelial lymphocytosis alone on duodenal biopsies is not sufficient to diagnose coeliac disease in the absence of villous atrophy and an inflammatory infiltrate in the lamina propria. Inflammatory bowel disease and pancreatic exocrine insufficiency are unlikely here.

Shah SC, Day LW, Somsouk M et al. Meta-analysis: antibiotic therapy for small intestinal bacterial overgrowth. *Aliment Pharmacol Ther.* 2013;38(8):925–934. Doi:10.1111/apt.12479.

## 23. C. Colestyramine

- Bile acid malabsorption (BAM) is common in patients with Crohn's disease especially in the context of distal ileal resection
- BAM usually responds to bile acid sequestrants such as colestyramine
- There is a dose–response relationship between the severity of BAM and the effect of bile acid sequestrants

The most likely diagnosis here is BAM. Resection of the distal ileum (usually >100 cm) prevents reabsorption of bile salts that subsequently enter the colon causing diarrhoea. BAM may also be caused by primary diseases of the terminal ileum, HIV infection, or defects in bile acid synthesis or transport mechanisms. Previous cholecystectomy and post-infectious diarrhoea may predict BAM.

The severity of BAM can be assessed by measuring seven-day retention of an orally administered, selenium-labelled bile acid (SeHCAT scan): 10%–15% retention = mild; 5%–10% = moderate; <5% = severe. The lower the retention, the more likely the patient is to respond to bile acid sequestrants (colestyramine, colesevelam, colestipol).

Recurrence of Crohn's disease or bacterial overgrowth is less likely. There is no consistent evidence for the use of mesalazine in the management of Crohn's disease.

Wilcox C, Turner J, Green J. Systematic review: the management of chronic diarrhoea due to bile acid malabsorption. *Aliment Pharmacol Ther.* 2014;39(9):923–939. Doi:10.1111/apt.12684.

## 24. C. NSAID metabolites

- Non-steroidal anti-inflammatory drug (NSAID) enteropathy classically presents with small bowel ulceration, abdominal pain, iron-deficiency anaemia and hypoalbuminaemia
- Patients may often deny taking NSAIDs
- Diaphragm-like structures in the small bowel are pathognomonic

The association between gastro-duodenal ulceration and NSAID use is well recognized but jejunum, ileum, and colon can also be affected. Aspirin appears to be less harmful than other NSAIDs at inducing small bowel damage. The signs and symptoms of NSAID enteropathy can be varied but typically include iron-deficiency anaemia, hypoalbuminaemia (from a protein-losing enteropathy), and small bowel ulceration. Abdominal pain may result from partial small bowel obstruction caused by diaphragm-like structures. These are rare, fibrotic structures causing luminal narrowing and are pathognomonic of the condition.

Establishing the diagnosis requires an index of suspicion based on clinical presentation. A careful history of NSAID ingestion has to be taken including prescribed and over-the-counter medications, combination medications (e.g. ibuprofen with caffeine and paracetamol). Patients may deny using

NSAIDs, and serum or urinary NSAID measurements may need to be considered to confirm the diagnosis. Acid-suppressants such as omeprazole and ranitidine do not protect against small bowel ulceration secondary to NSAIDs. Management of the condition involves cessation of NSAID intake and treatment of anaemia. Ulceration should resolve upon drug cessation. Obstructive symptoms secondary to diaphragm disease may require endoscopic dilatation or surgical resection of stricturoplasty.

Shin SJ, Noh CK, Lim SG et al. Non-steroidal anti-inflammatory drug-induced enteropathy. *Intest Res.* 2017;15(4):446–455. Doi:10.5217/ir.2017.15.4.446.

### 25. B. Bone marrow culture

- Enteric fever is characterized by fever and gastrointestinal involvement including abdominal pain, diarrhoea or constipation, and, rarely, intestinal perforation
- Blood, urine, and stool culture for microbiological diagnosis perform poorly compared with bone marrow culture

Typhoid and paratyphoid fever (collectively enteric fever) are caused by *Salmonella enterica* serovar typhi (formerly *Salmonella typhi*) and *Salmonella paratyphi* A, B, and C. Typical presentation includes fevers, rose spots and relative bradycardia or pulse–temperature dissociation. Later, gastrointestinal features predominate including abdominal pain (60%), diarrhoea or constipation (30%), and rectal bleeding (10%). Intestinal perforation from necrosis of ileocaecal Peyer's patches occurs in 10% of hospitalized patients. Laboratory investigations usually demonstrate leucopenia or leukocytosis, and mildly elevated LFTs. Transmission is faecal–oral and is endemic in South Asia, parts of South-East Asia, the Middle East, Central and South America, and Africa. Oral and parenteral vaccines are available for *Salmonella enterica* serovar typhi but are imperfect, with the oral vaccine offering a cumulative three-year efficacy of 50%. A microbiological diagnosis can be made by positive cultures of blood (40%), stool (37%), and urine (7%). Although invasive, bone marrow culture is positive in 90% of cases, making it the most sensitive diagnostic investigation, and it should be considered in complicated cases of suspected treatment failure due to antimicrobial resistance.

Parry CM, Wijedoru L, Arjyal A et al. The utility of diagnostic tests for enteric fever in endemic locations. *Expert Rev Anti Infect Ther.* 2011;9(6):711–725. Doi:10.1586/eri.11.47.

## QUESTIONS

1.  **A 40-year-old man with a 5-year history of Crohn's colitis was admitted to hospital with a severe flare necessitating intravenous hydrocortisone.**

    **Which pro-inflammatory cytokine is produced in higher amounts in Crohn's disease (CD) than ulcerative colitis (UC)?**

    A. IFN-γ

    B. IL-5

    C. IL-6

    D. IL-13

    E. TNF-α

2.  **A 33-year-old woman with a 15-year-history of ileocolonic CD attended for her follow-up appointment. She had no family history of inflammatory bowel disease (IBD) and nor did her husband. She was 33 weeks' pregnant and concerned about the risk of CD in her child.**

    **Which of the following percentages most accurately reflects the child's likelihood of developing CD?**

    A. 1%

    B. 10%

    C. 25%

    D. 30%

    E. 45%

*Best of Five MCQs for the European Specialty Examination in Gastroenterology and Hepatology.* Thomas Marjot, Colleen G C McGregor, Tim Ambrose, Aminda N De Silva, Jeremy Cobbold, and Simon Travis, Oxford University Press (2021). © Oxford University Press.
DOI: 10.1093/oso/9780198834373.003.0007

3. **A 29-year-old man was admitted with acute severe ulcerative colitis (ASUC) and required infliximab (IFX) after failing intravenous steroids. He was previously well and a non-smoker. During the ward round, he had several questions regarding his condition.**

   **Which of the following statements is most accurate?**

   A. Accelerated IFX dosing in hospitalized patients with UC reduces colectomy rate

   B. Approximately 30% of patients with ASUC will require a colectomy

   C. Approximately 40% of patients will require hospitalization because of ASUC

   D. Smoking increases the risk of recurrence of ASUC

   E. The presence of mucosal islands (areas of oedematous mucosa surrounded by deep ulceration) or colonic dilatation >5.5 cm on a plain abdominal radiograph is associated with colectomy in 50% of patients

4. **A 34-year-old man attended clinic with a new confirmed diagnosis of UC. He had several questions about UC.**

   **Regarding UC, which of the following statements is most accurate?**

   A. Around 25% of patients with pancolitis eventually have a colectomy

   B. At 10 years, disease extent progresses in less than 10% of patients with proctitis

   C. Maintenance 5-aminosalicylate (5-ASA) therapy reduces colorectal cancer (CRC) by 10%

   D. The incidence of CRC is 20% at 20 years and 40% at 30 years

   E. The relapse rate is 20% per year

5. **A 21-year-old woman presented to clinic with a one-week history of bloody diarrhoea eight times per day, with nocturnal motions and generalized abdominal pain. She had a long history of arthralgia in the hands and recurrent mouth ulcers. Her father had ankylosing spondylitis. Examination revealed aphthous mouth ulcers, a small ulcer in the right leg with a violaceous border, and mild right iliac fossa tenderness. Her temperature was 38°C, heart rate 110 beats per minute and blood pressure 100/60 mmHg.**

   **What is the most appropriate first investigation?**

   A. Colonoscopy

   B. Faecal culture

   C. Flexible sigmoidoscopy

   D. HLA-B27

   E. Magnetic resonance (MR) enterography

6. **A 52-year-old Afro-Caribbean man with a 13-year history of Crohn's colitis underwent a gastroscopy and colonoscopy. He was maintained on azathioprine.**

   Investigations:

   | | |
   |---|---|
   | Gastroscopy | Normal including biopsies |
   | Colonoscopy | Patchy inflammation in the left colon, normal terminal ileum. Biopsies consistent with Crohn's colitis in the descending and sigmoid colon. |

   **Which of the following most accurately represents this patient's Montreal classification?**

   A. AI LI BI

   B. A2 L2 BI

   C. A2 L4 B3

   D. A3 L2 B3

   E. A3 L3 B2

7. **A 22-year-old woman presents with a four-week history of abdominal pain, malaise, and bloody stools. She undergoes a flexible sigmoidoscopy with biopsies.**

   **Which histological feature has the highest predictive value for a diagnosis of UC over infective colitis?**

   A. Basal plasmacytosis

   B. Crypt abscess formation

   C. Granuloma formation

   D. Lamina propria hypercellularity

   E. Paneth cell metaplasia

8. **A 35-year-old woman with colonic CD presented complaining of perianal pain and rectal discharge.**

   Investigations:

   | | |
   |---|---|
   | Haemoglobin | 145 g/L |
   | White cell count (WCC) | $10.9 \times 10^9$/L |
   | Platelet count | $534 \times 10^9$/L |
   | Serum C-reactive protein (CRP) | 67 mg/L |

   **Which of the following statements is the most accurate?**

   A. Flexible sigmoidoscopy is useful in determining the management of perianal fistulae

   B. Ileocolonic CD has a higher rate of perianal disease

   C. Perianal disease presents late in the course of CD

   D. Perianal pain commonly occurs with isolated perianal fistulae

   E. Routine assessment of perianal fistulae includes pelvic magnetic resonance imaging (MRI), examination under anaesthesia (EUA), and anorectal ultrasound

9. **A 63-year-old lorry driver with a previous diagnosis of ileal CD and a perianal fistula attended the IBD specialist nurse clinic. On examination, his fistula was producing purulent fluid.**

   Investigations:

   | | |
   |---|---|
   | Haemoglobin | 178 g/L |
   | WCC | 8.9 × 10⁹/L |
   | Platelet count | 145 × 10⁹/L |
   | Serum C-reactive protein (CRP) | 35 mg/L |
   | Pelvic MRI | Inter-sphincteric perianal fistula; no abscess was demonstrated |
   | Flexible sigmoidoscopy | Quiescent disease |

   **Which of the following treatments is the most appropriate?**

   A. Defunctioning ileostomy

   B. IFX induction 5 mg/kg

   C. Intravenous ciclosporin 4–5 mg/kg/day

   D. Seton suture and antibiotics

   E. Total parenteral nutrition

10. **A 21-year-old student with a seven-month history of intermittent post-prandial abdominal pain and fatigue was referred with worsening of symptoms during her final exams. On further enquiry, she reported 3 kg of weight loss with no diarrhoea or anorexia. She had a previous history of irritable bowel syndrome (IBS). She was a non-smoker and had no family history of IBD.**

    Investigations:

    | | |
    |---|---|
    | Haemoglobin | 109 g/L |
    | Serum albumin | 33 g/L |
    | Serum C-reactive protein | 18 mg/L |

    **Which of the following would have the highest diagnostic yield for small bowel CD?**

    A. Capsule endoscopy (CE)

    B. CT enteroclysis

    C. Double-balloon enteroscopy

    D. Faecal calprotectin

    E. MR enterography

11. **A 26-year-old man with a five-month history of diarrhoea, abdominal pain, and fatigue was referred. On further enquiry, he reported 4 kg of weight loss. He had been a smoker, and had a family history of IBD.**

    Investigations:

    | | |
    |---|---|
    | Haemoglobin | 114 g/L |
    | Serum albumin | 35 g/L |
    | Serum C-reactive protein | 26 mg/L |

    **An abdominal ultrasound was performed in clinic.**

    **Which is considered the most consistent ultrasound finding in CD?**

    A. Altered echogenicity of the bowel wall

    B. Decreased peristalsis

    C. Enhanced mesenteric nodes

    D. Increased bowel wall thickness (BWT)

    E. Vascularity of the mesentery

12. **A 48-year-old man is diagnosed with UC and commenced on oral and rectal 5-ASA. After two weeks of treatment, he continues to experience loose stools three times per day with occasional blood. He is subsequently commenced on budesonide multimatrix (MMX).**

    **Which of the following statements is correct regarding budesonide MMX?**

    A. It is only recommended in those with extensive colitis

    B. It has high first-pass metabolism in the liver

    C. It is a topical rectal preparation

    D. It leads to double the rate of clinical improvement compared with mesalamine 2.4 g in mild–moderate UC

    E. The recommended dosing is 6 mg once daily for 16 weeks

13. **Following rescue therapy for ASUC, a 27-year-old man is subsequently maintained on 5 mg/kg IFX eight-weekly alongside 50 mg of azathioprine and 2.4 g mesalazine. He initially had complete resolution of symptoms but six months later he reported four times stools per day with occasional blood.**

    Investigations:

    | | |
    |---|---|
    | Serum C-reactive protein | 43 mg/l |
    | Faecal calprotectin | 800 µg/g |
    | IFX trough level | 2.6 µg/ml |
    | Antibodies to IFX | Undetectable |

    **What is the next most appropriate management step?**

    A. Change IFX to adalimumab

    B. Change IFX to vedolizumab

    C. Colectomy

    D. Continue IFX and restart oral corticosteroids

    E. Increase dose of IFX

14. **You review a 73-year-old man with steroid-dependent left-sided UC. You wish to counsel him regarding azathioprine.**

    **What would be this patient's approximate annual risk of incident lymphoma if commenced upon azathioprine?**

    A. 1 in 100

    B. 1 in 300

    C. 1 in 1,000

    D. 1 in 3,000

    E. 1 in 10,000

15. **A 78-year-old woman with pancolitis was admitted with bloody diarrhoea (11 times per day) with a pulse of 92 beats per minute and blood pressure 124/70 mmHg. On day three of intravenous corticosteroids, her stool chart reported four bloody stools in the past 24 hours. She denied abdominal pain. Her pulse was 72 beats per minute and temperature 37.4°C. Her background included heart failure (NYHA IV), morbid obesity, obstructive sleep apnoea (requiring nocturnal continuous positive airway pressure), and chronic obstructive pulmonary disease. She had investigations performed on day three of admission.**

    Investigations:

    | | |
    |---|---|
    | Haemoglobin | 90 g/L |
    | WCC | $10.4 \times 10^9$/L |
    | Platelet count | $550 \times 10^9$/L |
    | Serum C-reactive protein | 46 mg/L |
    | Cholesterol | 5.1 mmol/L |
    | Magnesium | 0.97 mmol/L |
    | Chest radiograph | Clear |
    | Abdominal radiograph | No evidence of toxic megacolon |

    **What is the most appropriate next step?**

    A. Continue intravenous corticosteroids and reassess in 48 hours

    B. IFX (5 mg/kg) induction regime

    C. Intravenous ciclosporin (2 mg/kg per day)

    D. Oral ciclosporin (5 mg/kg per day in divided doses)

    E. Subtotal colectomy

16. **A 35-year-old man was diagnosed with UC. His flexible sigmoidoscopy reported mild activity extending to 15 cm from the anus. His bowel frequency was two times per day with occasional rectal bleeding and mucus. His main concern was tenesmus and urgency. Examination was unremarkable.**

Investigations:

| | |
|---|---|
| Haemoglobin | 142 g/L |
| WCC | $6.1.0 \times 10^9$/L |
| Platelet count | $313 \times 10^9$/L |
| Serum C-reactive protein | 4 mg/L |
| Alanine transferase (ALT) | 17 U/L |
| Alkaline phosphatase (ALP) | 77 U/L |

**What treatment should be initiated?**

A. Mesalazine enema

B. Mesalazine suppository

C. Oral mesalazine

D. Oral prednisolone

E. Prednisolone enema

17. **A 34-year-old man underwent a proctocolectomy and ileal pouch-anal anastomosis for ulcerative pancolitis. There were no perioperative complications. Eight months later, he was reviewed in clinic and described a one-week history of increased frequency of non-bloody stools, abdominal cramping, tenesmus, and urgency.**

Investigations:

| | |
|---|---|
| Pouchoscopy | Mucosal oedema, friability, and loss of vascular pattern. Biopsy histology pending. |

**What is the most appropriate management?**

A. IFX

B. Mesalazine enema

C. Oral budesonide

D. Oral ciprofloxacin

E. VSL#3 probiotic

18. **A 43-year-old man with IBD attended the outpatient clinic asking if he could manage his disease with nutritional measures.**

    **Which of the following statements is most accurate?**

    A. Evidence supports dietary strategies in mild UC

    B. Good evidence supports a low-residue diet and avoiding insoluble fibre in stricturing CD

    C. Probiotics in the management of IBD have no evidence base

    D. The evidence base for elemental feed and polymeric diet is similar in CD

    E. Total parenteral nutrition and complete bowel rest are a useful adjunct to medical therapy in resistant CD

19. **A 35-year-old Caucasian woman with ileocolonic CD was admitted with worsening abdominal pain and diarrhoea. She was previously controlled on azathioprine. After a partial response to corticosteroids, she was commenced on adalimumab. She showed a good response after induction and was maintained on fortnightly doses. She was seen urgently in clinic with a five-month history of worsening symptoms, despite maintenance adalimumab.**

    Investigations:

    | | |
    |---|---|
    | Serum C-reactive protein (CRP) | 57 mg/L |
    | Faecal calprotectin | 256 µg/g |
    | Anti-drug antibodies | Positive |
    | Adalimumab level | Undetectable |

    **Which factor has been shown to predict low drug concentrations in adalimumab therapy?**

    A. Concomitant immunomodulator

    B. Disease duration

    C. Ex-smoker

    D. Male sex

    E. Obesity

20. **A 35-year-old man diagnosed with ileocaecal CD five years ago presented to the gastroenterology clinic with abdominal pain, nausea, and intermittent vomiting. His bowel frequency had reduced, going once every three days with loose stools. He took azathioprine 150 mg/day.**

Investigations:

| | |
|---|---|
| Haemoglobin | 135 g/L |
| Platelet count | $340 \times 10^9$/L |
| Serum C-reactive protein (CRP) | 10 mg/L |
| Albumin | 35 g/L |
| Colonoscopy | Partial loss of vascular pattern in the caecum and unpassable stricture at ileocaecal valve. Able to take terminal ileal biopsies. No ulcers or erosions. Colon biopsy series taken. |
| Histology | Normal terminal ileum. Ulceration at the ileocaecal valve with chronic inflammatory changes. Otherwise normal colon. |
| MR enterography | 6 cm stricture at the terminal ileum involving the ileocaecal valve with proximal dilatation of the small bowel. No evidence of fistula or abscess. Normal colon. |

## What is the most appropriate next step for this patient?

A. Addition of anti-tumour necrosis factor (anti-TNF) therapy

B. Endoscopic dilatation +/- stenting of ileocaecal valve

C. Prednisolone

D. Referral for ileocaecal resection

E. Referral for strictureplasty

21. **A 28-year-old man was admitted with ASUC. He was treated with intravenous hydrocortisone. On day three of admission, he complained of increasing abdominal pain. On examination, he had diffuse abdominal tenderness with rebound.**

Investigations and observations:

| | |
|---|---|
| Heart rate | 113 bpm |
| Temperature | 38.9 °C |
| Haemoglobin | 101 g/L |
| Serum sodium | 149 mmol/L |
| Serum potassium | 2.4 mmol/L |
| Serum phosphate | 0.56 mmol/L |
| Serum calcium | 1.59 mmol/L |
| Serum magnesium | 0.57 mmol/L |
| Serum albumin | 22 g/L |
| Abdominal radiograph | Loop of featureless transverse colon with a maximum diameter of 6.1 cm. |

**Which electrolyte abnormality should be corrected first to prevent further colonic dilatation?**

A. Hypernatraemia

B. Hypocalcaemia

C. Hypokalaemia

D. Hypomagnesaemia

E. Hypophosphataemia

22. **A 35-year-old man with CD presented to clinic with lower back pain.**

**What is the next most appropriate investigation to make a diagnosis?**

A. CRP

B. CT spine

C. HLA-B27 antigen

D. MRI pelvis

E. X-ray pelvis

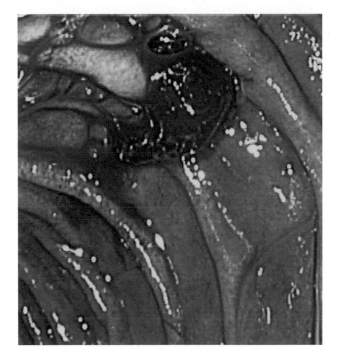

**Plate 1** Endoscopic image of the second part of the duodenum.

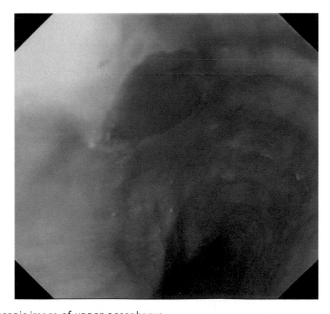

**Plate 2** Endoscopic image of upper oesophagus

Image courtesy of Prof Barbara Braden, Consultant Gastroenterologist, Oxford University Hospitals NHS Foundation Trust

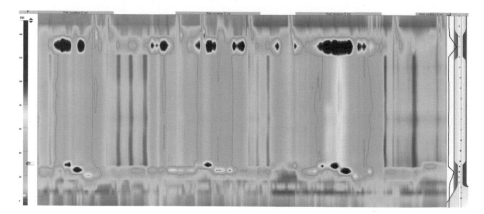

**Plate 3** Pressure topography plot obtained during high resolution oesophageal manometry

Image courtesy of Dr Tanya Miller, Principal Clinical Scientist in GI Physiology, Oxford University Hospitals NHS Foundation Trust

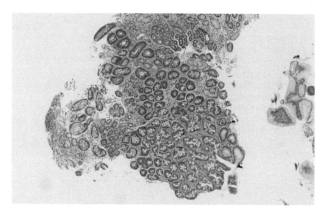

**Plate 4** Histology specimen from stomach body

Image courtesy of Dr Eve Fryer, Consultant Histopathologist, OUH NHS Foundation Trust, Oxford

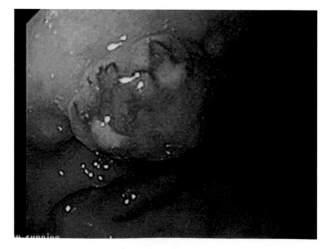

**Plate 5** Endoscopic image of lesion in stomach

Courtesy of Oxford University Hospitals NHS Foundation Trust

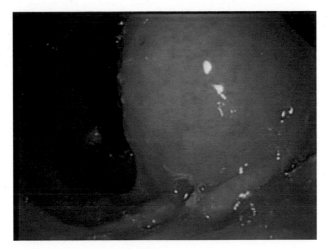

**Plate 6** Endoscopic view of stomach in retroflexion

Courtesy of Oxford University Hospitals NHS Foundation Trust

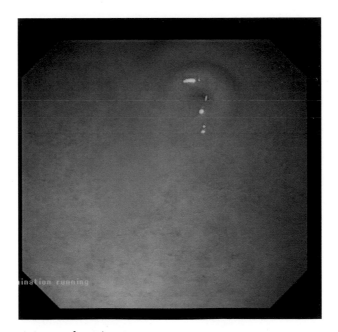

**Plate 7** Endoscopic image of gastric antrum

Image courtesy of Dr Tim Ambrose, Oxford University Hospitals NHS Foundation Trust

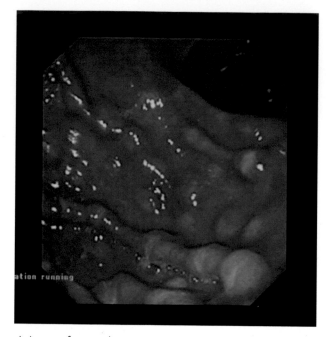

**Plate 8** Endoscopic image of stomach

Image courtesy of Dr Tim Ambrose, Consultant Gastroenterologist, Oxford University Hospitals NHS Foundation Trust

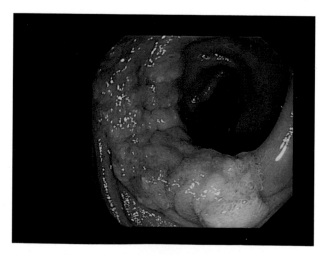

**Plate 9** Endoscopic image of second part of duodenum

Image courtesy of Dr Tim Ambrose, Oxford University Hospitals NHS Foundation Trust

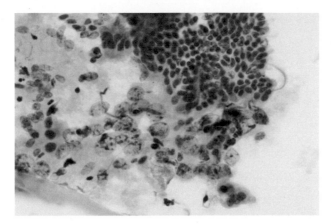

**Plate 10** Brush cytology specimen from biliary stricture

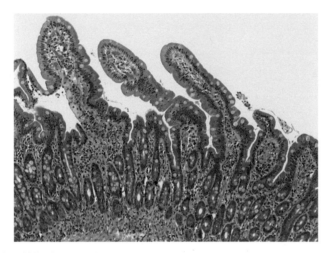

**Plate 11** Duodenal histology specimen

Image courtesy of Dept of Histopathology, Oxford University Hospitals NHS Foundation Trust

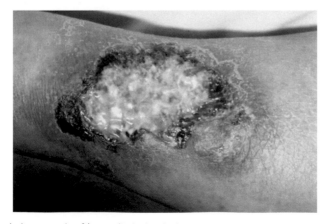

**Plate 12** Clinical photograph of lower limb skin lesion

Reproduced with permission from *Oxford Handbook of Medical Dermatology* (2 ed.), Susan Burge, Rubeta Matin, and Dinny Wallis, Figure 15.5, page 297, Oxford University Press, Oxford, UK, Copyright © 2016

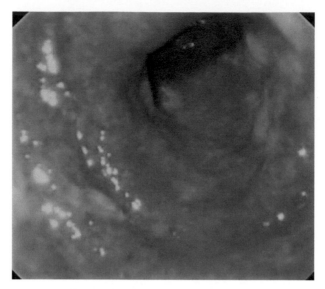

**Plate 13** Endoscopic image of sigmoid colon

Image courtesy of Dr Vincent Cheung, OUH NHS Foundation Trust, Oxford

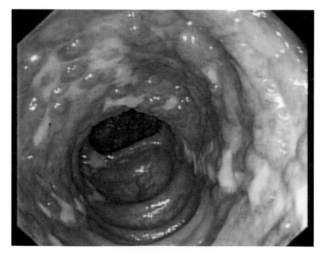

**Plate 14** Endoscopic image of sigmoid colon

Courtesy of Oxford University Hospitals

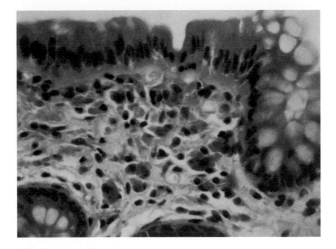

**Plate 15** Colonic histology specimen

Permission granted by Dr N. Ryley, Torbay Hospital; slides from his personal collection

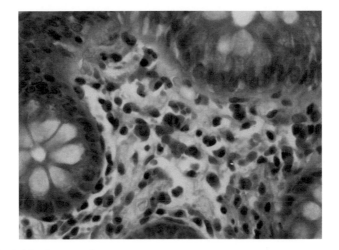

**Plate 16** Colonic histology specimen

Permission granted by Dr N. Ryley, Torbay Hospital; slides from his personal collection

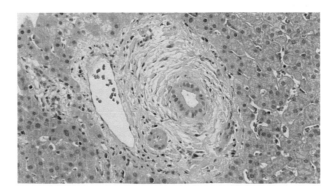

**Plate 17** Liver biopsy histology specimen

Image courtesy of Dr Eve Fryer, OUH NHS Foundation Trust, Oxford

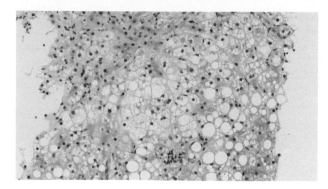

**Plate 18** Liver histology specimen

Image courtesy of Dr Eve Fryer, OUH NHS Foundation Trust, Oxford

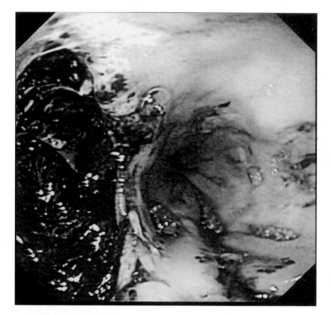

**Plate 19** Endoscopic image of oesophagus

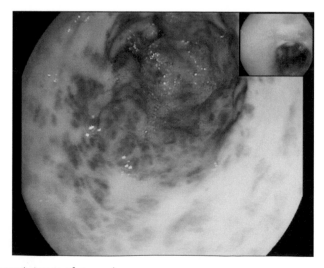

**Plate 20** Endoscopic image of stomach

23. **You reviewed a 23-year-old man in clinic with extensive UC for which he took mesalazine and azathioprine. He had been well in the past year and was clinically in disease remission. However, he showed you a new skin lesion on his left shin (Fig. 7.1).**

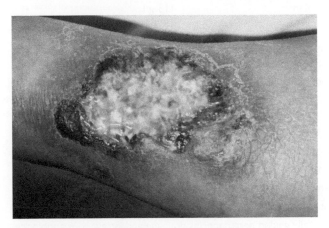

**Fig. 7.1** Clinical photograph of lower limb skin lesion. See also Plate 12

Reproduced with permission from *Oxford Handbook of Medical Dermatology* (2 ed.), Susan Burge, Rubeta Matin, and Dinny Wallis, Figure 15.5, page 297, Oxford University Press, Oxford, UK, Copyright © 2016

**Which statement regarding the likely diagnosis of this skin lesion is correct?**

A. It is usually associated with active bowel inflammation

B. It occurs more commonly in CD than UC

C. It never causes deep (sub-epidermal) inflammation

D. It occurs in 5%–10% of patients with UC

E. Lesions are often precipitated by trauma (pathergy)

24. **A 37-year-old man with CD presented to the emergency department with right iliac fossa pain and pyrexia. He had three previous ileal resections for stricturing disease in the past 10 years. He was taking azathioprine (1 mg/kg) once a day and an oral 5-ASA.**

Investigations:

| | |
|---|---|
| Haemoglobin | 113 g/L |
| WCC | 18 × 10⁹/L |
| Platelet count | 556 × 10⁹/L |
| Serum C-reactive protein (CRP) | 358 mg/L |
| Serum albumin | 24 g/L |
| CT abdomen and pelvis | Tethered loops of small bowel in the right iliac fossa with evidence of active disease and a 1 × 1 cm abscess in the region of the ileocaecal valve |

**What is the most appropriate next management step?**

A. Cessation of azathioprine and prescribing of intravenous antibiotics

B. Intravenous antibiotics and azathioprine 2 mg/kg once a day

C. Intravenous antibiotics and IFX induction regime

D. Laparotomy, ileocaecal resection, and end ileostomy

E. Radiologically guided percutaneous drainage and intravenous antibiotics

25. **A 59-year-old woman with quiescent CD, asthma, and hypertension presented to the emergency department with an acute febrile illness following her annual influenza vaccination. She complained of fever, malaise, headache, mouth ulcers, and arthralgia. The emergency department doctor noted the development of multiple erythematous and tender papules on her neck and at her immunization site.**

Investigations:

| | |
|---|---|
| Haemoglobin | 156 g/L |
| WCC | 15.9 × 10⁹/L |
| Platelet count | 365 × 10⁹/L |
| Serum albumin | 35 g/L |
| Serum C-reactive protein (CRP) | 67 mg/L |

Anti-neutrophil cytoplasmic antibodies:

| | |
|---|---|
| c-ANCA | Negative |
| p-ANCA | Weakly positive |
| PR3-ANCA | 8 U/mL (<10) |
| MPO-ANCA | 4 U/mL (<10) |

**Which of the following is the most likely diagnosis?**

A. Dermatitis herpetiformis

B. Erythema nodosum

C. *Mycobacterium tuberculosis*

D. Pyoderma gangrenosum (PG)

E. Sweet's syndrome

26. **An 18-year-old man with a childhood diagnosis of small bowel CD attended the emergency department with a painless, erythematous right eye. His vision was reported to be unchanged.**

    **What is the most likely diagnosis?**
    A. Anterior uveitis
    B. Episcleritis
    C. Intermediate uveitis
    D. Posterior uveitis
    E. Scleritis

27. **A 29-year-old with small bowel CD attended clinic. He was opening his bowels two to three times per day and reported mild right iliac fossa discomfort. His primary complaint was fatigue, which was having an impact on his work as a teacher.**

    Investigations:
    | | |
    |---|---|
    | Haemoglobin | 103 g/L |
    | MCV | 77 fL |
    | Platelet count | $475 \times 10^9$/L |
    | Ferritin | 85 µg/L |
    | Iron | 8.9 umol/L |
    | Serum albumin | 32 g/L |
    | Serum C-reactive protein (CRP) | 17 mg/L |

    **Which is not an indication for intravenous iron as first-line treatment in IBD patients with clinically active disease?**
    A. Patients on erythropoiesis-stimulating agents
    B. Patients with a previous intolerance to oral iron
    C. Patients with acute flare of disease
    D. Patients with Hb <100 g/L
    E. Patients with previous intestinal resection

28. **A 42-year-old man with UC enquired about colonoscopy surveillance for CRC. He was diagnosed with pancolitis 12 years ago. He took mesalazine 4 g daily for maintenance therapy. His paternal uncle and a first cousin had developed CRC. A colonoscopy performed two years ago for screening was macroscopically normal, but biopsies reported extensive colitis with moderate microscopic activity (Nancy Histology Index Grade 3).**

    **Regarding colonoscopy surveillance, which of the following statements is most accurate?**

    A. He is overdue a colonoscopy by one year

    B. Left-sided colitis at the time of diagnosis warrants a screening colonoscopy at five years

    C. Post-inflammatory polyps require annual surveillance

    D. Surveillance should be scheduled for one year's time

    E. The family history of CRC warrants five-yearly colonoscopy

29. **A 43-year-old man with a 12-year history of pancolitis was overdue colonoscopic surveillance. He enquired about his personal risk of CRC.**

    **With respect to CRC and IBD, which statement is most accurate?**

    A. IBD patients diagnosed with CRC are older than sporadic CRC patients

    B. Only IBD patients with a family history of CRC are at risk of developing malignancy

    C. Patients with Crohn's colitis have a higher risk of CRC than those with UC

    D. Risk factors associated with UC-related CRC include pancolitis and male sex

    E. Women have a preponderance to IBD-related CRC

30. **A paediatric gastroenterologist wrote to you, asking you to take over the care of a 16-year-old with two previous resections for small bowel CD. He was maintained on azathioprine and IFX.**

    **Which of the following statements is most accurate?**

    A. A joint paediatric-adult clinic, as part of a transition programme, is the ideal model

    B. A transition coordinator is only necessary for inter-hospital transfers

    C. Consultations with adolescent patients should focus on disease and its treatment, in order to avoid creating uncomfortable discussions about physical, emotional, educational, and sexual development

    D. Transfer of care is best achieved through a formal written handover

    E. Transition should occur on completion of education

31. **A 24-year-old woman with UC is very well controlled on azathioprine 100 mg/day and mesalazine 2 g/day. She discovers that she is 10 weeks pregnant and attends clinic concerned about her medications.**

    **What would be the best advice for this patient?**

    A. Continue current medications

    B. Halve the dose of azathioprine

    C. Stop azathioprine

    D. Stop azathioprine and mesalazine

    E. Stop mesalazine

32. **A 28-year-old lady with extensive UC was commenced on IFX 11 months previously because of active disease despite mesalazine and azathioprine therapy. She had subsequently been in clinical remission for the past eight months. She wished to consider starting a family imminently. She had not undergone any prior operations.**

    Investigations:

    | | |
    |---|---|
    | Colonoscopy | Quiescent colitis, no macroscopic or microscopic evidence of inflammation. |

    **What would be the most appropriate advice regarding discontinuing IFX?**

    A. Continue treatment throughout pregnancy and breastfeeding, even if in disease remission

    B. Stop three months prior to conception

    C. Stop as soon as conception known if remains in disease remission

    D. Stop at end of first trimester (approx. 12 weeks' gestation) if remains in disease remission

    E. Stop at end of second trimester (approx. 26 weeks' gestation) if remains in disease remission

33. **A 65-year-old woman with metastatic melanoma received four cycles of combination immunotherapy including ipilimumab (anti-CTLA-4) and nivolumab (anti-PD1), which commenced 50 days ago. She was referred with two days of watery, non-bloody stool (six times per day) and abdominal discomfort. She was taking methotrexate, folic acid, and naproxen for rheumatoid arthritis. She also recently completed a week's course of co-amoxiclav for a chest infection.**

Investigations:

| | |
|---|---|
| Haemoglobin | 130 g/L |
| Haematocrit | 44% |
| WCC | $10.0 \times 10^9$/L |
| Platelet count | $389 \times 10^9$/L |
| Erythrocyte sedimentation rate | 8 mm/hr |
| Albumin | 32 g/L |
| Serum C-reactive protein (CRP) | 9 mg/L |
| Flexible sigmoidoscopy | Patchy erythema and partial loss of vascular pattern with small superficial ulcers from rectum to splenic flexure (Fig. 7.2). |

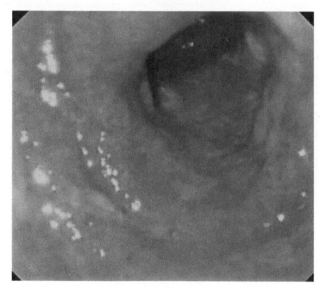

**Fig. 7.2** Endoscopic image of sigmoid colon. See also Plate 13
Image courtesy of Dr Vincent Cheung, Oxford University Hospitals NHS Foundation Trust

### Which is the most likely diagnosis?

A. *Clostridiodes difficile*-associated diarrhoea

B. Immunotherapy-associated colitis

C. Lymphocytic colitis

D. NSAID-associated enterocolitis

E. UC

34. **A 72-year-old woman presented to the emergency department. Twenty-four hours earlier, she developed acute onset, severe left-sided abdominal pain, rectal bleeding, and loose stools. The pain since reduced and was now more diffuse. Her medication included lisinopril for hypertension, bisoprolol for atrial fibrillation, and diclofenac for osteoarthritis. She finished one week of amoxicillin for a chest infection 10 days ago. Examination revealed a tender left lower quadrant with guarding.**

**Her temperature was 37.8°C, blood pressure 98/60 mmHg, pulse 105 beats per minute, respiratory rate 16, oxygen saturations 98% on room air.**

Investigations:

| | |
|---|---|
| Haemoglobin | 128 g/L |
| Platelet count | 365 × 10⁹/L |
| Serum C-reactive protein (CRP) | 10 mg/L |
| Serum albumin | 34 g/L |
| Lactate | 3.5 mmol/L |
| Faecal culture | Negative |
| CT abdomen and pelvis | Colitis from splenic flexure to the rectum |
| Flexible sigmoidoscopy | (Fig. 7.3) |

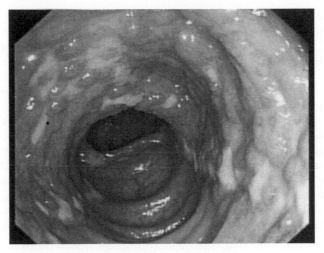

**Fig. 7.3** Endoscopic image of sigmoid colon. See also Plate 14
Courtesy of Oxford University Hospitals NHS Foundation Trust

**What is the most likely diagnosis?**

A. CD

B. Ischaemic colitis

C. NSAID-induced colitis

D. Pseudomembranous colitis

E. UC

35. **A 36-year-old woman presented with rectal bleeding, tenesmus, and mucus discharge three years after a temporary loop ileostomy for refractory colonic CD. After surgery, she was managed in the community without further symptoms or medical therapy. She underwent ileoscopy, at which the mucosa was macroscopically normal. At flexible sigmoidoscopy, a diagnosis of diversion colitis was made.**

    **What is the best management option?**

    A. Acetarsol suppositories

    B. Azathioprine

    C. Mesalazine enemas

    D. Oral corticosteroids

    E. Short-chain fatty acid enemas (SCFAs)

36. **A 65-year-old woman presented to her GP with a four-year history of watery diarrhoea.**

    **Her only comorbidity was depression, which was managed with sertraline.**

    Investigations:

    | | |
    |---|---|
    | Haemoglobin | 132 g/L |
    | WCC | 4.6 × 10⁹/L |
    | Platelet count | 470 × 10⁹/L |
    | MCV | 88.1 fL |
    | Serum sodium | 137 mmol/L |
    | Serum potassium | 3.8 mmol/L |
    | Serum urea | 7 mmol/L |
    | Serum creatinine | 89 µmol/L |
    | Anti-tissue transglutaminase antibodies | 9 U/ml |
    | Plasma thyroid-stimulating hormone | 3.4 mu/L |
    | Faecal microscopy, culture, and sensitivities | Negative |
    | Faecal elastase | 405 µg/g |
    | Colonoscopy | Normal |
    | Colonic histology | Pending |

    **Which of the following histological findings would be most in keeping with a diagnosis of collagenous colitis?**

    A. Focal active cryptitis

    B. Greater than 20 eosinophils per high-powered field

    C. Greater than 20 lymphocytes per 100 epithelial cells

    D. Preservation of crypt architecture

    E. Subepithelial collagen layer 6 µm in thickness

37. **An 82-year-old diabetic woman was referred to the acute medical take with severe diarrhoea and abdominal pain. She was a nursing home resident and had recently completed a course of clindamycin for a chronic infection of her third metatarsal. *Clostridiodes difficile* was confirmed.**

    **What is the overall sensitivity of glutamate dehydrogenase assay?**

    A. 78%

    B. 80%

    C. 85%

    D. 91%

    E. 96%

38. **A 19-year-old British man spent the summer working as a water-sports instructor in America. He had no medical background. On his return, he presented to his GP complaining of an intermittent patch of raised itchy skin, which appeared and disappeared in a matter of hours, at different sites on his back. He had had an area of inflamed skin between his toes while abroad. He attributed this to a fungal infection.**

    **He also complained of diarrhoea.**

    Investigations:

    | | |
    |---|---|
    | Haemoglobin | 156 g/L |
    | MCV | 92 fL |
    | WCC | $10.2 \times 10^9$/L |
    | Neutrophil count | $6.5 \times 10^9$/L |
    | Lymphocyte count | $1.7 \times 10^9$/L |
    | Eosinophil count | $1.6 \times 10^9$/L |
    | Basophil count | $0.04 \times 10^9$/L |
    | Platelet count | $420 \times 10^9$/L |
    | Faecal microscopy and culture | Negative × 3 |

    **Which treatment is the most appropriate?**

    A. Corticosteroids

    B. Filaricides

    C. Ivermectin

    D. Metronidazole

    E. Tiabendazole

39. **A 45-year-old software engineer in France presented with a seven-day history of bloody diarrhoea, no vomiting, and severe abdominal pain. He was opening his bowels seven times a day and had a temperature of 39°C.**

Investigations:

| | |
|---|---|
| Haemoglobin | 140 g/L |
| WCC | $15.1 \times 10^9$/L |
| Serum C-reactive protein (CRP) | 120 mg/L |
| Urea | 12.1 mmol/L |
| Creatinine | 130 µmol/L |

**Which organism is the most likely cause of this patient's symptoms?**

A. *Campylobacter jejuni*

B. *Clostridiodes difficile*

C. Norovirus

D. *Salmonella typhi*

E. Shigella

40. **A 32-year-old South African man recently moved to the UK and presented with a 12-day history of fevers and watery diarrhoea up to 20 times a day.**

Investigations:

| | |
|---|---|
| Haemoglobin | 100 g/L |
| WCC | $0.9 \times 10^9$/L |
| CD4+ lymphocyte count | 42/µL |
| Serum C-reactive protein (CRP) | 120 mg/L |
| Urea | 15.1 mmol/L |
| Creatinine | 120 µmol/L |
| HIV antibody | Positive |
| Flexible sigmoidoscopy | Erythema, loss of vascular pattern and multiple, well-defined, punched out ulcers throughout the left colon. |

**What is the best treatment option?**

A. Clarithromycin and ethambutol

B. Intravenous foscarnet

C. Intravenous ganciclovir

D. Nitazoxanide

E. Supportive care including intravenous fluids alone

41. **A 75-year-old man is referred by his GP with iron-deficiency anaemia. Because he is fit, active, and independent, with no other medical comorbidities, it is decided that an upper and lower gastrointestinal endoscopy is warranted.**

Investigations:

| | |
|---|---|
| Haemoglobin | 102 g/L |
| MCV | 72 fL |
| Iron level | 8.2 umol/L |
| Transferrin | 3.13 g/L |
| Transferrin saturation | 12% |
| Ferritin | 9 μmg/L |
| Gastroscopy | Normal |
| Duodenal biopsies | Normal |
| Colonoscopy | 1.5 cm pedunculated polyp in the transverse colon, snared and retrieved. |
| Histology | 15 mm tubulovillous adenoma with no low-grade dysplasia. |

**What is the most appropriate follow-up for this patient?**

A. Colonoscopy in one year's time

B. Colonoscopy in two years' time

C. Colonoscopy in three years' time

D. Colonoscopy in five years' time

E. No surveillance

42. **A 42-year-old male patient attended clinic. He was diagnosed with acromegaly in his early twenties. He did not complain of any bowel symptoms, but had read about an increased risk of developing CRC.**

**His screening colonoscopy at age 40 years demonstrated one 3 mm hyperplastic polyp that was completely excised from the sigmoid colon. He was otherwise healthy and his body mass index (BMI) was 25 kg/m$^2$.**

Investigations:

| | |
|---|---|
| Thyroid-stimulating hormone | 2.4 mU/L |
| Insulin-like growth factor-1 | 42.6 nmol/L |
| Fasting plasma glucose | 4.9 mmol/L |

**Which of the following is the most appropriate with regard to ongoing surveillance?**

A. Two-yearly colonoscopy

B. Three-yearly colonoscopy

C. Five-yearly colonoscopy

D. Ten-yearly colonoscopy

E. Annual colonoscopy

43. **A 35-year-old woman presented with a history of chronic diarrhoea. She was referred for a colonoscopy. Multiple polyps (around 50) were found in the ascending and transverse colon. You asked about her family history and she revealed that her great uncle died of bowel cancer and her nephew recently had bowel surgery for polyps. Both her parents, aged 65 and 70 years, and her two brothers, aged 45 and 42 years, were healthy.**

   **Which of the following is the most likely diagnosis?**

   A. Familial adenomatous polyposis

   B. Hereditary non-polyposis CRC

   C. Juvenile polyposis syndrome (JPS)

   D. MUTYH-associated polyposis (MAP)

   E. Peutz–Jeghers syndrome

44. **A 40-year-old female patient presented with a history of intermittent central abdominal pain. Examination revealed freckles on her lips, buccal mucosa, and eyelids. Her past medical history included breast cancer diagnosed a year ago.**

   **What would be the most appropriate next step?**

   A. Colonoscopy and genetic testing for breast cancer susceptibility gene 1 and breast cancer susceptibility gene 2

   B. Colonoscopy and genetic testing for serine/threonine kinase 11 gene mutation

   C. Colonoscopy and mammogram

   D. CT chest, abdomen, and pelvis

   E. Urgent colonoscopy

45. **A 56-year-old man attended for a colonoscopy for a change in bowel habit.**

   Investigations:

   | | |
   |---|---|
   | Colonoscopy | Multiple serrated polyps. 24 polyps counted in total; majority right sided (8 transverse, 6 ascending) with largest measuring 11 mm. All polyps measuring more than 5 mm were removed. |
   | Histology | A mix of sessile serrated lesions without dysplasia and hyperplastic polyps |

   **What surveillance interval would you recommend for this condition?**

   A. One year

   B. Three years

   C. Five years

   D. Endoscopic surveillance interval dependent on family history

   E. Surveillance timing stratified according to the presence of an associated genetic mutation

46. **A 35-year-old woman was diagnosed with dyssynergic defecation.**

    **Which of the following is the most effective treatment modality?**

    A.  Biofeedback therapy (BFT)

    B.  Botulinum toxin injection

    C.  Diet

    D.  Laxatives

    E.  Myectomy of the anal sphincter

47. **A 35-year-old woman complained of constipation for the past eight months. She was treated with movicol and sodium docusate at the maximum doses. This did not improve her symptoms.**

    **Which is the most appropriate next drug to try?**

    A.  Glycerol suppositories

    B.  Lactulose

    C.  Poloxamer drops

    D.  Prucalopride

    E.  Sodium phosphate enemas

48. **A 49-year-old woman complained of accidental leakage of solid and liquid stools for the past two years. There was no history of IBD. However, she had been diagnosed with IBS. She had smoked 20 cigarettes a day for 28 years. She had an episiotomy and vaginal forceps-assisted delivery at the age of 27 years. On examination, she was obese with a BMI 31 kg/m². She had reduced anal tone on digital rectal examination.**

    **What is the strongest risk factor for faecal incontinence (FI) in this woman?**

    A.  Episiotomy

    B.  Forceps-assisted delivery

    C.  High BMI

    D.  IBS

    E.  Smoking

**49. A 72-year-old woman underwent a colonoscopy because of abdominal bloating and discomfort. The colonoscopy revealed brownish discoloration of the colonic wall.**

Colonic histology              (Figs. 7.4 and 7.5)

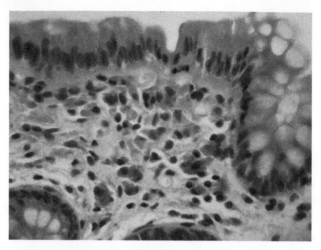

**Fig. 7.4** Colonic histology specimen. See also Plate 15

Permission granted by Dr N. Ryley, Torbay Hospital; slides from his personal collection

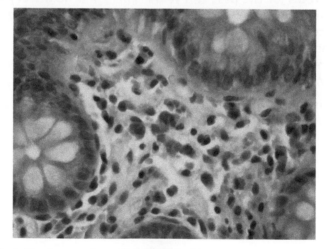

**Fig. 7.5** Colonic histology specimen. See also Plate 16

Permission granted by Dr N. Ryley, Torbay Hospital; slides from his personal collection

## The pigmentation found in the submucosa is most likely:

A.  Haemosiderin

B.  Iron sulphide

C.  Lipofuscin

D.  Melanin

E.  Silicate

50. **A 51-year-old woman presented with a history of constipation for two years. She opened her bowels every 4–5 days, passing hard and lumpy stool; she also complained of abdominal pain and bloating. She denied weight loss, fever, or bloody stools. There was no family history of IBD and she had no past medical history of note. She subsequently underwent a bowel transit study (Fig. 7.6).**

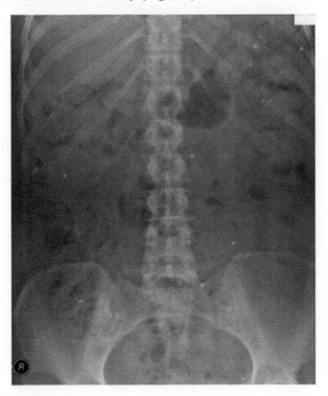

**Fig. 7.6** Bowel transit study

Investigations:

| | |
|---|---|
| Haemoglobin | 125 g/L |
| WCC | 5.6 × 10⁹/L |
| Platelet count | 290 × 10⁹/L |
| MCV | 88.1 fL |
| Serum sodium | 139 mmol/L |
| Serum potassium | 3.9 mmol/L |
| Serum urea | 6.7 mmol/L |
| Serum creatinine | 89 μmol/L |
| Anti-tissue transglutaminase antibodies | 9 U/mL |
| Plasma thyroid-stimulating hormone | 3.4 mU/L |
| Faecal microscopy, culture, and sensitivities | Negative |
| Faecal elastase | 405 μg/g |
| Colonoscopy | Normal |
| Colonic histology | Normal |
| Ano-rectal manometry | Normal |

**Which of the following is the most likely diagnosis?**

A.  Dyssynergic defecation

B.  Irritable bowel syndrome with predominant constipation (IBS-C)

C.  Normal-transit constipation

D.  Slow-transit constipation

E.  Slow-transit constipation and dyssynergic defecation

## 1. A. IFN-γ

- IBD is driven by dysregulated immune responses to environmental and microbial triggers
- IFN-γ and IL-2 are produced in higher amounts in CD when compared with UC

Immunological factors play an important role in the pathogenesis of IBD. Chronic intestinal inflammation is driven by a dysregulated immune response to environmental and microbial triggers. Cytokines are key mediators of cellular interactions in the intestine in both health and disease. Governed by cytokine networks, epithelial barrier function, host defence pathways, immune regulation, and tissue repair are key components of intestinal homeostasis. Disruption of these cytokine-guided networks can lead to inflammation, primarily by innate derived pro-inflammatory cytokines and subsequent IBD.

Exposure to foreign antigens leads to activation of naïve CD4+ cells that differentiate into either $T_h1$ cells, $T_h2$ cells, or $T_h17$ cells. $T_h1$ cells produce pro-inflammatory cytokines: IL-2, IL-6, IFN-γ and tumour necrosis factor-alpha (TNF-α). Production of IL2 differs in CD versus UC. Mucosal T-cells in CD produce more IL-2, suggesting a more significant response and T-cell function in CD. Increased production of IFN-γ is also seen in CD, however not UC, supported by evidence of increased levels of IL-12 and IL-18 (which induce IFN-γ) in CD. IL-6 is expressed in abundance in IBD mucosa. Its roles include immune cell activation, inhibition of apoptosis, and induction of $T_h17$ cell differentiation. Increased TNF-α activity weakens epithelial barrier function through alteration in epithelial integrity and apoptosis of intestinal epithelial cells. Compromise of the barrier function and microbial dysbiosis are key events in the initiation of IBD.

In UC, pro-inflammatory cytokines IL-5 and IL-13 (derived from Natural Killer T [NKT] cells) are produced in substantially higher amounts. In colitis, IL-12 and IL-23, produced by macrophages, drive pathogenic T-cell responses in part due to deficiencies in anti-inflammatory IL-10 and TGF-β pathways.

$T_h17$ cells participate in the inflammatory response by producing multiple cytokines, including IL-17 in conjunction with IL-21, IL-22, and IL-23. IL-17 leads to the induction of pro-inflammatory cytokines via stimulation of Th1 cells. Increased IL-17 expression is seen in most patients with IBD. However, it is consistently higher in those with CD than UC. IL-22 promotes epithelial repair and antimicrobial defence.

Friedrich M, Pohin M, Powrie F. Cytokine networks in the pathophysiology of inflammatory bowel disease. *Immunity.* 2019;50(4):992–1006. Doi: 10.1016/j.immuni.2019.03.017.

## 2. B. 10%

- The greatest risk factor for the development of IBD is an affected first-degree relative (FDR)
- Genetic susceptibility is greater in CD
- If only one parent has IBD, the risk is 9% and 6% for offspring CD and UC respectively

*Best of Five MCQs for the European Specialty Examination in Gastroenterology and Hepatology.* Thomas Marjot, Colleen G C McGregor, Tim Ambrose, Aminda N De Silva, Jeremy Cobbold, and Simon Travis, Oxford University Press (2021). © Oxford University Press.
DOI: 10.1093/oso/9780198834373.003.0007

There is strong evidence that genetic factors play an important role in determining susceptibility to IBD:

- Extensive genome-wide association studies (GWAS) have identified approximately 240 genes associated with pathogenesis or risk of IBD
- Nucleotide-binding oligomerization domain-containing protein 2 (NOD2) has shown the greatest association with fibrostenosing CD; NOD2 signalling is essential for bacterial recognition; in addition, it suppresses transcription of IL-10, a potent anti-inflammatory cytokine
- NOD2 gene variants are found primarily in patients of European or Ashkenazi Jewish descent
- IL23R, a gene encoding the receptor of pro-inflammatory cytokine IL-23, is associated with both CD and UC
- GWAS identified variants in ATG16L1 and IRGM, two genes involved in autophagy, in association with CD
- Human leucocyte antigen (HLA) genes have also been implicated with disease susceptibility and severity in both UC and CD; this region is also implicated as a region subject to epigenetic dysregulation in IBD; the most consistent HLA allelic associations involve the HLA class II loci, with variants playing a more important role in UC than CD
- Genetic factors are more common in patients with early onset disease; causal mutations have been identified in several cases of very early onset IBD; approximately 50 single genes causing monogenic forms of IBD have been identified, such as IL10R and XIAP

Data from family studies, twin studies, and GWAS describe the heritability of IBD:

- The greatest risk factor is an affected FDR; siblings of an affected individual are at highest risk
- Genetic susceptibility is more frequently identified in patients with CD (9%–15%) than in those with UC (6%–9%)
- In CD, the rate of concordance for identical twins has been reported to be as high as 53%; in UC, the concordance rate is lower (6%–17%)
- The lifetime risk to offspring of two parents with IBD exceeds 30%; if only one parent has IBD, the risk is 9% in parental CD and 6% in parental UC

Mirkov M, Verstock B, Cleynen. Genetics of inflammatory bowel disease: beyond NOD2. *Lancet Gastroenterol Hepatol.* 2017;2:224–234. Doi: 0.1016/S2468-1253(16)30111-X.

### 3. B. Approximately 30% of patients with ASUC will require a colectomy

- Thirty-three per cent of patients with ASUC will require colectomy
- Accelerated dose IFX (>5 mg/kg) is no more effective than standard dose IFX
- Seventy-five per cent of patients with colonic dilatation on plain abdominal X-ray will require colectomy

Fifteen to twenty per cent of patients with UC will require hospital admission with acute severe ulcerative colitis (ASUC). In ASUC, intravenous steroids are the mainstay of therapy. However, 30%–40% of patients will require rescue therapy and approximately 33% will ultimately require colectomy. Important indications for colectomy are failure of medical therapy, suspected perforation, refractory bleeding, and toxic megacolon. The presence of mucosal islands (areas of oedematous mucosa surrounded by deep ulceration) or colonic dilatation (diameter of ≥ 5.5 cm or caecum >9 cm) are associated with colectomy in up to 75% of patients.

IFX as a single dose (5 mg/kg) is an effective rescue therapy in patients with acute severe colitis refractory to intravenous steroids. Accelerated dose IFX (>5 mg/kg) appears to be no more effective than standard dose IFX and may be associated with higher 30-day colectomy rates.

Smoking cessation in patients with UC is associated with an increase in hospital admissions and disease activity.

Dinesen LC et al. The pattern and outcome of acute severe colitis. *J Crohns Colitis.* 2010;4:431–437. Doi: 10.1016/j.crohns.2010.02.001.

## 4. A. Around 25% of patients with pancolitis eventually have a colectomy

- 50% of individuals with UC flare each year
- Proctitis extends in 10% of patients over 10 years

Among individuals with UC, around 50% have a flare each year. Early relapse or active disease in the first two years confers a worse disease course subsequently. Around 25% of patients with pancolitis will eventually require a colectomy. Progression from proctitis to extensive colitis occurs in 10% of patients over 10 years. The cumulative incidence of CRC or dysplasia is 8% at 20 years and 16% at 30 years. Meta-analysis suggests a 50% risk reduction for CRC in patients taking 5-ASAs.

Lamb C et al. BSG consensus guidelines on the management of inflammatory bowel disease in adults. *Gut.* 2019;68(Suppl 3):s1–s106. Doi: 10.1136/gutjnl-2019-318484.

## 5. B. Faecal culture

- In patients presenting with acute diarrhoea, faecal culture must not be overlooked
- Bacterial intestinal infection is associated with an increased risk of future IBD

Although this case could represent an index presentation of IBD with a relevant family history and possible extra-intestinal manifestations (EIMs; mouth ulcers and PG), infection must always excluded. Endoscopic investigation and small bowel imaging may be necessary but basic initial investigations, such as a plain abdominal film and faecal culture, should not be overlooked. A positive faecal culture, however, does not necessarily exclude a diagnosis of underlying IBD, with up to 20% of patients presenting with a first attack of IBD-related colitis having concurrent positive microbiologic investigations. Bacterial intestinal infections have also been implicated as a possible trigger for initiation and/or exacerbation of future IBD. The association of HLA-B27 with axial spondylarthritis is seen in IBD but to a lesser degree than in idiopathic ankylosing spondylitis, and its presence has no diagnostic role in this presentation or in the diagnosis of IBD-related arthropathies.

Nielson HL, Dalager-Pedersen M et al. Risk of inflammatory bowel disease after Campylobacter jejuni and Campylobacter concisus infection: a population-based cohort study. *Scand J Gastroenterol.* 2019 Mar;54(3):265–272. Doi: 10.1080/00365521.

## 6. B. A2 L2 B1

CD is difficult to classify meaningfully because it is such a heterogenous disease. The Montreal Classification was developed by the Working Party for the 2005 World Congress of Gastroenterology in Montreal to better subclassify clinical phenotypes—namely, disease extent and behaviour (Box 7.1). A revision of the 2000 Vienna Classification, the Montreal Classification's key modifications advocate:

- the introduction of an early age of onset category
- allowing for co-classification of location L4 (upper gastrointestinal involvement)
- the inclusion of a modifier for perianal disease

---

**Box 7.1** Summary of revised 'Montreal classification' of Crohn's disease

**Age at diagnosis (A)**

A1 16 years or younger
A2 17–40 years
A3 Over 40 years

**Location (L)**

L1 Terminal ileum
L2 Colon
L3 Ileocolon
L4 Upper GI (modifier)

**Behaviour (B)—Perianal disease modifier (p)**

B1 Nonstricturing, nonpenetrating
B2 Stricturing
B3 Penetrating
B2p Stricturing + perianal
B3p Penetrating + perianal

Box reproduced from: Silverberg MS, Satsangi J et al. Toward an integrated clinical, molecular and serological classification of inflammatory bowel disease: Report of a Working Party of the 2005 Montreal World Congress of Gastroenterology. *Can J Gastroenterol*. 2005;19:5A—36A. DOI: 10.1155/2005/269076

---

Silverberg MS, Satsangi J et al. Toward an integrated clinical, molecular and serological classification of inflammatory bowel disease: Report of a Working Party of the 2005 Montreal World Congress of Gastroenterology. *Can J Gastroenterol*. 2005;19:5A–36A. Doi: 10.1155/2005/269076.

## 7. A. Basal plasmacytosis

- Basal plasmacytosis gives the highest predictive value for a diagnosis of UC over infective colitis
- Acute disease activity is defined by neutrophil mediated injury to the mucosa leading to cryptitis and crypt abscess formation
- Chronic mucosal injury, including mucosal atrophy, crypt distortion, and Paneth cell metaplasia, may still be seen in quiescent disease

Basal plasmacytosis is the presence of a lymphoplasmacytic infiltrate between the crypt bases and the *muscularis mucosae*, and is recognized as the earliest feature with the highest predictive value for a diagnosis of UC. Presence of basal plasmacytosis is useful in differentiating between the index presentation of UC (63%) and infectious colitis (6%), but not CD (62%). Granuloma formation is characteristic of CD. Paneth cell metaplasia reflects chronicity. The remaining options are also observed in infectious colitis.

Active disease is defined as neutrophil-mediated epithelial injury limited to the mucosa. This includes neutrophils invading crypt epithelium leading to cryptitis and collections of neutrophils within crypt lumens forming crypt abscesses. The inflammatory infiltrate is diffuse and the severity increases characteristically towards the rectum. While Paneth cells are a normal component of the right colon, their presence in the left colon is a metaplastic process, due to chronic crypt architectural distortion.

Quiescent disease is defined by the lack of mucosal neutrophils although chronic mucosal injury including mucosal atrophy, crypt distortion, and Paneth cell metaplasia may persist.

Magro et al. European Society of Pathology (ESP); European Crohn's and Colitis Organisation (ECCO). European consensus on the histology of inflammatory bowel disease. *J Crohns Colitis*. 2013 Nov;7(10):827–851. Doi: 10.1016/j.crohns.2013.06.001.

## 8. A. Flexible sigmoidoscopy is useful in determining the management of perianal fistulae

- Presence of concomitant rectosigmoid inflammation is of prognostic and therapeutic significance
- Perianal pain is highly predictive of an abscess
- The sensitivity and specificity of either pelvic MRI or EUS is increased when combined with EUA

Perianal fistulae affect up to half of CD patients, and are most common in colonic disease affecting the rectum, where rates exceed 90%. Perianal disease can occur before, with, or after intestinal CD. Perianal pain is strongly predictive of the presence of an abscess.

The management of fistulae in CD should include the following:

- Defining and mapping the anatomy of the fistula; determining which organs are affected; Parks Classification (Fig. 7.7) is one of the various tools for classifying perianal fistulae in CD
- Assessing for concurrent active disease
- Identification or exclusion of local sepsis (abscess)
- Assessment of general status including nutrition and quality of life

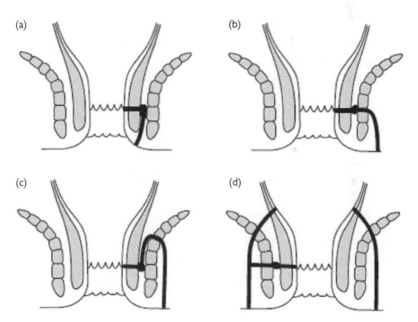

**Fig. 7.7** Park's classification; A, inter-sphincteric anal fistula; B, transphincteric anal fistula; C, supra-sphincteric anal fistula; D, extra-sphincteric anal fistula

Reproduced from Parks AG, Gordon PH and Hardcastle JD, 'A classification of fistula-in-ano', *British Journal of Surgery*, 63, pp. 1–12, 1976, with permission from Wiley and British Journal of Surgery Society Ltd. doi: 10.1002/bjs.1800630102

Contrast-enhanced pelvic MRI is a useful first-line investigation for assessment of perianal fistulizing CD. It is not always necessary because simple fistulae may not require imaging. MRI has the additional benefits of non-ionizing radiation and being non-invasive. EUA is the gold standard investigation with a reported sensitivity of 90%. EUA requires a specialist colorectal surgeon and allows for therapeutic management. Provided rectal stenosis is excluded, endoscopic anorectal ultrasound (EUS) is equivalent to pelvic MRI and a useful alternative modality. The specificity and sensitivity of both imaging modalities are increased when combined with EUA. Endoscopy is essential for determining whether concurrent medical management is required with surgical management of fistulae, because treatment is rarely successful in untreated active CD.

Gionchetti P, Dignass A et al. Third European evidence-based consensus on the diagnosis and management of Crohn's Disease 2016: Part 2: Surgical management and special situations. *J Crohns Colitis.* 2017, 135–149. Doi: 10.1093/ecco-jcc/jjw169.

### 9. D. Seton suture and antibiotics

- Perianal fistulae should be classified as either simple or complex (Table 7.1)
- Asymptomatic simple fistulae in CD do not require treatment whereas symptomatic simple perianal fistulae often require combination treatment with seton placement and antibiotics
- In complex perianal fistulizing disease, anti-TNF agents can be used first line provided adequate surgical drainage has been achieved (where indicated)

**Table 7.1** Classification of fistulae

| Simple fistula | Complex fistula |
| --- | --- |
| Superficial perianal or ano-vaginal | Trans-sphincteric perianal |
| Inter-sphincteric perianal or ano-vaginal | Supra-sphincteric perianal |
| | Extra-sphincteric perianal |
| | Enterocutaneous |
| | Entero-enteric |
| | Enterovesical |
| | Recto-vaginal |

The European Crohn's and Colitis Organisation (ECCO) consensus states that symptomatic simple perianal fistulae warrant treatment. First-line management favours seton placement in combination with antibiotics (metronidazole and/or ciprofloxacin). Evidence for antibiotics demonstrates efficacy in improving symptoms. However, it rarely induces healing.

Although there are currently no randomized controlled trials (RCTs) primarily assessing the effect of thiopurines in perianal disease, secondary end-point data from a meta-analysis of five RCTs favour the efficacy of thiopurines in both closing and maintaining closure of perianal fistula. Anti-TNFs may be used as third-line management in recurrent, refractory simple fistulae. However, data is limited.

In complex perianal fistulizing disease, anti-TNFs (IFX or adalimumab) may be used as first-line therapy following effective surgical drainage when necessary. The ACCENT II and CHARM trials demonstrated efficacy for IFX and adalimumab, respectively, in inducing and maintaining closure of perianal fistulae.

Limited evidence exists for ciclosporin. Total parenteral nutrition can be a useful adjunct in the management of complex fistulae. Abscesses due to internal fistulae mandate early surgical intervention.

Sands BE, Anderson FH et al. Infliximab maintenance therapy for fistulising Crohn's disease. *NEJM* 2004;350(9):876–885. Doi: 10.1056/NEJMoa030815.

### 10. A. Capsule endoscopy (CE)

- Ileocolonoscopy with biopsies is the first-line investigation to establish a diagnosis of CD
- Cross-sectional imaging (MRI and CT enterography) are adjuncts to colonoscopy to detect and stage inflammatory, obstructive, and fistulizing CD
- The diagnostic yield of CE in small bowel disease is superior to other modalities (small bowel enteroscopy/small bowel follow through)

Currently, the diagnosis of CD involves an analysis of clinical, radiological, endoscopic, and histopathological results. Contrast-enhanced radiography is used to localize the extent, severity, and distribution of disease. CT scanning provides cross-sectional images for assessing mural and extramural involvement. Ileocolonoscopy with multiple biopsies remains the first-line investigation in diagnosing CD. Endoscopy enables direct visualization of the mucosa and histopathological correlation. Ultrasonography and MRI are adjuncts that provide alternative cross-sectional images in populations in whom radiation exposure is a concern.

CE has emerged successfully as a non-invasive test in the diagnostic armamentarium of IBD, and may be considered to be the gold standard for diagnosing small bowel IBD. It has demonstrated superior performance compared with other modalities in its ability to detect early small bowel CD, especially when ileocolonoscopy is negative or unsuccessful. It has a 30% incremental yield over other imaging modalities in non-stricturing CD. CE has a high negative predictive value for small bowel CD. A recent meta-analysis also found a high incremental yield of CE over other modalities, both in patients with suspected symptoms of CD, and in those with established non-stricturing CD being evaluated for small bowel recurrence.

Gomollon F, Dignass A et al. Third European evidence-based consensus on the diagnosis and management of Crohn's Disease 2016: Part 1: Diagnosis and medical management. *J Crohns Colitis.* 2017, 3–25. Doi: 10.1093/ecco-jcc/jjw168.

### 11. D. Increased bowel wall thickness (BWT)

- Increased BWT and vascularity are diagnostic sonographic findings for CD

Utilization of intestinal ultrasound (IUS) in the diagnosis and monitoring of CD is increasing (Fig. 7.8, Table 7.2). The most widely accepted diagnostic criterion for IBD diagnosis is increased bowel wall thickening with increased vascularization. Several studies have also demonstrated a relation between BWT and disease activity scores such as the CD activity index and Harvey Bradshaw index.

Maaser C, Sturm A et al. ECCO-ESGAR Guideline for diagnostic assessment in IBD Part 1: Initial diagnosis, monitoring of known IBD, detection of complications. *J Crohn's Colitis.* 2019;13(2):144-164. Doi: 10.1093/ecco-jcc/jjy113.

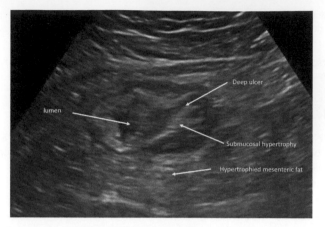

**Fig. 7.8** Inflamed segment of distal ileum on ultrasound

Image courtesy of Dr Andrew Slater, Consultant Radiologist, Oxford University Hospitals NHS Foundation Trust

**Table 7.2** Sonographic features of Crohn's disease

| Mural changes | Extramural changes | Complications |
|---|---|---|
| Increased bowel wall thickness | Thickened and hyperechoic mesentery | Narrowed lumen/stenosis |
| Altered echogenicity of the bowel wall | Vascularity of the mesentery* | Abscesses |
| Loss of normal wall stratification | Enlarged mesenteric nodes | Fistulae |
| Increased color doppler signal* | Mesenteric fat hypertrophy | |
| Decrease in/lack of peristalsis | | |
| Prominent submucosal layer | | |

*with the use of contrast enhanced ultrasound

Data from Maaser C, Sturm A et al. ECCO-ESGAR Guideline for diagnostic assessment in IBD Part 1: Initial diagnosis, monitoring of known IBD, detection of complications. *J Crohn's Colitis.* 2019;13(2):144-164. Doi: 10.1093/ecco-jcc/jjy113

## 12. B. It has high first-pass metabolism in the liver

- Budesonide MMX (9 mg/day for eight weeks) can be used in mild to moderately active UC
- Budesonide has low systemic bioavailability due to high first-pass hepatic metabolism, limiting steroid side effects compared with prednisolone

Budesonide is now well established in the treatment of IBD. The local activity of budesonide in the colonic mucosa is the key to its efficacy. Budesonide undergoes 90% hepatic first-pass metabolism limiting systemic bioavailability and minimizing steroid-related adverse effects compared with equivalent doses of prednisolone. Standard budesonide formulations release the drug only in the distal ileum and proximal colon, and so are not optimally designed for the distribution of UC. To improve release, budesonide can therefore be coupled with a colonic release system (MMX) that provides targeted drug delivery to the entire colon.

While budesonide MMX and mesalazine 2.4 g are equivalent in treating mild–moderate active UC, for those not controlled with oral 5-ASA, additional budesonide MMX 9 mg/day induces clinical, endoscopic, and histological remission at week eight more frequently than placebo. It can be considered as an alternative to escalation to conventional corticosteroids.

Travis SPL et al. Once-daily budesonide MMX in active, mild-to-moderate ulcerative colitis: results from the randomised CORE II study. *Gut.* 2014;63:433. Doi: 10.1136/gutjnl-2012-304258.

### 13. E. Increase dose of IFX

- Therapeutic drug monitoring can help establish cause of secondary loss of response to anti-TNF therapy
- Low trough anti-TNF levels with absence of antibodies is most likely due to inadequate dosing
- Clinical relapse despite adequate trough levels and the absence of anti-TNF antibodies may represent inflammation driven by TNF-independent pathways, and switching medication class should be considered

When a patient develops symptoms suggestive of secondary loss of response, the clinician must first assess compliance and then assess whether symptoms are attributable to active IBD. This often necessitates a combination of endoscopy, CRP, faecal calprotectin, and imaging. Once inflammation is confirmed and other causes of symptoms have been excluded, therapeutic drug monitoring can help establish the reason for loss of response. In patients with subtherapeutic anti-TNF levels and the absence of antibodies, the most likely cause of symptoms is inadequate dosing and dose intensification may be tried. If antibodies are detected, immunogenicity may be causing the loss of response and therefore switching to an alternative anti-TNF agent or adding an immunomodulator are suitable options. Patients with adequate trough levels and absence of antibodies may have inflammation not driven by TNF-mediated pathways, and therefore switching to a drug with a different mechanism of action may improve control of disease activity.

Roda G et al. Loss of response to anti-TNFs: definition, epidemiology, and management. *Clin Transl Gastroenterol.* 2016 Jan;7(1):e135. Doi: 10.1038/ctg.2015.63.

### 14. B. 1 in 300

- Azathioprine is an immunomodulator commonly prescribed for steroid refractory/dependent IBD
- Azathioprine use is associated with a two- to five-fold increased incidence of lymphoma
- Given the increased risks of lymphoma, myelosuppression and hepatotoxicity, caution is advised in the prescription of azathioprine in older patients

Azathioprine is a prodrug used as an immunomodulator in IBD. It exerts its immunosuppressive effect via metabolism to the active compound 6-thioguanine, which inhibits purine and protein synthesis in lymphocytes. Indications in IBD include the requirement of ≥2 courses of oral corticosteroids within a 12-month period. A therapeutic response is typically observed after three months.

Azathioprine is metabolized to mercaptopurine, which is subsequently metabolized to three compounds:

1. 6-methyl-mercaptopurine (inactive), catalysed by thiopurine methyltransferase (TPMT)
2. Thiourate (inactive), catalysed by xanthine oxidase
3. 6-thioguanine nucleotides (active metabolite), catalysed by hypoxanthine-guanine-phosphoribosyltransferase

Approximately 11% of people have low TPMT activity and 0.3% have negligible activity, risking toxic accumulation of 6-thioguanine and subsequent myelosuppression. Similarly, caution should be used in the prescription of xanthine oxidase inhibitors (e.g. allopurinol, febuxostat).

Approximately 25% of patients treated with thiopurines develop side effects (Table 7.3)

**Table 7.3** Side effects of thiopurines

| Dose dependent | Dose independent |
|---|---|
| • Bone marrow suppression<br>• Hepatotoxicity: acute (transaminitis or acute cholestatic injury) or chronic (nodular regenerative hyperplasia, veno-occlusive disease, or peliosis hepatitis) | • Gastrointestinal intolerance: nausea, vomiting, and anorexia<br>• Pancreatitis<br>• Non-melanoma skin cancer<br>• Lymphoma |

There is a two- to five-fold increased risk of lymphoma in IBD patients treated with thiopurines. Co-prescription with an anti-TNF agent (e.g. IFX) increases this risk further. Importantly, lymphoma risk decreases upon discontinuation.

Yearly lymphoma incidence increases with advancing age. In the 70–74 year age group, it is approximately 1 in 1,000 in the general population, increasing to 1 in 300 for those on azathioprine. Given the additional increased risk of liver toxicity and myelosuppression with advancing age, azathioprine in elderly patients should be used with caution.

Kotlyar DS, Lewis JD et al. Risk of lymphoma in patients with inflammatory bowel disease treated with azathioprine and 6-mercaptopurine: a meta-analysis. *Clin Gastroenterol Hepatol.* 2015 May;13(5):847–858.e4. Doi: 10.1016/j.cgh.2014.05.015.

## 15. C. Intravenous ciclosporin (2 mg/kg per day)

- The Oxford day 3 criteria predict failure to respond to intravenous corticosteroids
- Those meeting the criteria have an 85% chance of coming to colectomy
- IFX and ciclosporin have similar efficacy as rescue therapies

This patient has ASUC as defined by the Truelove and Witts criteria:

Bloody stool frequency of ≥ 6 per day plus any of

- Tachycardia (>90 bpm)
- Temperature (>37.8°C)
- Haemoglobin <10.5 g/dL
- Elevated ESR (or CRP) >30

The Oxford day 3 criteria predicts failure to respond to intravenous corticosteroids by assessing stool frequency and/or CRP at day three.

- Stool frequency ≥ 9 or
- CRP ≥ 45 mg/L and a stool frequency of 3–8 per 24 hours

Those meeting these criteria have an 85% chance of coming to colectomy during that admission. Prolonged intravenous corticosteroids are unhelpful. Instead, second-line ('rescue') therapy is required. Ciclosporin and IFX are both recognized rescue therapies with placebo-controlled evidence supporting their use and RCTs demonstrating similar efficacy (Table 7.4).

**Table 7.4** Choice of rescue therapy in acute severe ulcerative colitis

| Factors favouring infliximab | Factors favouring ciclosporin |
|---|---|
| • Hypocholesterolaemia (<3 mmol/L) or hypomagnesaemia (<0.5 mmol/L)—increased risk of neurotoxicity with ciclosporin <br> • Hyperkalaemia or hypertension <br> • Epilepsy <br> • Renal/hepatic impairment | • Shorter half-life—if more likely to need colectomy; will clear the system quicker <br> • Azathioprine-naïve patients <br> • History of tuberculosis, Hepatitis B, multiple sclerosis or heart failure (NYHA III or IV) |

NYHA: New York Heart Association

IFX is relatively contraindicated in this elderly patient with severe heart failure. Older patients requiring emergency colectomy have poorer surgical outcomes. Ciclosporin (2 mg/kg intravenous infusion over six hours) as a bridge to thiopurines or vedolizumab is the best option here. Vedolizumab is a particularly attractive option in older patients because it provides gut-specific immunosuppression and negates the risk of systemic immunosuppression and malignancy seen with anti-TNFs and thiopurines.

Travis S et al. Predicting the need for colectomy in severe ulcerative colitis: a critical appraisal of clinical parameters and currently available biomarkers. *Gut.* 2011 Jan;60(1):3–9. Doi: 10.1136/gut.2010.216895.

### 16. A. Mesalazine enema

- Mesalazine suppositories are effective for proctitis but may be ineffective for disease extending beyond 10 cm when liquid enemas are preferred
- Patients who cannot retain enemas because of rectal irritability should be treated with mesalazine foam preparations
- Topical steroids should be prescribed to patients who have an inadequate response, or who are intolerant to topical mesalazine

Topical mesalazine (5-aminosalicylic acid or 5-ASA) is first-line induction and maintenance therapy for proctitis. The remission rate can be as high as 90% and provides a quicker response than oral preparations. Mesalazine suppositories are effective for proctitis. However, their use in more proximal disease is limited by insufficient spread of active drug beyond the rectum. For active disease beyond 10 cm, mesalazine liquid enemas can have therapeutic benefit up to the splenic flexure. It is important to recognize patient acceptability of topical preparations and adherence may be limited by retention discomfort, prolonged bed rest, or difficulties in self-administration. Rectal mesalazine foam enemas may be better tolerated.

Two meta-analyses concluded that topical mesalazine is more effective than topical steroids in achieving clinical, endoscopic, and histological remission. Topical steroids should be prescribed to patients who have an inadequate response, or who are intolerant to topical mesalazine.

Combined therapy has been shown to work more effectively than oral or topical mesalazine therapy alone. Given that this patient has mildly active proctosigmoiditis with normal bloods, oral mesalazine or steroid therapy are not indicated at present. Refractory proctitis may require treatment with systemic steroids, and immunosuppressive and/or biological therapy.

Bryant R et al. Conventional drug therapy for inflammatory bowel disease. *Scand J Gastroenterol.* 2015 50(1),90–112. Doi: 10.3109/00365521.2014.968864.

## 17. D. Oral ciprofloxacin

- Acute pouchitis is common following ileal pouch anal anastomosis (IPAA) for UC and most patients respond to a short course of oral antibiotics
- Chronic pouchitis is uncommon and alternative causes of pouch dysfunction should be considered
- The probiotic VSL#3 reduces incidence of acute pouchitis one year after surgery and prevents relapse of chronic pouchitis in remission

Proctocolectomy with IPAA is the procedure of choice for patients with UC requiring surgical intervention. This patient has developed acute pouchitis, a non-specific inflammation of the ileal reservoir and the most common complication following IPAA for UC occurring in up to 60% of patients. Pouchitis is rare in patients having IPAA for familial adenomatous polyposis.

Symptoms of pouchitis include increased faecal frequency, abdominal cramping, urgency, tenesmus, and pelvic discomfort. Pouchoscopy with mucosal biopsy is required to confirm the diagnosis. Endoscopic findings include patchy mucosal erythema, friability, loss of vascular pattern, haemorrhage, and erosions. Ninety per cent of acute pouchitis diagnoses respond to a short course of ciprofloxacin or metronidazole with the former having a better side effect profile.

Five to ten per cent of patients develop chronic pouchitis (>4 weeks) requiring longer courses of combined antibiotic therapy with or without oral budesonide. Other causes of pouch dysfunction must be considered including infection, peri-pouch sepsis, pre-pouch ileitis, pouch intussusception, pouch volvulus, and irritable pouch syndrome. Refractory cases of chronic pouchitis may require biologic therapy or surgery.

The probiotic VSL#3 can help prevent relapse of chronic proctitis in remission and reduce incidence of acute pouchitis within the first year after surgery.

Magro F, Gionchetti P et al. Third European evidence-based consensus on diagnosis and management of ulcerative colitis. Part 1: Definitions, diagnosis, extra-intestinal manifestations, pregnancy, cancer surveillance, surgery, and ileo-anal pouch disorders. *J Crohns Colitis.* 2017 Jun;11(6):649–670. Doi: 10.1093/ecco-jcc/jjx008.

## 18. D. The evidence base for elemental feed and polymeric diet is similar in CD

- Exclusive enteral nutrition (EEN) is as effective as corticosteroids at inducing remission in paediatric CD populations
- There is no evidence for dietary strategies in UC
- Patients with stricturing CD should consider limiting dietary fibre intake

In CD, EEN has been shown to be as effective as corticosteroids at inducing remission (73% of paediatric populations). There is a paucity of robust evidence for EEN as a therapeutic strategy in adults. However, some evidence suggests that it can be effective at inducing remission even in the presence of complications. Therefore, when tolerated, EEN has a role when corticosteroid avoidance is desired. The efficacy of elemental feed and a polymeric diet in CD is similar.

Evidence for a low-residue diet in stricturing CD is lacking, although it is a safe and common-sense measure. Supplementation with enteral or parenteral nutrition may be required to meet nutritional requirements. There is no evidence for total parenteral nutrition to induce remission in CD as a sole therapy or adjunct.

There is no evidence for dietary strategies in UC. However, there is evidence for the use of the probiotic VSL#3 in pouchitis, and some evidence for its role in the maintenance and treatment of UC. *E. coli* Nissle 1917 has a similar efficacy to mesalazine for UC remission maintenance.

Lamb C et al. BSG consensus guidelines on the management of inflammatory bowel disease in adults. *Gut.* 2019;0:1–106. Doi: 10.1136/gutjnl-2019-318484.

## 19. E. Obesity

- Obesity at baseline is predictive of low adalimumab drug concentrations at week 14
- Concomitant immunomodulator use significantly reduces immunogenicity

The personalised anti-TNF therapy in CD (PANTS) was a prospective, observational UK-wide study enrolling anti-TNF naïve patients (aged ≥6 years) with active luminal CD. Patients received either IFX or adalimumab and were evaluated for 12 months or until drug withdrawal. Demographic data, disease phenotype, previous medical and Crohn's related surgeries were recorded. At every visit, disease activity, adverse events (AEs), drug and total anti-drug antibody concentrations were also measured. Treatment failure endpoints included primary non-response (PNR) at week 14, non-remission at week 54, and AEs leading to drug withdrawal.

PNR occurred in 23.8% (n=1,241) of patients and non-remission at week 54 occurred in 63.1% (n=1,211). The only factor independently associated with PNR was low drug concentration at week 14 (IFX: OR 0.35 [95% CI 6.9–19.9], p=0.00038; adalimumab: 0.13 [0.06–0.28], p<0.0001); the optimal week 14 drug concentrations associated with remission at both weeks 14 and 54 were 7 mg/L for IFX and 12 mg/L for adalimumab.

The proportion of patients who developed anti-drug antibodies (immunogenicity) was higher for IFX than adalimumab (62.8% and 28.5%, respectively). For both drugs, suboptimal week 14 drug concentrations predicted immunogenicity, and the development of anti-drug antibodies predicted subsequent low drug concentrations. Combination immunomodulator significantly mitigated the risk of developing anti-drug antibodies and was the main protective factor against immunogenicity.

In multivariable analyses, lower albumin concentrations at week 14 were independently associated with week 14 drug concentration for IFX, whereas obesity was independently associated with week 14 and 54 drug concentrations for adalimumab. Time to immunogenicity was associated with smoking for IFX-treated patients. Male sex and disease duration were not significantly associated with low drug concentrations.

Kennedy NA, Heap GA et al. Predictors of anti-TNF treatment failure in anti-TNF-naïve patients with active luminal Crohn's disease: a prospective, multicentre, cohort study. *Lancet Gastroenterol Hepatol.* 2019;4(5):341–353. Doi: 10.1016/S2468-1253(19)30012-3.

## 20. D. Referral for ileocaecal resection

- ECCO guidelines advise that surgery is the preferred option in patients with localized ileocaecal CD with obstructive symptoms but no significant active inflammation
- In extensive disease with long strictured bowel segments where resection would compromise the effective small bowel length, non-conventional strictureplasties may be attempted

An ileocaecal resection is most appropriate in a fibrotic Crohn's stricture without evidence of active inflammation. Endoscopic dilatation +/- stenting is generally reserved for accessible strictures <5 cm.

Patients who have lost ≥10% body mass in a three-month period are considered significantly malnourished to benefit from pre-operative nutritional optimization to reduce post-operative complications. In patients requiring surgery (usually as an emergency) while significantly malnourished, a staged procedure, which includes resection of the diseased segment with formation of a stoma, followed by delayed restoration of continuity, is recommended. Early ambulation and extended VTE prophylaxis are also recommended for 28 days in patients with IBD post-operatively.

Bemelman et al. ECCO-ESCP consensus on surgery for Crohn's Disease. *J Crohns Colitis.* 2018 Jan 5;12(1):1–16. Doi: 10.1093/ecco-jcc/jjx061.

### 21. D. Hypomagnesaemia

- 'Toxic megacolon' is defined as total or segmental non-obstructive dilatation of the colon (diameter of ≥ 5.5 cm or caecum >9 cm), associated with systemic toxicity
- Magnesium deficiency exacerbates potassium wasting by increasing distal potassium secretion
- Daily potassium replacement of at least 60 mmol/L is necessary in ASUC

'Toxic megacolon' is defined as total or segmental non-obstructive dilatation of the colon >5.5 cm diameter or >9 cm in the caecum alongside systemic toxicity. Risk factors include hypokalaemia, hypomagnesaemia, bowel preparation, opioids, non-steroidal anti-inflammatory drugs, anti-cholinergics, and anti-diarrhoeals.

Early diagnosis and treatment of ASUC reduces the incidence of toxic megacolon. Toxic megacolon increases the risk of perforation where colectomy has been inappropriately delayed, and carries a mortality risk of up to 50%.

Intravenous fluids and electrolyte replacement are required in the management of ASUC to prevent dehydration and electrolyte imbalance. Potassium supplementation of at least 60 mmol/day is necessary. Magnesium deficiency is frequently associated with hypokalaemia. Magnesium deficiency exacerbates potassium wasting by increasing distal luminal potassium secretion.

Autenrieth DM, Baumgart DC. Toxic megacolon. *Inflamm Bowel Dis.* 2012 Mar;18(3):584–591. Doi: 10.1002/ibd.21847.

### 22. D. MRI pelvis

- Diagnosis of axial arthritis in IBD requires clinical features of inflammatory low back pain alongside MRI findings
- 20%–50% of IBD patients have radiological evidence of sacroiliitis but progressive disease occurs in only 1%–10%
- A multidisciplinary approach and early consideration of anti-TNF therapy is preferential for those who are refractory to, or intolerant of, NSAIDS

Radiological evidence of sacroiliitis is observed in 20%–50% of IBD patients but progressive, destructive ankylosing spondylitis occurs in only 1%–10%. Conversely, 70% of patients with idiopathic ankylosing spondylitis have microscopic evidence of gut inflammation but with evolution to IBD occurring in only 7%. Diagnosis of axial spondyloarthritis in IBD is based on the clinical features of inflammatory low back pain associated with MRI or radiographic features of sacroiliitis. MRI is the best imaging modality with the ability to identify inflammation prior to bony abnormalities. The ECCO guidelines recommend early MRI assessment for patients aged <40 years with back pain lasting more than three months. The association of HLA-B27 with axial spondylarthritis is seen in IBD, but to a lesser degree than in idiopathic AS [≈70% vs 94%] making it a less reliable diagnostic test.

Short-term treatment for axial arthritis includes physiotherapy and NSAIDs. However, NSAIDs are not a long-term option in IBD so patients with axial arthritis should be jointly managed with a rheumatologist.

Harbord M et al. The first European evidence-based consensus on extra-intestinal manifestations in inflammatory bowel disease. *J Crohns Colitis.* 2016 Mar;10(3):239–254. Doi: 10.1093/ecco-jcc/jjv213.

### 23. E. Lesions are often precipitated by trauma (pathergy)

- PG occurs in approximately 0.6%–2.1% patients with UC
- PG is one of the EIMs of IBD not classically associated with disease activity

- Treatment of moderate to severe PG includes systemic immunosuppression (corticosteroids and/or anti-TNF therapy)

The lesion (Fig. 7.1) is most in keeping with PG. PG is one of the neutrophilic dermatoses (a group that also includes erythema nodosum and Sweet's syndrome). PG can present as single or multiple erythematous papules or pustules. If untreated, necrosis of the dermis leads to development of deep ulcers (which can expose tendons and bone) containing purulent, but usually sterile, material. PG lesions occur most commonly on the shins or around a surgical stoma. It is seen more commonly in UC (0.6%–2.1% of patients) than CD, and is one of the EIMs of IBD not classically associated with disease activity. Other EIMs independent of disease activity include anterior uveitis, type 2 peripheral arthropathy, and primary sclerosing cholangitis (PSC). PG is more common in young to middle-aged adults, and has a slight female preponderance. Lesions often occur at sites of trauma (pathergy).

The aim of treatment is to achieve rapid healing prior to significant deep ulceration. In mild disease, topical agents such as corticosteroids or tacrolimus (0.03%–0.3% strength) can be used. Moderate to severe disease may require systemic immunosuppression including corticosteroids, ciclosporin, and/or anti-TNF therapy. A recent RCT demonstrated a 90% response rate with IFX in PG lesions.

Harbord M, Annese V et al. First European evidence-based consensus on extra-intestinal manifestations in inflammatory bowel disease. *J Crohns Colitis.* 2016 Mar;10(3):239–254. Doi: 10.1093/ecco-jcc/jjv213.

### 24. A. Cessation of azathioprine and prescribing of intravenous antibiotics

- Immunomodulator therapy should be temporarily withheld until the resolution of active infection

The ECCO guidelines state that this patient should be managed with intravenous antibiotics and percutaneous or surgical drainage (if amenable), followed by consideration of a delayed surgical resection. In this case, it is likely that the abscess is too small to drain, even percutaneously.

This patient has active disease that requires treatment. However, there is no consensus as to when it is safe to start further immunosuppression. The ECCO guidelines support withholding immunomodulator therapy temporarily until the resolution of active infection.

Rahier JF, Magro F et al. Second European evidence-based consensus on the prevention, diagnosis and management of opportunistic infections in inflammatory bowel disease. *J Crohns Colitis.* 2014;8:443–468. Doi: 10.1016/j.crohns.2013.12.013.

### 25. E. Sweet's syndrome

- Sweet's syndrome is a type of acute neutrophilic dermatosis
- It is a rare EIM of IBD
- It is associated with female gender, colonic disease, and other EIMs

This patient described the onset of an acute febrile illness associated with pathergy at the immunization site—this is Sweet's syndrome. Sweet's syndrome, also known as 'acute febrile neutrophilic dermatosis' was first described by Robert Sweet in 1964. It is characterized by rapidly evolving tender, red inflammatory papules, usually affecting the upper limbs, face, or neck, together with a fever. Oral ulcers may be present and a ¼ experience arthralgia.

Sweet's syndrome is associated with pathergy and can occur as a rare EIM of IBD. The rash is associated with active IBD in most. However, it may precede the onset of luminal symptoms. There is a strong female preponderance and predilection for patients with colonic disease and other EIMs.

Investigations:

- Raised inflammatory markers (WCC, ESR, and CRP)
- p-ANCA may be present
- Skin punch biopsy demonstrates a pathognomonic angiocentric, vessel-based dermal neutrophilic infiltrate

Treatment commonly involves topical or systemic corticosteroids with rapid resolution of symptoms. Potassium iodide, colchicine, and dapsone may also have a role. The use of IFX should be considered in resistant cases.

Vaz A, Kramer K et al. Sweet's syndrome in association with Crohn's disease. *Postgrad Med J.* 2000;76(901):713–714. Doi: 10.1136/pmj.76.901.713.

## 26. B. Episcleritis

- Episcleritis is the most common ocular extraintestinal manifestation of IBD and is associated with disease activity
- Painless visual loss in a patient with IBD could represent posterior uveitis and is an ophthalmological emergency

The history does not mention pain or visual disturbance. Therefore, episcleritis is most likely. Ocular complications of IBD occur in up to 6% of cases. Risk factors for developing ocular involvement include female sex and the presence of an arthropathy in CD. Episcleritis (2%–5%) is the most common ocular EIM followed by uveitis (0.5%–3.5%).

Episcleritis is a painless hyperaemia of the sclera without visual disturbance. It appears to be more associated with disease activity when compared with other ocular EIMs. It is usually self-limiting. If not, it responds to topical corticosteroids, analgesics, and effective treatment of intestinal disease.

Scleritis is inflammation of deep scleral vessels, causing erythema, ocular pain, and visual disturbance. It is characteristically worse at night. Systemic treatment is required, usually with NSAIDs (with caution in active IBD), systemic steroids, or immunosuppressants.

'Uveitis' is defined as inflammation of the uveal tract, middle layer of the eye and choroid. It can be anterior, affecting the iris with or without the ciliary body, posterior, affecting the choroid and the retina, or intermediate between the ciliary body and the retina. Anterior uveitis is the most common and has a more insidious onset. Uveitis runs a course independent of intestinal disease, and presents as an acute painful eye, with visual disturbance that can progress to blindness if it is not managed promptly with corticosteroids and, if refractory, with ciclosporin, thiopurines, or anti-TNF agents. Urgent referral to an ophthalmologist is required.

Troncoso L, Biancardi A et al. Ophthalmic manifestations in patients with inflammatory bowel disease: a review. *World J Gastroenterol.* 2017;23(32):5836–5848. Doi: 10.3748/wjg.v23.i32.5836.

## 27. E. Patients with previous intestinal resection

- Iron supplementation is recommended in all IBD patients when IDA is present
- Ferritin <30 μg/L (in absence of inflammation) and <100 μg/L (in presence of inflammation) is indicative of iron deficiency

Anaemia is the most common extraintestinal manifestation of IBD. Iron deficiency accounts for the majority of cases. The impact of anaemia on quality of life is significant. Identification, investigation, and treatment of anaemia is important. Development of anaemia may relate to disease activity and/ or complications of IBD. A complete full blood count, CRP, and iron studies are required to detect anaemia. Interpretation of the ferritin level is important in the context of inflammation. In the absence of inflammation, a ferritin <30 µg/L is consistent with iron deficiency. However, in the presence of inflammation (biochemical or clinical), serum ferritin levels may be high despite empty iron stores.

Intravenous iron should be considered as first-line treatment in IBD patients with iron deficiency and:

- clinically active disease
- Hb <100 g/L
- previous intolerance to oral iron
- those who need erythropoiesis-stimulating agents

Previous intestinal resection is not an indication for intravenous iron first line. One must consider alternative causes for anaemia, such as B12 and folate deficiency, in patients with extensive small bowel resection.

Intravenous iron is safe, effective, and well tolerated in IBD patients. The goal of iron supplementation is to normalize haemoglobin levels and iron stores. The estimation of iron need is based on baseline haemoglobin and body weight.

Dignass A, Gasche C et al. European consensus on the diagnosis and management of iron deficiency and anaemia in inflammatory bowel diseases. *J Crohns Colitis*. 2015 Mar;9(3):211–222. Doi: 10.1093/ecco-jcc/jju009.

## 28. A. He is overdue a colonoscopy by one year

- Screening colonoscopy should be performed 10 years after the onset of disease
- Higher-risk patients require annual surveillance
- Risk of colitis-associated colorectal cancer (CACRC) increases with time

The British Society of Gastroenterology guidelines recommend a screening colonoscopy after 10 years of disease (dated from the time of symptom onset, not diagnosis), ideally while in remission. Pan-colonic dye spraying with targeted biopsy of abnormal areas is recommended. If dye spray is unavailable, two to four random biopsies should be performed every 10 cm of the colon and rectum. The surveillance interval is determined by the latest endoscopic and histological findings.

Extensive colitis with moderate activity warrants annual surveillance according to guidelines. The risk of (CACRC) increases with time (8% and 16% after 20 and 30 years, respectively). The presence of persistent histological inflammation is a substantial driver of risk. This patient should have had a screening colonoscopy the previous year. His family history does not affect his surveillance interval as they are non-FDRs.

Cairns SR et al. Guidelines for colorectal cancer screening and surveillance in moderate and high risk groups. *Gut*. 2010 May;59(5):666–689. Doi: 10.1136/gut.2009.179804.

## 29.  D. Risk factors associated with UC-related CRC include pancolitis and male sex

- CRC risk is highest in UC patients with dysplasia on colonic biopsies
- Risk factors for UC-related CRC include male sex, young age of disease onset, and extensive disease
- Patients with IBD diagnosed with CRC are younger than non-IBD-related CRC patients

Patients with IBD are at an increased risk of developing CRC. CRC risk is highest in patients with UC with dysplasia on colonic biopsies. Disease duration and extent, family history of CRC, and the presence of PSC in UC are strictly related to CRC risk. Risk factors for UC-related CRC include male sex, young age of disease onset, and extensive colitis. PSC is a major risk factor for CRC in IBD patients, more so in UC. PSC–UC patients are five times more likely to develop CRC.

Although the prevalence of cancer is increasing, the risk of dying from CRC has decreased. The excess CRC risk for those with CD is 1.9 and UC 2.4 [standardized international ratio]. CRC patients with IBD tend to be younger at cancer diagnosis than their non-IBD counterparts.

Annese V, Beaugerie L et al. European evidence-based consensus: inflammatory bowel disease and malignancies. *J Crohns Colitis*. 2015, 945–965. Doi: 10.1093/ecco-jcc/jjv141.

## 30.  A. A joint paediatric-adult clinic, as part of a transition programme, is the ideal model

- Transition is the purposeful, planned movement of adolescents to adult-orientated health care
- Education of patients should be age-appropriate and addressed at least one year before transfer
- Transfer to adult care preferably occurs during stable remission

'Transition' is defined as the purposeful, planned movement of adolescents with chronic medical conditions into adult-orientated healthcare systems. The point of handover of care is referred to as 'transfer'. Transfer should be considered a part of, and not necessarily the end of, transition.

Paediatric and adult IBD services may be separated by hospital and location. A copy of the paediatric notes and/or a detailed written handover from the paediatric team is a vital resource. However, whenever possible, a joint paediatric-adult clinic to facilitate transition is the ideal model. It is recommended that all trusts have a coordinator for planning transitional care, and a defined policy. Transition should be a process that occurs gradually over time, and at a time determined to be appropriate on an individual case-by-case basis. In adult services, patients are expected to take responsibility for their own health care, and will be expected to ask questions and represent themselves. This can present a challenge for patients and parents alike, and should be managed sensitively.

Personal development is a key element of paediatric care and is often overlooked by adult gastroenterologists. Sexual development and maturation may be delayed in adolescents with IBD. Discussion regarding the impact of IBD on young people's development, psychosocial, physical, and sexual, should be made available in adult services.

Van Rheenen P, Aloi M et al. ECCO topical review on transitional care in inflammatory bowel disease. *J Crohns Colitis*, 2017;1032–1038. Doi: 10.1093/ecco-jcc/jjx010.

### 31. A. Continue current medications

- One third of pregnant patients with IBD think their medication is harmful to their unborn child
- Active inflammation in pregnancy is associated with low birthweight and preterm delivery
- Azathioprine and mesalazine are safe to use in pregnancy

IBD is highly prevalent in young individuals and reproductive issues frequently arise. Patients with IBD voluntarily have fewer children than the general population because negative views about foetal health and fertility. Over a third of pregnant patients consider their IBD medication harmful to their unborn children. Young women with IBD should therefore be offered routine education and counselling about pregnancy-related issues. Controlling disease activity is important to foetal health with moderate–severe activity linked to low birthweight and pre-term delivery.

Thiopurines (azathioprine and 6-mercaptopurione) can cross the placenta and metabolites can be determined in foetal red blood cells. While there are cases of low birthweight, spontaneous miscarriage, and preterm birth, meta-analysis of controlled trials has reported no increased risk for adverse pregnancy outcome in IBD patients treated during pregnancy with thiopurines. Furthermore, following up children exposed to thiopurines *in utero* has revealed no developmental or immunologic abnormalities at four years. Thiopurines are therefore considered safe to use in pregnancy. Low-dose excretion occurs into breast milk for four hours following ingestion. Therefore, consider advising expressing and wasting milk during this time period.

5-ASAs can be continued safely in pregnancy with meta-analyses demonstrating no increased risk for miscarriage or preterm birth. One study has shown a slight increased rate of congenital abnormalities with 5-ASA although it is likely confounded by the effect of active CD. Sulfasalazine treatment interferes with folate absorption. Therefore, supplementation with higher dose folic acid (2 mg/day of folate) is recommended.

van der Woude CJ et al. European Crohn's and Colitis Organization. The second European evidenced-based consensus on reproduction and pregnancy in inflammatory bowel disease. *J Crohns Colitis*. 2015 Feb;9(2):107–124. Doi: 10.1016/j.crohns.2010.07.004.

### 32. E. Stop at end of second trimester (approx. 26 weeks' gestation) if remains in disease remission.

- Active IBD is associated with preterm birth and low birthweight—therefore, conception during disease remission is advised
- If anti-TNF therapy is stopped in the third trimester or continued beyond the second trimester, the baby should avoid live vaccines for at least the first six months of life

It is important to defer pregnancy, whenever possible, until disease remission is achieved because active IBD is associated with preterm birth and low birthweight. A third of patients in disease remission will flare during pregnancy, similar to non-pregnant patients over the same time period. Active disease should be treated aggressively during pregnancy, noting that, with the exception of methotrexate, IBD medications are not proven to be associated with adverse pregnancy outcomes or congenital abnormalities.

Anti-TNF agents cross the placenta and remain detectable within the baby 2–7 months after discontinuation. To limit the transport of anti-TNF to the foetus, therapy is best discontinued around gestational weeks 24–26, unless maternal disease activity indicates that it should be continued. This is a matter for careful discussion between an experienced IBD specialist and the parents. When anti-TNF therapy is continued beyond the second trimester or stopped in the third trimester, the baby should avoid live vaccinations (e.g. rotavirus, MMR, and chickenpox vaccines) until at least six months after birth.

The combination of thiopurine and anti-TNF treatment during pregnancy has been shown to increase infections during the first year of childhood (RR 1.5, 95% CI 1.08–2.09).

van der Woude CJ, Ardizzone S et al. The second European evidenced-based consensus on reproduction and pregnancy in inflammatory bowel disease. *J Crohns Colitis*. 2015, 107–124. Doi: 10.1093/ecco-jcc/jju006.

### 33. B. Immunotherapy-associated colitis

- Immunotherapy-associated colitis can happen weeks after immunotherapy (median seven weeks)
- Endoscopic appearances may be variable; biopsies should be taken even in the absence of macroscopic colitis
- Prompt treatment with steroids is paramount

The history of combination immunotherapy and timescale to onset of diarrhoea makes immunotherapy-associated colitis the most likely diagnosis. Immunotherapy works by inhibiting the checkpoints of the immune system. Gastrointestinal immune-related adverse effects (GI-irAE) are commonly recognized. Checkpoint inhibitors are used to treat cancers including metastatic melanoma and lung cancer. The risk of immunotherapy-associated colitis is increased in patients receiving combination versus single agent therapy.

Diarrhoea is the most common symptom of GI-irAE, but patients may also report abdominal pain, nausea or vomiting, and rectal bleeding. Median onset of diarrhoea is 5–7 weeks. Baseline investigations should include bloods and faecal MC&S/CDT. Early sigmoidoscopy with biopsy in the acute setting is recommended. The endoscopic picture (Fig. 7.9) can vary in terms of

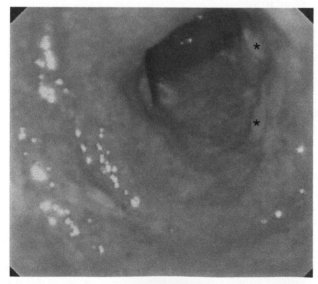

**Fig. 7.9** Flexible sigmoidoscopy image showing complete loss of vascular pattern and erosions (black asterisk) in the sigmoid colon

Image courtesy of Dr Vincent Cheung, Oxford University Hospitals NHS Foundation Trust distribution of colitis, presence of erosions/ulcers, loss of vascular pattern, and bleeding. Cases without macroscopic inflammation can have microscopic inflammation and present with severe clinical features. If nausea, vomiting, and anorexia predominate, then an gastroscopy with biopsies is indicated to rule out isolated immunotherapy-related gastritis.

Moderate to severe immunotherapy-associated colitis warrants prompt treatment. Delay in treatment may lead to death with intestinal perforation (1% of patients treated with high-dose ipilimumab). Treatment includes prednisolone 0.5–1 mg/kg/day or, in severe cases, intravenous methylprednisolone 1 mg/kg/day. If there is no improvement within 3–5 days, then IFX 5 mg/kg should be considered, which can be repeated two weeks later if needed).

Soularue E, Lepage P et al. Enterocolitis due to immune checkpoint inhibitors: a systematic review. *Gut.* 2018 Nov;67(11):2056–2067. Doi: 10.1136/gutjnl-2018-316948.

## 34. B. Ischaemic colitis

- Ischaemic colitis may result in systemic inflammatory response syndrome (SIRS)
- Fluid resuscitation is important in ischaemic colitis to prevent shock, which can lead to multiorgan failure
- Surgery may be considered if there is radiological evidence of perforation, generalized peritonitis, or continuing haemorrhage

The acute onset makes IBD and NSAID-induced colitis less likely. Recent antibiotics increase the risk of *Clostridioides difficile*-associated diarrhoea. However, there are no pseudomembranes to suggest pseudomembranous colitis. The endoscopic appearances, together with the risk factors of hypertension and atrial fibrillation, make ischaemic colitis the most likely diagnosis.

Causes can be physiological (e.g. heart failure, atherosclerosis, SIRS, atrial fibrillation, concurrent malignancy) or iatrogenic (e.g. pharmacological [chemotherapy, sex hormones, cardiac glycosides, interferon, diuretics, vasopressors, statins], abdominal aortic aneurysm repair, or bowel preparation for colonoscopy).

Raised serum lactate results from hypoperfusion and systemic dysfunction rather than indicating gastrointestinal ischaemia *per se*. It is, nonetheless, useful for monitoring progress during resuscitation.

Factors associated with severity that may not resolve with conservative treatment include:

- Right-sided distribution of colitis
- Male sex
- Lack of rectal bleeding
- Renal dysfunction
- Colonic strictures
- Peritonitis

The endoscopic image of the sigmoid colon in the question (Fig. 7.3) shows pale mucosa, longitudinal ulceration, and pseudopolyps.

Brandt LJ et al. ACG clinical guideline: epidemiology, risk factors, patterns of presentation, diagnosis, and management of colon ischemia. *Am J Gastroenterol.* 2015 Jan;110(1):18–44. Doi: 10.1038/ajg.2014.395.

### 35. E. Short-chain fatty acid enemas (SCFAs)

- Diversion colitis may occur early or late post-defunctioning
- Of those with histological evidence, only up to one third have symptoms
- Treatment may involve SCFA enemas, corticosteroid, or mesalazine enemas. Restoration of gut continuity is the only definitive treatment.

The diagnosis of diversion colitis can occur within a few months or after three years following defunctioning. The majority of patients have histological evidence, but it is not mandatory for the diagnosis. Of those with histological evidence, only up to one third have symptoms. Symptoms may include tenesmus, anorectal pain, mucous discharge, and rectal bleeding.

Diversion colitis is thought to occur as a result of deficiency of SCFAs. Unabsorbed carbohydrates entering the colon are metabolized by bacteria to SCFAs, such as butyric acid, that provide nutrition for the colonic mucosa. Butyrate is an oxidative substrate for colonocytes. Evidence suggests that SCFAs relax vascular smooth muscle and their deficiencies may result in a relative ischaemia to colorectal mucosa. Diversion colitis may therefore respond to SCFA enema treatment. Corticosteroid enemas and mesalazine may also have a role. Treatment is not urgent because many cases resolve spontaneously.

This patient has quiescent CD. Therefore, medical therapy is not indicated. Surgical options should also be considered. Restoration of continuity and faecal stream provides definitive treatment.

Tominaga K, Kamimura K et al. Diversion colitis and pouchitis: a mini-review. *World J Gastroenterol.* 2018;24(16):1734–1747. Doi: 10.3748/wjg.v24.i16.1734.

### 36. D. Preservation of crypt architecture

- Right-sided and transverse colon biopsies give the highest diagnostic yield in microscopic colitis
- An increase in the colonic mucosal subepithelial collagen layer is indicative of collagenous colitis
- Treatment with budesonide is effective although a third may relapse

Microscopic colitis can be divided into two subgroups—collagenous and lymphocytic colitis. Presentation is with watery, secretory, non-bloody diarrhoea. Onset can be sudden or gradual. Medications including proton pump inhibitors (PPIs), NSAIDs, and Selective Serotonin Reuptake Inhibitor (SSRIs) are common causes. Forty per cent of patients may have concomitant autoimmune disease such as coeliac disease or thyroid dysfunction.

Diagnosis is based on histology. Macroscopic findings at colonoscopy will be normal. Pancolonic biopsies need to be taken because there is a significant false-negative rate (40%) if only the left colon is biopsied. Right-sided and transverse colon biopsies give the highest yield.

*Histological findings*

- Collagenous colitis:
  - Intact crypt architecture
  - Increase in the colonic mucosal subepithelial collagen layer
  - A collagen band >10 μm thick, usually type I or III collagen, rather than type IV (normal measurement 2–5 μm)
- Lymphocytic colitis:
  - Increased numbers of intraepithelial lymphocytes
  - Absence of increased subepithelial collagen layer
  - >20 lymphocytes per 100 epithelial cells

By contrast, the histological lymphocyte count in normal, IBD, and infectious colitis specimens is 4–5 lymphocytes per 100 epithelial cells.

Management includes removal of offending medication, whenever possible, and investigation for co-existent coeliac disease. For mild symptoms, anti-diarrhoeal agents such as loperamide can be used first and, if symptoms are severe, a course of budesonide may help. However, if corticosteroids are ineffective, other therapies such as 5-ASAs and thiopurines may be required. The patient can be reassured that, although relapse may occur, there is no association with the development of malignancy: colonoscopic surveillance is not necessary.

Boland K, Nguyen G. Microscopic colitis: a review of collagenous and lymphocytic colitis. *Gastroenterol Hepatol (N Y)*. 2017 Nov;13(11): 671–677. PMID: 29230146.

## 37. E. 96%

- Glutamate dehydrogenase (GDH) antigen testing is a rapid screening tool that determines whether a patient is colonized with *Clostridioides difficile* or not

*Clostridioides difficile (C. difficile)* is a gram-positive bacillus that colonizes the gut following transmission via the faecal–oral route and disruption of the gut flora, usually following a course of antibiotics. There is a relatively high carrier population, especially in hospitals and care institutions.

The organism produces two exotoxins—toxin A (enterotoxin) and toxin B (cytotoxin). These are responsible for the colonic inflammation leading to diarrhoea and potentially pseudomembranous colitis. Certain strains may not produce toxin A, leading to false-negative results.

In clinical practice, several different laboratory tests are available to diagnose *C. difficile*. Different laboratory tests are often used in combination to confirm the diagnosis.

### Glutamate dehydrogenase (GDH) antigen testing

- GDH is an enzyme produced by all strains of *C. difficile*, whether toxin or non-toxin producing. A rapid test that determines whether a patient is colonized or not, in view of its high negative predictive value (98.4%–100%), it serves as a rapid screening test. The overall sensitivity of the GDH assay is 96%.
- Another initial screening test is the *nucleic acid amplification test (NAAT)*; if either are positive, further analysis can be performed.

### Cytotoxin testing

- This can follow a positive GDH screening test to determine whether or not the strain of *C. difficile* is toxin producing. This can be done by means of the following:
  - *Cell culture cytotoxicity assay*: High sensitivity although it is expensive and time consuming. If positive, however, it does not require a second confirmatory test.
  - *Enzyme immunoassay (EIA)*: Detect toxins A and B. It is quicker and simpler than the cytotoxin assay, but has a higher rate of false negatives.
  - *Polymerase chain reaction*: Rapid test with high sensitivity and specificity.

### Anaerobic faecal culture

- This is not routinely used: it takes a long time to obtain results, and it does not differentiate between toxin- and non-toxin-producing strains.

A positive cell-culture cytotoxin assay as a stand-alone test can confirm the diagnosis.

Guery B, Galperine T et al. Clostridioides difficile: diagnosis and treatments. *BMJ*. 2019 Aug;20;366:l4609. Doi: 10.1136/bmj.l4609.

### 38. C. Ivermectin

- Peripheral blood eosinophilia is indicative of strongyloidiasis
- Larva currens—a migratory, pruritic rash is pathognomonic of chronic infection
- Unlike most intestinal helminth infections, strongyloidiasis can be chronic

This patient is suffering from strongyloidiasis due to infection with the nematode, *Strongyloides stercoralis*. Although common in the tropics or subtropics, *S. stercoralis* is also found in southern Europe and the USA.

*S. stercoralis* infects humans through contact with soil containing the larvae. The life cycle of *S. stercoralis* includes autoinfection via the gastrointestinal tract. Therefore, a state of chronic strongyloidiasis can occur.

Infection with *S. stercoralis* may be asymptomatic (60%) or mild. Chronic infection may give a pathognomonic rash described as '*larva currens*'—a creeping eruption caused by subcutaneous migration of the larvae. It is raised and itchy like a wheal, transient, and usually develops on the trunk of the body. Other symptoms of chronic strongyloidiasis include abdominal pain, intermittent diarrhoea, weight loss, and rarely a dry cough or wheeze if the larvae migrate to the lungs.

Diagnosis is difficult. However, peripheral blood eosinophilia is indicative. Three stool samples for microscopy and *S. stercoralis* serology should be sent from those with a compatible history. Faecal microscopy has a low sensitivity (50%) due to intermittent larval excretion. However, it remains the gold standard.

A rare complication of *S. stercoralis* is hyperinfection syndrome. This occurs when the chronically infected patient becomes immunosuppressed. This triggers widespread dissemination of filariform larvae into tissues, with the risk of bacterial infection as they migrate through the bowel wall. Features may include bloody diarrhoea, bowel perforation, gram-negative septicaemia, pulmonary exudates, or meningoencephalitis.

Treatment is with anti-helminth agents (such as ivermectin) and supportive therapy.

Greaves D, Coggle S et al. Strongyloides stercoralis infection. *BMJ*. 2013;347. Doi: 10.1136/bmj.f4610.

### 39. A. Campylobacter jejuni

- *Campylobacter* is the most common bacterial cause of acute gastroenteritis in Europe
- It typically causes one week of fevers, diarrhoea +/− blood and significant abdominal pain
- *Campylobacter* infection is typically self-limiting although antibiotics have a modest impact on duration of symptoms and may be used in severe cases

In Europe, *Campylobacter* has been the most commonly reported gastrointestinal bacterial pathogen over the past 10 years. This is followed by infection with *Salmonella*, *C difficile*, Shiga-toxin/verocytotoxin-producing *Escherichia coli* (STEC/VTEC) and *Shigella*. Contact with contaminated poultry meat accounts for 80% of cases. Incubation period is three days and acute illness is characterized by seven days of cramping, periumbilical abdominal pain, which may mimic appendicitis, and diarrhoea. Bloody stools are observed in 15% of patients. Late onset complications following *Campylobacter* infection include reactive arthritis (2%) and Guillain-Barré syndrome (0.1%).

Most *Campylobacter* infections are self-limiting requiring supportive management alone. Antibiotics shorten the duration of intestinal symptoms by 1.3 days. However, because of their limited efficacy and antimicrobial resistance, their use should be limited to those with, or at risk of, severe disease (e.g. elderly or immunosuppressed patients). Norovirus is the most common cause of infectious intestinal disease overall, and has a shorter disease course of two days with non-bloody diarrhoea and vomiting. *C difficile* is relatively rare outside a healthcare setting with only 25% of cases diagnosed in the community. Bloody diarrhoea is also uncommon in *C difficile* infection.

European Centre for Disease Prevention and Control. Campylobacteriosis. In: ECDC. Annual epidemiological report for 2016. Stockholm: ECDC; 2018.

### 40. C. Intravenous ganciclovir

- Cytomegalovirus (CMV) colitis is a rare cause of diarrhoea in HIV-infected patients and CD4$^+$ lymphocyte count <50 cells/microlitre
- First line treatment of CMV colitis is with intravenous ganciclovir

CMV gastrointestinal disease is a serious complication of acquired immunodeficiency syndrome (AIDS), occurring at CD4+ <50 cells/microlitre, and it has fortunately become rare in the era of potent antiretroviral therapy (ART). Most clinical disease occurs in individuals previously infected with CMV and represents re-activation of latent infection. CMV colitis is characterized by low-grade fever, weight loss, anorexia, abdominal pain, and debilitating diarrhea. Haemorrhage and perforation can be life-threatening complications. Mucosal ulceration is seen at endoscopy and characteristic intranuclear and intracytoplasmic inclusions are found in histology samples. Most heavily immunosuppressed patients will have positive CMV serology that does not indicate end-organ involvement. Intravenous ganciclovir is the first-line treatment for CMV colitis that can be converted to oral valganciclovir to allow outpatient management typically for 3–6 weeks. Intravenous foscarnet has a significant side effect profile (renal impairment and seizures) but can be used as second-line therapy in cases of ganciclovir toxicity (myelosuppression) or resistance. ART should also be introduced. However, those with comorbid CMV retinitis should receive two weeks of CMV treatment prior to ART to reduce the risk of intraocular inflammation secondary to immune reconstitution. Cryptosporidiosis and disseminated mycobacterium avium complex disease are both causes of diarrhoea in HIV-infected patients, and can be treated with nitazoxanide and clarithromycin plus ethambutol respectively.

Yerushalmy-Feler A, Padlipsky J, Cohen S. Diagnosis and management of CMV colitis. *Curr Infect Dis Rep.* 2019 Feb 15;21(2):5. Doi: 10.1007/s11908-019-0664-y.

### 41. E. No surveillance

- Colonoscopic surveillance is not indicated in patients not meeting criteria for high-risk features at baseline colonoscopy
- The average lead time for progression of an adenoma to cancer is 10 years
- No surveillance is recommended if life expectancy is less than 10 years or if patient is older than 75 years

For further information on this subject, please refer to figure 1 from the British Society of Gastroenterology, the Association of Coloproctology of Great Britain and Ireland and Public Health England published consensus guidelines in 2019 regarding surveillance following adenoma removal. You can find the article in full here: https://www.bsg.org.uk/wp-content/uploads/2019/09/201.full_.pdf

Rutter MD, East J et al. BSG/SCPGBI/PHE Post-polypectomy and post-colorectal cancer resection surveillance guidelines. *Gut* 2020;69(2):201–223. Doi:10.1136/gutjnl-2019-319858.

## 42. B. Three-yearly colonoscopy

Patients with acromegaly:

- These patients are at increased risk of developing CRC
- Specific colorectal screening is required, which differs from other CRC screening programmes
- Colonoscopic screening should start at the age of 40 years (unless there are colonic symptoms at an earlier age)
- If an adenoma is found at first screening, or serum insulin-like growth factor-1 levels are elevated above the maximum of the age-corrected normal range, colonoscopic screening should be offered three-yearly
- If the initial colonoscopy is negative, or hyperplastic polyps are found, or the growth hormone/insulin-like growth factor-1 levels are normal, screening should be offered every 5–10 years
- Colonoscopy is required, rather than sigmoidoscopy, because a significant number of adenomas and carcinomas are right-sided
- Colonoscopy can be technically more difficult because of the increased bowel length, loop complexity, and poor bowel preparation. This can lead to a higher number of complications, and patients need to be counselled about this

Cairns SR, Scholefield JH, Steele RJ et al. Guidelines for colorectal cancer screening and surveillance in moderate and high risk groups (update from 2002). *Gut*. 2010;59(5):666–689. Doi: 10.1136/gut.2009.179804.

## 43. D. MUTYH-associated polyposis (MAP)

- MAP is an autosomal recessive condition
- Colorectal surveillance should commence at 18–20 years old; if surgery is not undertaken, then annual surveillance is recommended
- Upper GI surveillance should be considered at 35 years old

All except MAP are due to dominant transmission of a gene defect associated with a susceptibility to CRC and other cancer types.

- The MutY human homologue (MYH) gene is located on chromosome 1p and is one of three identified genes involved in base-excision repair
- MYH, discovered in 2002, encodes for MUTYH glycosylase, which is involved in oxidative DNA damage repair
- MAP is inherited in an autosomal-recessive pattern.
- It accounts for less than 0.4%–3% of all CRCs; the population prevalence of heterozygotes is 1:100
- The lifetime risk of a homozygous person developing CRC is estimated to be 100% at 60 years
- The number of colonic polyps found in MAP can vary significantly from thousands to fewer than 100
- CRC in MAP is more likely to be right sided and synchronous
- Upper gastrointestinal polyps have been seen, albeit rarely. The lifetime risk of developing duodenal cancer is around 4%
- An increased incidence of breast cancer has been seen in female bi-allelic mutation carriers
- Heterozygotes may have a slightly increased risk of CRC compared with the general population

*Management*

- Colonoscopy surveillance should start at 18–20 years on an annual basis using dye-spray colonoscopy for patients who are bi-allelic MUTYH carriers
- It is recommended that upper gastrointestinal surveillance is started at 35 years old
- Depending on the number of polyps found and the degree of dysplasia, prophylactic colectomy should be considered
- Breast screening should be considered because there may be an increased risk of developing breast cancer

Monahan K, Dunlop M et al. *Guidelines for the management of hereditary colorectal cancer from the British Society of Gastroenterology (BSG)/ Association of Coloproctologists of Great Britain and Ireland (ACPGBI)/ United Kingdom Cancer Genetics Group (UKCGG). Gut* 2020;69(3):411–444. Doi: 10.1136/gutjnl-2019-319915.

## 44. B. Colonoscopy and genetic testing for serine/threonine kinase 11 gene mutation

- Peutz-Jeghers syndrome (PJS) is an autosomal dominant hamartomatous polyposis syndrome
- PJS is associated with a substantial risk of GI-related and breast cancers
- Surveillance by gastroscopy, colonoscopy, and video capsule endoscopy (VCE) should commence at age eight years in asymptomatic patients with PJS

PJS is an autosomal dominant syndrome characterized by harmartomatous polyps in the GI tract and mucocutaneous pigmentation of the lips, oral mucosa, and perianal region. Its prevalence is between 1 in 8.300 and 1 in 29,000. The common germline mutation is *STK11* (aka *LKB1*) located on chromosome 19p. Approximately 40%–80% of patients with PJS have no detectable pathogenic mutation in *STK11*.

### Diagnostic criteria

This is based on any one of the following:
- ≥2 histologically confirmed PJ polyps
- Any number of PJ polyps detected in one individual who has a family history of PJS in a close relative
- Characteristic mucocutaneous pigmentation in an individual who has a family history of PJS in a close relative
- Any number of PJ polyps in an individual who also has characteristic mucocutaneous pigmentation
- A pathogenic variant in STK11

Features such as hamartomatous polyps or characteristic mucocutaneous pigmentation should lead to genetic evaluation. If PJS is confirmed, all FDRs should be tested.

In an asymptomatic patient with PJS, gastrointestinal surveillance by gastroscopy, colonoscopy, and VCE commence at the age of eight years. We recommend that small bowel surveillance should continue three yearly. If baseline colonoscopy and OGD are normal, then they can be safely deferred until age 18 years. However, if polyps are found at baseline examination, then they should be repeated three yearly. Earlier investigation of the GI tract should be performed in symptomatic patients.

### Surveillance for PJS

PJS is associated with a substantial risk of colon, stomach, pancreatic, and breast cancers. However, the malignant potential of the PJS polyp is unclear.

- In an asymptomatic patient, colonoscopy, gastroscopy, and VCE is indicated at eight years of age. Small bowel surveillance should continue three yearly
- If baseline colonoscopy and OGD are normal, then they can be safely deferred until age 18 years; however, if polyps are found at baseline examination, then they should be repeated three yearly
- Earlier investigation of the GI tract should be performed in symptomatic patients
- Elective polypectomy to prevent polyp-related complications (e.g. intussusception, bleeding) is recommended

Monahan K, Dunlop M et al. *Guidelines for the management of hereditary colorectal cancer from the British Society of Gastroenterology (BSG)/Association of Coloproctologists of Great Britain and Ireland (ACPGBI)/ United Kingdom Cancer Genetics Group (UKCGG). Gut* 2020;69(3):411–444. Doi: 10.1136/gutjnl-2019-319915.

## 45. A. One year

- Serrated polyposis syndrome (SPS) is diagnosed phenotypically
- Annual surveillance colonoscopy should be offered to all SPS patients until the colon has been cleared of all lesions >5 mm in size
- FDRs of patients with SPS should be offered an index colonoscopy at age 40 years and five-yearly surveillance thereafter dependent on polyp burden

This patient has SPS. A diagnosis of SPS should be phenotypically driven because no single causative gene has been identified. Individuals should fulfil the phenotypic criteria as defined by the World Health Organization in 2019 for a diagnosis of SPS to be made (Box 7.2).

---

**Box 7.2** Updated World Health Organization clinical criteria for the diagnosis of serrated polyposis 2019

Criterion 1

At least 5 serrated lesions/polyps proximal to the rectum all being ≥ 5 mm in size, with 2 or more ≥ 10 mm in size

Criterion 2

More than 20 serrated lesions/polyps of any size distributed throughout the large bowel, with at least 5 proximal to the rectum

Note: Any histological subtype of serrated lesion/polyp (hyperplastic polyp, sessile serrated lesion without or with dysplasia, traditional serrated adenoma, and unclassified serrated adenoma) is included in the final polyp count. The polyp count is cumulative over multiple colonoscopies.

---

The prevalence of SPS in the West is 1:3,000. However, this may be an underestimate because the awareness of this condition continues to increase among clinicians. The overall lifetime risk of CRC is approximately 7%–10% with an increased risk in FDRs of patients with SPS. There is a degree of phenotypic overlap with other intestinal polyposis syndromes (e.g. MAP, attenuated Familial adenomatous polyposis [FAP]). If the patient is under 50 or there are multiple affected relatives or dysplasia in the polyp, one should exclude other polyposis syndromes with gene panel testing prior to making a definitive diagnosis of SPS.

Colonoscopic surveillance should be performed yearly once the colon has been cleared of all lesions >5 mm in size. If no polyps ≥10 mm in size are identified at subsequent surveillance examination, the interval can be extended to two yearly. FDRs of patients with SPS should be offered an index colonoscopy at age of 40 years or 10 years prior to the diagnosis of the index case. Thereafter, surveillance examination should occur five-yearly unless polyp burden dictates earlier assessment.

Monahan K, Dunlop M et al. *Guidelines for the management of hereditary colorectal cancer from the British Society of Gastroenterology (BSG)/ Association of Coloproctologists of Great Britain and Ireland (ACPGBI)/United Kingdom Cancer Genetics Group (UKCGG). Gut* 2020;69(3):411–444. Doi: 10.1136/gutjnl-2019-319915.

### 46. A. Biofeedback therapy (BFT)

• BFT is superior to other treatment modalities for dyssynergic defecation

BFT is an instrument-based learning process: it employs equipment to record a patient's bodily activities and then provides feedback to the patient as a sensory (visual, auditory, or verbal) response. It was first used in chronic constipation due to dyssynergia defecation to rehabilitate anorectal function.

BFT requires active engagement. Therefore, preserved cognition and motivation are prerequisites to treatment. Sessions last approximately one hour and a typical course of BFT may include 5–10 sessions.

BFT has been shown to be efficacious in reducing dyssynergia and laxative use in patients with dyssynergic defecation. Other treatment modalities, listed below, have limited benefit in comparison.

*Treatment modalities*
• Avoiding constipating medications
• Increasing fibre (optimal intake is 20–30 g daily) and fluid intake
• Exercise
• Timed toilet training
• Laxatives
• Myectomy of the anal sphincter helps only 10%–30% of patients
• Using botulinum toxin injections to paralyse the anal sphincter muscle and reverse the anal spasm shows no improvement

In constipation that is refractory to medical therapy, surgery can be an option, including colectomy, ileostomy, or ileorectal anastomosis.

Narayanan S, Bharucha A. A practical guide to biofeedback therapy for pelvic floor disorders. *Curr Gastroenterol Rep.* 2019 Apr 23;21(5):21. Doi: 10.1007/s11894-019-0688-3.

### 47. D. Prucalopride

• Prucalopride is a selective 5-hydroxytryptamine type 4 receptor (5-HT$_4$) agonist
• Its use is licensed for women with chronic constipation in whom at least two different classes of laxatives, at the highest tolerated dose for minimum 6 months, have failed to be effective

Prucalopride is an 5-HT$_4$ agonist: it has a stimulating effect on colonic motility. Transit studies show that prucalopride increases gastric emptying, and small bowel and colonic transit.

Robust evidence has demonstrated the efficacy of prucalopride in severe constipation. Three large, randomized controlled Phase III trials showed a significant improvement in bowel function in up to 69% of patients treated over three months.

Its use is recommended for the treatment of chronic constipation in women:

- who have been treated with at least two different classes of laxatives at the highest tolerated dose for at least six months
- in whom current treatment has failed to provide adequate relief
- for whom invasive treatment for constipation is being considered

If it is not effective after four weeks, appraisal of continued use should be considered.

The most common side effects are headaches, abdominal pain, nausea, and diarrhoea, and these seem to be apparent early after starting treatment with prucalopride.

Tack J, Muller-Lissner S et al. Diagnosis and treatment of chronic constipation—a European perspective. *Neurogastroenterol Motil.* 2011 Aug;23(8):697–710. Doi: 10.1111/j.1365-2982.2011.01709.x.

## 48. D. IBS

- FI is a common and unreported symptom
- IBS, diarrhoea, and prior cholecystectomy are the strongest independent risk factors for FI in middle-aged women

'Faecal incontinence' is defined as any involuntary loss of faeces that causes a social or hygienic problem. It is a common symptom that is often under-reported because of social stigma. Around 0.5%–1.0% of adults suffer from regular FI that affects their quality of life. A common error is to assume that a single cause is responsible for a patient's symptoms.

Baseline assessment includes:

- Taking a relevant medical and obstetric history
- Discussing the patient's bowel habit
- Considering faecal loading or treatable causes of diarrhoea (e.g. IBD or IBS)
- Considering red flag symptoms for gastrointestinal cancer
- Performing a general examination and assessing for neurological sequalae of disc prolapse/ cauda equina syndrome
- Performing a rectal examination and assessing for rectal prolapse, third-degree haemorrhoids, and anal sphincter injury, including obstetric and other trauma
- If appropriate, performing a cognitive assessment

According to a population-based case–control study conducted by the Mayo Clinic, diarrhoea, IBS, and prior cholecystectomy are the strongest independent risk factors for FI in middle-aged women. The mean age of onset of FI in this group was 55 years. Less strong risk factors are a high BMI, current smoking, rectocoele, and urinary stress incontinence. In contrast to being a risk factor for postpartum FI, obstetric events on their own, such as vaginal delivery, forceps-assisted delivery, and episiotomy, did not predict delayed FI.

Bharucha AE, Zinsmeister AR, Schleck CD et al. Bowel disturbances are the most important risk factors for late-onset fecal incontinence: a population-based case–control study in women. *Gastroenterology.* 2010;139:1559–1566. Doi: 10.1053/j.gastro.2010.07.056.

## 49. C. Lipofuscin

- Melanosis coli is caused by chronic laxative use
- The pigment in melanosis coli is lipofuscin
- Melanosis coli is more common in the proximal colon

The pigment in melanosis coli is lipofuscin, not melanin as the name may imply. Long-term use of laxatives, typically from the anthranoid group, such as senna, cause melanosis coli. Anthraquinones have a toxic effect on the epithelial cells of the colon; damage caused to intracellular components is phagolysed. The products of this phagolysis are then found within the cells as lipofuscin. These cells are phagocytosed by macrophages that can later be found in the mucosa and submucosa of the colon. This commonly affects the proximal colon, which is thought to be related to the distribution of macrophages in the colon. Melanosis coli may occur within a few months of chronic laxative use. It is asymptomatic and often an incidental finding at colonoscopy. Treatment is cessation of causative laxative.

Brown bowel syndrome is also a brown discoloration of the colon due to lipofuscin deposition. Unlike melanosis coli, the lipofuscin deposits are found in the tunica muscularis but not in the mucosa. An association between brown bowel syndrome, malabsorptive conditions, and vitamin E deficiency has been reported.

Aluminium, silicon, and magnesium are found in Peyer's patches in melanosis ilei. Haemosiderin in the lamina propria of the ileum has been found in a patient with melanosis ilei after chronic ingestion of iron.

Nesheiwat Z, Al Nasser Y. Melanosis Coli. [Updated 2020 Jan 15]. In: StatPearls [Internet]. Treasure Island (FL): StatPearls Publishing; 2020 Jan. Available at: https://www.ncbi.nlm.nih.gov/books/NBK493146/

## 50. D. Slow-transit constipation

- Presence of ≥6 markers in the colon on transit study is diagnostic of slow bowel transit
- Constipation is more common in women
- Secondary causes of constipation include drugs, and neurological and metabolic disorders

A colonic transit study measures whole gut transit time (primarily colon) via the ingestion of radio-opaque markers. The study is inexpensive, simple, and safe. The patient ingests a single capsule containing 24 markers on day 1, followed by a plain abdominal film on day 6 (120 hours later). In patients with normal transit time, fewer than 5 markers remain in the colon. The presence of ≥6 markers scattered throughout the colon is diagnostic of slow bowel transit. In dyssynergic defecation, ≥6 markers are found in the rectosigmoid region, with near normal transit of markers through the rest of the colon.

### Primary or functional constipation

Constipation is common and polysymptomatic. The prevalence of chronic constipation ranges from 2% to 28%. Constipation is more common in women, with an estimated female:male ratio of 2.2:1. Its prevalence increases with advancing age. Chronic constipation has a significant impact on quality of life and is a major cause of psychological distress.

Three subtypes of primary or functional constipation are known. However, overlaps exist.
- *Slow-transit constipation* is characterized by prolonged delay of the transit time of stool throughout the colon
- *Dyssynergic defecation* (also known as 'anismus', 'pelvic floor dyssynergia', or 'outlet obstruction') is difficulty in expelling, or inability to expel, stool from the anorectum
- Irritable bowel syndrome with predominant constipation (IBS-C) is characterized by symptoms of constipation, with discomfort or pain as a prominent feature

*Rome IV diagnostic criteria for IBS*

- Recurrent abdominal pain on average at least one day/week in the past three months, associated with two or more of the following:
  - related to defecation and/or
  - associated with a change in frequency of stool and/or
  - associated with a change in form (appearance) of stool
- In IBS-C, more than one-fourth (25%) of bowel movements with Bristol Stool Scale Types 1-2

*Secondary causes of constipation*

- Colonic pathology (e.g. stricture, cancer, anal fissure, proctitis, rectocoele)
- Metabolic pathology (e.g. hypercalcaemia, hypothyroidism, diabetes mellitus)
- Neurological disorders (e.g. parkinsonism, spinal cord lesions)
- Psychiatric disorders
- Drugs (e.g. opioids)
- Diet and behavioural lifestyle

Drossman D. Functional gastrointestinal disorders: history, pathophysiology, clinical features, and Rome IV. *Gastroenterology*. 2016 Feb;19. pii: S0016-5085(16)00223-7. Doi: 10.1053/j.gastro.2016.02.032.

# chapter 8

# LIVER DISORDERS

## QUESTIONS

1. **A 65-year-old man with known Child-Pugh A alcohol-related cirrhosis was admitted with abdominal pain.**

   Investigations:
   CT triple phase liver — 5 × 5 cm mass in right liver lobe enhancing vividly during late arterial phase and becoming hypoattenuating in the portal venous phase.

   **After multidisciplinary team discussion, the man was referred for transarterial chemoembolization (TACE), which required access to the hepatic arterial blood supply.**

   **From which artery does the common hepatic artery (HA) directly arise?**

   A. Aorta

   B. Coeliac axis

   C. Left gastric artery

   D. Right gastric artery

   E. Superior mesenteric artery

2. **The confluence of which structures lead to the formation of the structure marked in the image (Fig. 8.1)?**

   A. Inferior mesenteric vein and splenic vein

   B. Left and right hepatic duct

   C. Left and right hepatic duct and cystic duct

   D. Superior mesenteric artery and splenic artery

   E. Superior mesenteric vein and splenic vein

*Best of Five MCQs for the European Specialty Examination in Gastroenterology and Hepatology.* Thomas Marjot, Colleen G C McGregor, Tim Ambrose, Aminda N De Silva, Jeremy Cobbold, and Simon Travis, Oxford University Press (2021). © Oxford University Press.
DOI: 10.1093/oso/9780198834373.003.0008

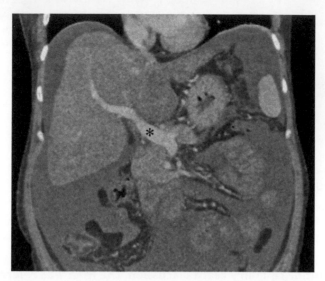

**Fig. 8.1** CT abdomen

Courtesy of Dr Shahana Shahid, OUH NHS Foundation Trust

3. **A 43-year-old woman was admitted with new onset jaundice and abdominal distension. She went on to have a transjugular liver biopsy with measurement of portal pressures.**

   **What hepatic venous pressure gradient would be compatible with clinically significant portal hypertension?**

   A. 5 mmHg

   B. 6 mmHg

   C. 8 mmHg

   D. 9 mmHg

   E. 10 mmHg

4.  **A 52-year-old man with type 2 diabetes was recently diagnosed with non-alcoholic steatohepatitis (NASH) with cirrhosis. He currently has no clinical features of decompensation. His screening gastroscopy demonstrated two columns of oesophageal varices that flattened completely upon insufflation of air. There was mild portal hypertensive gastropathy, but no gastric varices.**

    **Which is the most appropriate regarding further surveillance and treatment?**

    A.  Prescribe non-selective beta blocker (e.g. Propranolol) and no further varices surveillance required
    B.  Repeat gastroscopy in one year, without current primary prophylaxis for varices
    C.  Repeat gastroscopy in 2–3 years, without current primary prophylaxis for varices
    D.  Repeat gastroscopy only in the event of hepatic decompensation, without current primary prophylaxis for varices
    E.  Repeat gastroscopy with endoscopic variceal ligation (EVL) in 4–6 weeks.

5.  **A 58-year-old woman came to clinic to discuss the results of a recent liver biopsy that confirmed cirrhosis due to autoimmune hepatitis (AIH). She had not previously had a gastroscopy.**

    Investigations:
    | | |
    |---|---|
    | Serum alanine aminotransferase (ALT) | 32 U/L |
    | Serum aspartate transaminase (AST) | 38 U/L |
    | Serum bilirubin | 21 µmol/L |
    | Serum albumin | 34 g/L |
    | International normalized ratio (INR) | 1.1 |
    | Platelet count | 178 × 10⁹/L |

    **Which additional investigation result would be best used to avoid screening gastroscopy for varices for one year?**

    A.  Absence of ascites on transabdominal ultrasound
    B.  Enhanced liver fibrosis (ELF) score of 10.6
    C.  Hepatic venous pressure gradient (HVPG) measurement of 11 mmHg
    D.  Liver stiffness reading of 18.4 kPa
    E.  Spleen diameter of 12.5 cm on transabdominal ultrasound

6.  **A 46-year-old man with cirrhosis had his first screening gastroscopy, which showed small gastro-oesophageal varices.**

    **Which of the following is the strongest predictor for the progression from small to large varices?**

    A.  Alcohol aetiology of cirrhosis
    B.  Female sex
    C.  HVPG 10 mmHg
    D.  NASH aetiology of cirrhosis
    E.  Spider naevi

7. **A 40-year-old man with cirrhosis and known oesophageal varices presented to hospital with haematemesis.**

   **Which of the following statements regarding the resuscitation of patients with cirrhosis and VH is most accurate?**

   A. Hyponatraemia is a recognized side effect of terlipressin

   B. Optimal timing for diagnostic endoscopy is at 12–24 hours after presentation

   C. Packed red blood cells should be transfused when haemoglobin falls below 9 g/dL

   D. Platelet transfusion in severe thrombocytopaenia (platelet count <50 × 10$^9$/L) helps prevent re-bleeding

   E. Severe coagulopathy (INR >4) should be corrected with recombinant factor VII or fresh frozen plasma

8. **A 44-year-old woman from Pakistan presented to the emergency department with new ascites.**

   Investigations:

   | | |
   |---|---|
   | Haemoglobin | 120 g/L |
   | White cell count | 9.6 × 10$^9$/L |
   | Platelet count | 150 × 10$^9$/L |
   | Serum bilirubin | 30 µmol/L |
   | Serum ALP | 120 U/L |
   | Serum ALT | 25 U/L |
   | Serum creatinine | 75 µmol/L |
   | Serum albumin | 30 g/L |
   | Serum Ca 125 | 200 U/mL |
   | Ascitic fluid white cell count | 100 cells/mm$^3$ (75% neutrophils) |
   | Ascitic fluid albumin | 15 g/L |
   | Ascitic fluid protein | 20 g/L |
   | Ascitic fluid Gram stain | No organisms |

   **What is the most likely diagnosis?**

   A. Cirrhosis

   B. Gynaecological malignancy

   C. Heart failure

   D. Nephrotic syndrome

   E. Tuberculosis

9. **A 59-year-old man with NASH cirrhosis and diuretic-intolerant ascites presented to the emergency department with abdominal pain. On examination, he had tense ascites and diffuse abdominal tenderness. He had a temperature of 38°C, heart rate 105 beats per minute and blood pressure 90/59 mm/Hg. He was treated empirically with intravenous ceftriaxone and a diagnostic paracentesis was performed.**

Investigations:

| | |
|---|---|
| Ascitic fluid cell count | 1,555 cells/mm³ (90% neutrophils) |
| Ascitic fluid culture at 24 hours | *Clostridium perfringens* |
| | *Bacteroides vulgatus* |
| | *Enterococcus faecalis* |

### What is the next best approach to management?

A. Continue ceftriaxone and add metronidazole

B. Continue ceftriaxone and repeat diagnostic paracentesis in 48 hours

C. Give 1.5 g/kg human albumin solution

D. Perform large volume paracentesis

E. Request computed tomography (CT) abdomen and pelvis

10. **A 53-year-old woman with alcohol-related cirrhosis was admitted with hepatic encephalopathy (HE). Her medications were lactulose 20 ml three times a day and carvedilol 3.75 mg once a day.**

Investigations:

| | |
|---|---|
| Serum sodium | 130 mmol/L |
| Serum potassium | 4.7 mmol/L |
| Serum urea | 1.6 mmol/L |
| Serum creatinine | 90 µmol/L |
| Serum creatinine five days previously | 40 µmol/L |
| Serum bilirubin | 50 µmol/L |
| Serum ALT | 30 U/L |
| Serum ALP | 150 U/L |
| Serum albumin | 20 g/L |
| INR | 1.4 |
| Haemoglobin | 13 g/L |
| Liver ultrasound | Irregular liver edge, moderate ascites, normal portal vein flow, spleen 15 cm |
| Renal ultrasound | Normal |
| Full septic screen | Negative |

### What is the most appropriate next management step for the patient's renal dysfunction?

A. Infusion of crystalloid 1L over eight hours

B. Large volume paracentesis with human albumin replacement.

C. Monitor renal function

D. Terlipressin (1 mg four times a day)

E. Twenty per cent human albumin solution (1 g/kg) for two consecutive days

11. **A 54-year-old man with alcohol-related cirrhosis was admitted with acute kidney injury (AKI). Forty-eight hours into his admission, he was diagnosed with hepatorenal syndrome–acute kidney injury (HRS-AKI) and started on terlipressin 1 mg every six hours and 40 g of human albumin daily.**

    Investigations:

    | | |
    |---|---|
    | Baseline serum creatinine | 40 µmol/L |
    | Peak serum creatinine before terlipressin | 102 µmol/L |
    | Serum creatinine after 48 hours of terlipressin | 94 µmol/L |

    **What would be the next most appropriate management step?**

    A. Continue current doses of terlipressin and human albumin

    B. Continue terlipressin 1 mg every 6 hours and increase human albumin to 80 g daily

    C. Increase terlipressin to 2 mg every six hours and continue 40 g human albumin daily

    D. Noradrenaline infusion

    E. Renal replacement therapy

12. **Which of the following is the earliest feature in the pathogenesis of HRS-AKI?**

    A. Activation of the renin–angiotensin–aldosterone system (RAAS)

    B. Reduced cardiac output

    C. Renal vasoconstriction

    D. Splanchnic arterial vasodilation

    E. Systemic inflammatory response syndrome

13. **Which of the following investigations would most favour a diagnosis of acute tubular necrosis (ATN) over hepatorenal syndrome (HRS)?**

    A. Low fractional excretion of sodium (<1%)

    B. Low fractional excretion of urea (<35%)

    C. Normal renal ultrasound scan

    D. Urinary muddy brown casts

    E. Urinary protein >500 mg in 24 hours

14. **Which of the following statements is correct regarding ammonia in HE?**

    A. An elevated blood ammonia has no prognostic significance in patients with acute liver failure (ALF)

    B. An elevated blood ammonia has no prognostic significance in patients with cirrhosis

    C. An elevated blood ammonia >150 µg/dL is diagnostic for HE in patients with cirrhosis

    D. Delay in laboratory measurement of ammonia in a venous sample leads to high false-negative rates

    E. Rifaximin has no impact on circulating ammonia levels

15. **Which of the following is correct regarding the natural history of hepatocellular carcinoma (HCC)?**
    A. A high serum Hepatitis B virus (HBV) DNA level is not a risk factor for HCC
    B. Approximately half the cases of NASH-related HCC arise in non-cirrhotic patients
    C. HCC surveillance can be stopped in patients with hepatitis C virus (HCV) cirrhosis who achieve sustained virologic response (SVR)
    D. Ten per cent of patients with cirrhosis will develop HCC during their lifetime
    E. There is a low rate of HCC recurrence post-treatment with curative intent in patients with HCV cirrhosis who achieve SVR with direct-acting antivirals (DAAs)

16. **A 62-year-old man with compensated cirrhosis due to HCV was diagnosed with HCC. He was asymptomatic and had unlimited exercise tolerance. Sustained viralogical response was achieved three years previously.**

    Investigations:

    | | |
    |---|---|
    | Magnetic resonance imaging (MRI) liver | 28 mm HCC lesion in segment 5 and 18 mm HCC lesion in segment 7; no macroscopic vascular invasion or extrahepatic spread; portosystemic collaterals; no ascites |
    | Gastroscopy | Grade 1 oesophageal varices |
    | Serum alpha fetoprotein | 54 ng/ml |
    | MELD | 8.5 |

    **What would be the preferred management approach for this patient?**
    A. Liver transplantation (LT)
    B. Palliative chemotherapy (e.g. oral Sorafenib)
    C. Radiofrequency ablation
    D. Surgical resection
    E. Transarterial embolization

17. **A 38-year-old woman was referred to clinic after a 6 cm liver mass was identified incidentally on a CT kidneys, ureters, and bladder. She had a body mass index (BMI) of 32 kg/m², no other co-morbidities and was taking the oral contraceptive pill (OCP).**

    Investigations:

    | | |
    |---|---|
    | CT liver triple phase | Well-demarcated mass with early enhancement in the arterial phase before iso-attenuation in the portal venous phase |
    | MRI liver | Hyperintense lesion on T1 and T2 weighted imaging, with early enhancement with gadolinium. |

    **Following discussion at the multi-disciplinary meeting, what would be the most appropriate recommendation?**

    A. Discharge, no follow-up needed

    B. Lifestyle changes and repeat MRI in six months

    C. Referral for LT

    D. Surgical resection

    E. Transarterial embolization

18. **A 36-year-old man with alcohol-related cirrhosis presented to the emergency department with haematemesis. On examination, he had moderate ascites and Grade 2 encephalopathy. A gastroscopy showed three columns of Grade 3 varices, which were banded. His oral intake remained inadequate on the ward for 48 hours after the procedure.**

    Investigations:

    | | |
    |---|---|
    | Haemoglobin | 97 g/L |
    | White cell count | 11.5 × 10⁹/L |
    | Platelet count | 89 × 10⁹/L |
    | Serum bilirubin | 163 μmol/L |
    | Serum ALP | 213 U/L |
    | Serum ALT | 79 U/L |
    | Prothrombin time | 29 seconds |

    **What is the most appropriate nutritional management?**

    A. Nasogastric feeding

    B. Nasojejunal feeding

    C. Oral nutritional supplements

    D. Parenteral nutrition

    E. Trial of low protein oral nutrition for further 24 hours

**19. A 24-year-old woman had blood tests after her mother tested positive for HBV. She had no symptoms or signs of chronic liver disease.**

Investigations:

| | |
|---|---|
| Serum bilirubin | 15 µmol/L |
| Serum ALT | 86 U/L |
| Serum creatinine | 65 µmol/L |
| Haemoglobin | 120 g/L |
| Platelet count | $214 \times 10^9$/L |
| HBsAg | Positive |
| HBeAb | Positive |
| HBeAg | Negative |
| HBV DNA | 21,000 IU/ml |
| HCV antibody | Negative |
| Hepatitis D (HDV) antibody | Negative |
| HIV antibody | Negative |
| Ultrasound abdomen | Normal |

**What is the best next step in her management?**

A. Liver biopsy and start treatment with tenofovir if evidence of cirrhosis

B. Start treatment with tenofovir

C. Transient elastography (TE) and no treatment if liver stiffness measurement (LSM) <6 kPa with follow-up in one year with repeat ALT, HBV DNA, and TE

D. TE and start treatment with pegIFNα if LSM >9 kPa.

E. TE and start treatment with tenofovir if LSM >12 kPa.

**20. A 35-year-old Vietnamese man was referred to clinic after his primary care doctor investigated abnormal LFTs and subsequently found him to be positive for HBsAg.**

Investigations:

| | |
|---|---|
| HBsAg | Positive |
| HBeAg | Positive |
| HBV DNA | 230,000 IU/mL |
| Serum ALT | 99 U/L |
| Liver stiffness | 8.2 kPa |

**What should be the main goal of antiviral treatment?**

A. Loss of HBeAg

B. Loss of HBsAg

C. Normalization of ALT

D. Reduction in liver stiffness <7 kPa

E. Suppression of HBV DNA

21. **A 76-year-old woman was recently diagnosed with diffuse large B-cell Lymphoma. She was about to be started on R-CHOP chemotherapy and has some pre-treatment blood tests.**

    Investigations:

    | | |
    |---|---|
    | Serum ALT | 34 U/L |
    | Serum bilirubin | 4 umol/L |
    | HBsAg | Positive |
    | HBeAg | Negative |
    | HBeAb | Positive |
    | HBV DNA | 310 copies/ml |
    | Liver stiffness | 3.4 kPa |

    **What is the next most appropriate approach to her management?**

    A. Advise haematologist to avoid Rituximab

    B. Pre-emptive approach with monthly blood tests and to start treatment if HBV DNA >2,000 copies/ml or ALT >upper limit of normal (ULN)

    C. Prophylaxis with entecavir throughout R-CHOP treatment and for 6 months after its discontinuation

    D. Prophylaxis with entecavir throughout R-CHOP treatment and for 12 months after its discontinuation

    E. Prophylaxis with entecavir throughout R-CHOP treatment and for 18 months after its discontinuation

22. **Which of the following combinations is a pangenotypic treatment regimen for HCV?**

    A. Grazoprevir, elbasvir

    B. Sofosbuvir, ledipasvir

    C. Sofosbuvir, ledipasvir, ribavirin

    D. Sofosbuvir, velpatasvir

    E. Velpatasvir, ledipasvir, ribavirin

23. **A 61-year-old man with HCV cirrhosis developed progressive jaundice, ascites, and encephalopathy, and was listed for LT.**

    **What is the best approach to treating his HCV infection with DAAs?**

    A. Treat with DAAs post-LT if MELD ≥18–20 and time to transplantation likely to be <6 months

    B. Treat with DAAs post-LT if MELD <18-20 irrespective of likely time until transplantation

    C. Treat with DAAs post-LT irrespective of MELD and waiting time

    D. Treat with DAAs pre-LT if MELD ≥18–20 and time to transplantation likely to be <6 months

    E. Treat with DAAs pre-LT irrespective of MELD and waiting time

24. **A 50-year-old man with known untreated chronic HBV infection (CHB) was referred to hepatology clinic with worsening LFTs and malaise. He recently returned to the UK from a four-week trip to Thailand where he reported having unprotected sex with a sex-worker. His examination was unremarkable.**

Investigations:

| | |
|---|---|
| Haemoglobin | 145 g/L |
| White cell count | $5 \times 10^9$/L |
| Platelet count | $190 \times 10^9$/L |
| Serum ALT | 600 U/L |
| Serum bilirubin | 25 µmol/L |
| Serum creatinine | 84 µmol/L |
| HBsAg | Positive |
| HBeAg | Negative |
| HBeAb | Positive |
| HDV RNA | Detectable |
| HBV DNA | 1,900 U/L |
| HCV Ab | Negative |
| HIV antibody | Negative |
| Liver ultrasound | Normal |
| Liver stiffness | 8.7 kPa |

**What is the most appropriate approach to his management?**

A. No change to management

B. Referral for LT assessment

C. Treatment with combination of nucleoside reverse transcriptase inhibitors (NRTIs) and non-nucleoside reverse transcriptase inhibitors (NNRTIs) for 48 weeks

D. Treatment with Peg-IFNα for 48 weeks

E. Treatment with tenofovir for 48 weeks

25. **A 66-year-old woman had a liver biopsy performed as part of her work-up for abnormal LFTs.**

Investigations:

| | |
|---|---|
| Liver biopsy | A dense infiltrate of immune cells in the lobules and within the portal tracts with prominent interface hepatitis. There is a predominance of plasma cells, as well as some lymphocytes, and the presence of hepatic rosette formation and emperipolesis. There is some steatosis (40%), bridging fibrosis with nodule formation, and Ishak fibrosis score 6/6. |

**How would you treat this patient?**

A. Azathioprine 100 mg daily

B. Budesonide 9 mg daily and azathioprine 50 mg daily

C. Observe with repeat liver biochemistry in three months' time.

D. Prednisolone 40 mg daily

E. Ursodeoxycholic acid (UDCA) 500 mg twice a day

**26. A 31-year-old man presented with three weeks of lethargy and arthralgia.**

Investigations:

| | |
|---|---|
| Serum ALT | 710 U/L |
| Serum ALP | 210 U/L |
| Serum bilirubin | 50 μmol/L |
| Platelet count | 233 × 10⁹/L |
| Antinuclear antibody (ANA) | Positive 1:40 |
| Liver kidney microsomal antibody | Positive 1:40 |
| IgG | 28 g/L |
| HCV Ab | Negative |
| HBsAg | Negative |
| Hepatitis E IgM | Negative |
| Hepatitis A IgM | Negative |
| Liver biopsy histology | Interface hepatitis with lymphoplasmocytic-rich infiltrate in portal tracts extending into the lobule. |

**Which of the following carries the lowest weighting in the simplified diagnostic criteria of the International Autoimmune Hepatitis Group?**

A. Absence of viral hepatitis

B. ANA or SMA ≥1:40

C. IgG >1.1 × ULN

D. Liver histology typical of AIH

E. LKM ≥1:40

**27. A 40-year-old woman with AIH, previously treated with prednisolone and azathioprine for three years, and who has been in complete biochemical remission for one year on azathioprine monotherapy, asks whether her treatment can be stopped.**

**Which of the following is true?**

A. Biochemical remission for over one year is associated with a better outcome in those who discontinue treatment

B. Immunosuppressive treatment should be continued for at least five years

C. Relapse commonly occurs within the first year of treatment withdrawal

D. The majority of patients will stay in remission without maintenance therapy

E. There is no role for repeat liver biopsy prior to withdrawal of treatment

28. **A 38-year-old woman complained of one year of lethargy. She had a history of Raynaud's phenomenon and gastro-oesophageal reflux. Her medications were omeprazole 40 mg and the OCP. She recently had a course of trimethoprim for a urinary tract infection. Clinical examination was unremarkable.**

Investigations:

| | |
|---|---|
| Serum bilirubin | 13 μmol/L |
| Serum ALP | 211 U/L |
| Serum ALT | 55 U/L |
| Serum albumin | 39 g/L |
| Full blood count | Normal |
| INR | 0.9 |
| ANA | Negative |
| Antinuclear cytosplasmic antibody | Negative |
| Anti-mitochondrial antibody | Positive |
| Anti-smooth muscle antibody | Negative |
| IgA | 0.9 g/L |
| IgG | 10.1 g/L |
| IgM | 3.5 g/L |
| HBV/HCV | Negative |
| Liver ultrasound | Normal |

**What is the most likely diagnosis?**

A. Cholelithiasis

B. Drug-induced liver injury (DILI)

C. Non-alcoholic fatty liver disease (NAFLD)

D. Primary biliary cholangitis (PBC)

E. Primary sclerosing cholangitis

29. **A 53-year-old woman presented with fatigue and pruritis. She had a history of hypothyroidism and 'minor liver function test elevations' one year previously. She drank no alcohol and was a non-smoker. On clinical examination, she had xanthelasma, borderline hepatomegaly, and excoriation marks over her limbs.**

Investigations:

| | |
|---|---|
| Serum bilirubin | 17 µmol/L |
| Serum ALP | 256 U/L |
| Serum ALT | 67 U/L |
| Serum albumin | 35 g/L |
| Full blood count | Normal |
| INR | 1.0 |
| ANA | Positive, 1:320, nuclear dot pattern |
| Anti-mitochondrial antibody | Negative |
| Anti-smooth muscle antibody | Negative |
| Anti-sp100 | Positive |
| Anti-gp210 | Negative |
| IgA | 1.5 g/L |
| IgG | 12 g/L |
| IgM | 4.1 g/L |
| HBsAg | Negative |
| HCV antibody | Negative |
| Ultrasound upper abdomen | Normal |

**What would be the next best step?**

A. Liver biopsy

B. MRCP

C. Serum autotaxin levels

D. Start UDCA 13–15 mg/kg/day

E. Start UDCA 15–20 mg/kg/day

30. **A 31-year-old man with PBC presented one year after starting UDCA 500 mg twice a day. His baseline alkaline phosphatase (ALP) prior to starting UDCA was 401 U/L. He was asymptomatic, had normal clinical examination, and was taking no other medications. His weight was 70 kg.**

Investigations:

| | |
|---|---|
| Serum bilirubin | 21 µmol/L |
| Serum ALP | 321 U/L |
| Serum ALT | 80 U/L |
| Serum albumin | 37 g/L |
| Liver ultrasound | Normal |

**How would you manage this patient?**

A. Consider second-line therapy with obeticholic acid (OCA)

B. Continue current management

C. Increase UDCA to 750 mg twice a day

D. Refer for early consideration of LT

E. Stop UDCA

31. **A 35-year-old woman with PBC attended clinic. Her medications were UDCA 1,000 mg once a day and OCA 10 mg once a day. She had been on OCA for one year and her ALP prior to OCA was 423 U/L. She was asymptomatic with normal clinical examination and weighed 70 kg.**

    Investigations:

    | | |
    |---|---|
    | Serum ALT | 75 U/L |
    | Serum ALP | 338 U/L |
    | Serum bilirubin | 35 μmol/L |
    | Serum albumin | 37 g/L |

    **How would you counsel her regarding her prognosis?**

    A. Good prognostic group because her ALP has reduced by >15% from baseline on OCA

    B. Good prognostic group because she is asymptomatic, female, and less than 45 years old

    C. Poor prognostic group because her ALP is above 2 × ULN and her bilirubin is above the ULN.

    D. Poor prognostic group because she is female and her albumin is <40 g/L.

    E. Referral for LT is required

32. **A 31-year-old man with ulcerative pancolitis attended clinic to discuss his up-to-date investigations after finding abnormal liver function tests six months previously.**

    Investigations:

    | | |
    |---|---|
    | Serum bilirubin | 18 μmol/L |
    | Serum ALP | 432 IU/L |
    | Serum ALT | 85 IU/L |
    | Haemoglobin | 134 g/L |
    | White cell count | $8 \times 10^9$/L |
    | Platelet count | $210 \times 10^9$/L |
    | ANA | Positive 1:160 |
    | Antineutrophilic cytoplasmic antibody | Positive (p-ANCA) |
    | Anti-mitochondrial antibody | Negative |
    | Anti-smooth muscle antibody | Negative |
    | Anti-sp100 | Negative |
    | Anti-gp210 | Negative |
    | IgA | 1.45 g/L |
    | IgG | 16.7 g/L |
    | IgM | 1.59 g/L |
    | Liver ultrasound | Normal liver, biliary tree and gallbladder; no cholelithiasis |

    **What would be the best next step?**

    A. ERCP

    B. Liver biopsy

    C. MRCP

    D. Repeat liver biochemistry in six months' time

    E. Serum copper and caeruloplasmin

**33. A 40-year-old man presented with abnormal liver biochemistry. He was asymptomatic.**

Investigations:

| | |
|---|---|
| Serum ALT | 78 IU/L |
| Serum ALP | 327 IU/L |
| Serum bilirubin | 17 µmol/L |
| Serum albumin | 39 g/L |
| Liver ultrasound | Normal liver echotexture, normal biliary tree, and gallbladder |
| MRCP | Normal |
| Liver biopsy histology | (See Fig. 8.2) |

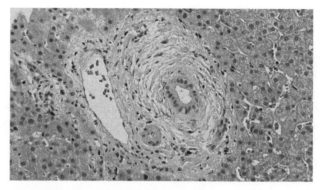

**Fig. 8.2** Liver biopsy histology specimen. See also Plate 17

Image courtesy of Dr Eve Fryer, OUH NHS Foundation Trust, Oxford

**What is the diagnosis?**

A. AIH

B. Classical primary sclerosing cholangitis

C. PBC

D. Primary sclerosing cholangitis (PSC)/AIH overlap

E. Small-duct PSC

**34. A 56-year-old man with PSC was followed up in clinic. He complained of increasing pruritus affecting his hands, feet, and back, fluctuating during the day and typically worse after a hot bath. Blood tests revealed cholestatic liver biochemistry with preserved synthetic function.**

**Which of the following options is true regarding pruritus in this case?**

A. Pruritus is not an indication for LT

B. Pruritus usually gets worse as liver disease progresses and end-stage liver disease ensues

C. Rifampicin causes drug-induced hepatitis and significant liver dysfunction in 5% of patients

D. There is an extensive evidence base for use of cholestyramine as first-line treatment for cholestatic itch

E. UDCA can cause paradoxical worsening of pruritus in cholestatic liver disease

35. **Which one of the following blood results usually remains unchanged throughout pregnancy?**

    A. Alkaline phosphatase

    B. α-fetoprotein

    C. Bilirubin

    D. Immunoglobulin G

    E. Platelet count

36. **A 28-year-old woman who was 32 weeks' pregnant presented with worsening pruritis. Initially, this was confined to her palms and soles but progressed to affect her entire body. Her husband commented that she had become yellow over the last week. On examination, she was jaundiced with widespread excoriations.**

    Investigations:

    | | |
    |---|---|
    | Haemoglobin | 108 g/L |
    | White cell count | $10.4 \times 10^9$/L |
    | Platelet count | $160 \times 10^9$/L |
    | Bilirubin | 74 µmol/L |
    | ALP | 306 IU/L |
    | ALT | 106 IU/L |
    | Prothrombin time | 14.5 seconds |
    | Serum bile acids | 70 µmol/L |

    **What is the most appropriate first-line treatment for this patient?**

    A. Chlorphenamine

    B. Cholestyramine

    C. Prednisolone

    D. Rifampicin

    E. UDCA

37. **A 41-year-old primigravida women who was 33 weeks' pregnant presented with right upper quadrant pain, headache, and vomiting. Her antenatal care to date had been unremarkable. On examination, she was tender over the right upper quadrant and there was mild peripheral oedema. She was afebrile with a heart rate was 105 bpm and blood pressure of 152/92 mmHg.**

Investigations:

| | |
|---|---|
| Haemoglobin | 88 g/L |
| White cell count | $13.4 \times 10^9$/L |
| Platelet count | $76 \times 10^9$/L |
| Blood film | Spherocytosis with schistocytes present; no platelet clumps |
| Serum bilirubin | 40 µmol/L |
| Serum ALT | 381 IU/L |
| Serum ALP | 204 IU/L |
| Prothrombin time | 15 seconds |
| Serum LDH | 805 mmol/L |
| Urine dipstick protein | 3+ |
| Liver ultrasound | Hepatomegaly, no biliary dilatation; non-obstructing gallstones |

**Which is the most likely diagnosis?**

A. Acute fatty liver of pregnancy (AFLP)

B. Gallstones

C. Haemolysis, elevated liver enzymes, and low platelets (HELLP) syndrome

D. Hyperemesis gravidarum

E. Pre-eclampsia

38. **What is the estimated global population prevalence of NAFLD?**

A. 5%

B. 10%

C. 25%

D. 40%

E. 50%

39. **A 49-year-old woman was referred to clinic for evaluation of abnormal liver enzymes and moderate steatosis on liver ultrasound. She did not drink alcohol, had a BMI of 32.6 kg/m² and a past medical history of type 2 diabetes. She was subsequently diagnosed with NAFLD.**

    **Which test result would be most predictive of advanced (bridging) fibrosis on liver biopsy?**

    A. APRI score 0.404

    B. AST:ALT 0.63

    C. ELF score 10.76

    D. FIB4 score 1.18

    E. NAFLD fibrosis score -0.058

40. **A 37-year-old man presented to the emergency department with a paracetamol overdose. What is the toxic metabolite most responsible for liver injury?**

    A. Acetaminophen

    B. Glutathione

    C. Glycoaldehyde

    D. N-acetyl-p-benzoquinoneimine (NAPQI)

    E. Sulphydyl

**41. A 35-year-old-man presented with a three-day history of malaise, right upper quadrant pain and jaundice. He denied any paracetamol use.**

Investigations:

| | |
|---|---|
| Haemoglobin | 135 g/L |
| White cell count | $7 \times 10^9$/L |
| Platelet count | $192 \times 10^9$/L |
| Serum bilirubin | 256 µmol/L |
| Serum ALT | 1,685 IU/L |
| Serum ALP | 187 IU/L |
| Serum urea | 5 mmol/L |
| Serum creatinine | 160 µmol/L |
| INR | 7 |
| Arterial pH | 7.31 |
| Serum lactate | 4 mmol/L |
| Serum acetaminophen level | 0 mcg/ml |
| CT liver | Mild hepatomegaly; heterogeneous enhancement of liver parenchyma in portal venous phase; normal ducts; normal hepatic vein and portal vein flow; no splenomegaly |

**Which of the following is most likely to prompt emergency LT according to King's College criteria?**

A. Arterial pH 7.31

B. Bilirubin 256 µmol/L

C. Creatinine 160 µmol/L

D. INR 7

E. Lactate 4 mmol/L

**42. Which of the following medications is most associated with intrinsic versus idiosyncratic drug-induced liver injury?**

A. Acetaminophen

B. Amoxicillin-clavunalate

C. Halothane

D. Isoniazid

E. Phenytoin

**43. Which of the following is most likely to cause a predominantly cholestatic pattern of drug-induced liver injury?**

A. Flucloxacillin

B. Green tea

C. Ipilimumab

D. Isoniazid

E. Phenytoin

44. **A 65-year-old man with previous LT for alcohol-related cirrhosis is maintained on cyclosporin immunosuppression.**

    **The introduction of which of the following is likely to require an increase in his daily dose of cyclosporin?**
    A. Carbamazepine
    B. Clarithromycin
    C. Grapefruit juice
    D. Ketoconazole
    E. Ritonavir

45. **Which of the following statements regarding Wilson's disease (WD) is correct?**
    A. D-penicillamine is well tolerated with few recognized side effects
    B. It does not cause ALF
    C. It is caused by mutations of the ATP7B gene
    D. Serum ceruloplasmin within the normal range excludes the diagnosis
    E. Twenty-five per cent of patients present beyond the fourth decade of life

46. **A 28-year-old non-smoking man was found to have panlobular emphysema, advanced hepatic fibrosis, and panniculitis. A non-invasive liver screen was performed and a diagnosis of alpha-1-antitrypsin deficiency (A1ATD) was ultimately made.**

    **What is his genotype most likely to be?**
    A. Pi*MM
    B. Pi*MZ
    C. Pi*SS
    D. Pi*SZ
    E. Pi*ZZ

47. **A 39-year-old Caucasian man was referred with a history of right upper quadrant pain and deranged LFTs.**

    Investigations:
    | | |
    |---|---|
    | Serum bilirubin | 11 µmol/L |
    | Serum ALT | 75 IU/L |
    | Serum ALP | 80 IU/L |
    | Serum ferritin | 750 µg/L |
    | Transferrin saturation | 38% |

    **What is the most likely cause for his hyperferritinaemia?**
    A. C282Y heterozygote
    B. C282Y homozygote
    C. C282Y/H63D
    D. Metabolic syndrome
    E. Mutations in HAMP gene (encoding hepcidin)

48. **Which of the following statements regarding the treatment of hereditary haemochromatosis (HH) is correct?**

    A. Arthralgia does not improve with phlebotomy

    B. Cirrhosis is a contraindication to phlebotomy

    C. Iron chelators (e.g. deferoxamine) should always be used alongside phlebotomy

    D. Phlebotomy should aim to maintain a haemoglobin below the lower limit of normal.

    E. The benefit of phlebotomy on mortality has been proven in randomized controlled trials (RCTs)

49. **Which of the following is an absolute contraindication to LT?**

    A. Age 70 years

    B. Aspergillus chest infection

    C. Hepatorenal syndrome

    D. Mastectomy for locally advanced breast cancer five years previously

    E. Portal vein thrombosis (PVT)

50. **A 57-year-old woman was reviewed on the ward five days after LT for NASH cirrhosis. Initially, she had no evidence of graft dysfunction and liver ultrasound with Doppler of hepatic vessels on day one following her operation was satisfactory. She had a low-grade fever (37.6°C) and a hypoglycaemic episode two hours previously.**

    Investigations:

    | | |
    |---|---|
    | Serum ALT | 1,232 IU/L |
    | Serum ALP | 265 IU/L |
    | Serum bilirubin | 78 µmol/L |
    | Prothrombin time | 18 seconds |
    | Serum lactate | 2.8 mmol/L |

    **What is the most likely diagnosis?**

    A. Bile leak

    B. Hepatic artery thrombosis (HAT)

    C. Ischaemic cholangiopathy

    D. Post-transplant lymphoproliferative disorder

    E. PVT

## 1. B. Coeliac axis

- TACE is first-line therapy for Barcelona clinic liver cancer (BCLC) stage B HCC
- TACE involves injection of a chemoembolic emulsion into the tumour's hepatic arterial blood supply
- The common HA arises directly from the coeliac axis

This patient most likely has intermediate HCC (BCLC stage B) defined by a large (>5 cm) unresectable or multinodular lesion without macrovascular invasion and extrahepatic metastases in a patient with a performance status 0 and maintained liver function (Child-Pugh Pugh A/B). For BCLC stage B disease, TACE is considered first-line therapy and carries a median survival of around three years. TACE involves rapid injection of a viscous chemoembolic emulsion into the tumour's blood supply after passing a catheter into the right or left HA.

The hepatic arterial blood supply originates from the coeliac axis, which arises from the anterior aspect of the aorta at vertebral level T12. After ~1 cm, it then trifurcates into the left gastric, common hepatic and splenic arteries. The common HA then gives off the gastroduodenal artery before dividing into the right and left hepatic arteries that supply respective lobes of the liver. The right HA supplies liver segments I, V, VI, VII, and VIII, and the left HA supplies segments II, III, and IV.

Postembolization syndrome in which tissue ischaemia causes self-limiting nausea, abdominal pain, and fever occurs in 2%–7% following TACE. Transient hepatic decompensation occurs in <20% but only a minority of patients develop irreversible liver failure.

The European Association for the Study of the Liver (EASL) Clinical Practice Guidelines: management of hepatocellular carcinoma. *J Hepatol*. 2018 Jul;69(1):182–236. Doi: 10.1016/j.jhep.2018.03.019.

## 2. E. Superior mesenteric vein and splenic vein

- The portal vein is formed by the confluence of the superior mesenteric and splenic veins
- Varices are dilated end-organ veins that have the propensity to bleed and are formed by dilatation of portal venous tributaries
- Shunts are dilated collateral channels that connect the portal and systemic vascular beds and predispose to HE

The portal vein is formed at the confluence of the superior mesenteric and splenic vein behind the head of the pancreas and forms 70% of the blood supply to the liver. Other tributaries of the portal vein include the cystic and the left and right gastric veins. Portal hypertension leads to two modes of vascular remodelling: i) dilatation of portal venous tributaries leading to varices that have the propensity to bleed, and ii) development of collaterals connecting the portal and systemic vascular beds, which can dilate, causing 'shunts' that predispose to HE. Oesophageal varices arise

*Best of Five MCQs for the European Specialty Examination in Gastroenterology and Hepatology.* Thomas Marjot, Colleen G C McGregor, Tim Ambrose, Aminda N De Silva, Jeremy Cobbold, and Simon Travis, Oxford University Press (2021). © Oxford University Press. DOI: 10.1093/oso/9780198834373.003.0008

from dilation of the anterior and posterior oesophageal venous tributaries of the left gastric vein. Gastric varices result from enlargement of peripheral venous tributaries of the left gastric, short gastric, and gastro-epiploic veins. Varices outside the oesophagus and stomach are deemed 'ectopic' and can occur in the rectum (superior haemorrhoidal vein), retroperitoneum (gonadal, lumbar, or paraduodenal veins) or around a surgical stoma (due to venous communication between relocated mesenteric veins and cutaneous veins).

Pillai AK, Andring B, Patel A et al. Portal hypertension: a review of portosystemic collateral pathways and endovascular interventions. *Clin Radiol*. 2015 Oct;70(10):1047–1059. Doi: 10.1016/j.crad.2015.06.077.

## 3. E. 10 mmHg

- Clinically significant portal hypertension (CSPH)is defined as an HVPG ≥10 mmHg and is a pre-requisite for the development of varices
- Reducing HVPG to below 12 mmHg or >20% from baseline is associated with reduced risk of variceal bleeding, ascites, and mortality
- HVPG ≥10 mmHg increases the risk of decompensation after resection of HCC

Catheterization of the hepatic vein and measurement of the HVPG is the currently favoured method for determining portal venous pressure. HVPG is calculated as the difference between the wedged hepatic venous pressure (by balloon occlusion of the hepatic vein) and the free hepatic venous pressure. Access to the hepatic vein is usually via the jugular vein and measurements can therefore also be performed alongside trans-jugular liver biopsy.

HVPG values can be classified as normal (1–5 mmHg), preclinical sinusoidal portal hypertension (6–9 mmHg), and CSPH (≥10 mmHg) which is a pre-requisite for the development of varices. Further elevation to ≥12 mmHg is associated with ascites and variceal bleeding. Longitudinal studies have demonstrated that HVPG reduction to ≤12 mmHg with either drug therapy or secondary to improvement of liver disease prevents variceal bleeding. If a target of <12 mmHg cannot be achieved, a reduction of ≥20% from baseline is also associated with a reduced risk of first variceal bleeding, re-bleeding, ascites, and mortality.

CSPH is also an independent risk factor for the development of HCC in cirrhosis. Furthermore, in patients with well-compensated cirrhosis, HVPG ≥10 mmHg markedly increases the risk of hepatic decompensation within three months post-resection. Surgical resection for HCC should therefore be reserved for those with HVPG <10 mmHg.

Bosch J, Abraldes JG, Berzigotti A et al. The clinical use of HVPG measurements in chronic liver disease. *Nat Rev Gastroenterol Hepatol*. 2009 Oct;6(10):573–582. Doi: 10.1038/nrgastro.2009.149.

## 4. B. Repeat gastroscopy in one year without current primary prophylaxis for varices

- Patients with small varices on index gastroscopy, without red wale signs or Child-Pugh B/C cirrhosis, should undergo a repeat gastroscopy at one year.
- Those with high-risk features should receive non-selective beta blockers (NSBB)
- Patients with medium–large varices should receive primary prophylaxis with either NSBB or EVL

Oesophageal varices are present in 30%–40% of patients with compensated cirrhosis at diagnosis. Therefore, screening for varices with gastroscopy or non-endoscopic surrogate markers of portal hypertension is recommended for all patients diagnosed with cirrhosis.

This patient has oesophageal varices that collapse easily on insufflation (small, or Grade 1), no high-risk endoscopic stigmata, and no features of decompensation. Therefore, repeat gastroscopy in one year is the most appropriate answer. Some associations such as the British Society for

Gastroenterology recommend more urgent repeat gastroscopy if patients with cirrhosis develop hepatic decompensation due to the accelerated risk of variceal haemorrhage (VH).

Patients with medium–large varices (Grades 2–3) are at increased risk of haemorrhage and require primary prophylaxis. This is achieved through either NSBB or EVL depending on local expertise and patient preference.

NSBB prescription for patients with small oesophageal varices is an uncertain area. A recent RCT demonstrated a reduced progression to large varices with carvedilol vs placebo (20.6% vs. 38.6%; p=0.04). NSBB could therefore be considered in patients with small varices. The EASL Baveno VI position statement recommends their use in patients with small varices and red wale signs or Child-Pugh B/C cirrhosis.

de Franchis et al. Report of the Baveno VI Consensus Workshop: stratifying risk and individualizing care for portal hypertension. *J Hepatol.* 2015 Sep;63(3):743–752. Doi: 10.1016/j.jhep.2015.05.022.

### 5.  D. Liver stiffness reading of 18.4 kPa

- In compensated cirrhosis, the point prevalence for varices requiring primary prophylaxis is 10%–15%
- The Baveno VI criteria can be used to safely avoid screening gastroscopy for varices
- Tests relevant to the Baveno VI criteria should be measured yearly for ongoing risk stratification

Historically, all patients diagnosed with cirrhosis were referred for varices screening via gastroscopy. In compensated cirrhosis, the prevalence of any varices is 30%–40%, and of high-risk varices requiring primary prophylaxis only 10%–15%. The majority of screening gastroscopies therefore result in an unnecessary invasive investigation.

In 2015, the Baveno VI consensus report made recommendations regarding non-invasive parameters to avoid the need for screening gastroscopy in patients with cirrhosis. In these criteria, patients with compensated cirrhosis, platelet count >150 × 10⁹/L and LSM (via transient elastography) <20 kPa are recommended to safely avoid screening gastroscopy. It is suggested that these Baveno VI criteria are measured annually. Subsequent studies have shown that only 2%–5% of patients who meet the Baveno VI criteria would have high-risk varices requiring treatment.

A HVPG ≥10 mmHg is a prerequisite for the development of varices and, although patients with a measurement of <10 mmHg can safely avoid screening gastroscopy, it is an invasive investigation and not readily available in all hospitals.

de Franchis et al. Report of the Baveno VI Consensus Workshop: stratifying risk and individualizing care for portal hypertension. *J Hepatol.* 2015 Sep;63(3):743–752. Doi: 10.1016/j.jhep.2015.05.022.

### 6.  A. Alcohol aetiology of cirrhosis

- A baseline HVPG >10 mmHg is the strongest predictor of future development of gastro-oesophageal varices (GOV)
- Child-Pugh B/C cirrhosis, alcohol aetiology, and endoscopic red wale signs predict the transformation from small to large varices
- Large varices, Child-Pugh B/C cirrhosis, and red wale signs predict the future risk of (VH)

GOV are present in approximately 50% of patients with cirrhosis and their presence correlates with the severity of liver disease being found in 40% and 86% of Child-Pugh A and Child-Pugh C patients respectively. Patients with cirrhosis but without varices at baseline develop them at a rate of 8% per annum with the strongest predictor for development being a HVPG >10 mmHg, termed 'clinically significant portal hypertension'. Patients with small varices develop large varices at a rate of 8% per annum with the main risk factors for this progression being Child-Pugh B/C cirrhosis, alcohol aetiology, and the presence of red wale marks (longitudinal dilated venules) endoscopically. Increasing variceal size is clinically important because VH in the first year is best predicted by the presence of large varices (15% vs 5% with small varices). Severity of liver disease and red wale signs also predict VH, which occurs only once HVPG exceeds 12 mmHg. Treatment strategies that reduce HVPG <12 mmHg or >20% from baseline (e.g. beta blockers) lower the risk of recurrent VH, further decompensation events, and death.

A small body of historic data has shown an association of cutaneous vascular spider naevi with the presence of varices, large varices, and VH. But no longitudinal data exists to show that their presence at baseline predicts the development or progression of varices over time.

Garcia-Tsao G, Sanyal AJ, Grace ND et al. Prevention and management of gastroesophageal varices and variceal haemorrhage in cirrhosis. *Hepatology*. 2007 Sep;46(3):922–938.

## 7. A. Hyponatraemia is a recognized side effect of terlipressin

- For most patients with VH, a restrictive packed red cell transfusion strategy should be employed aiming for haemoglobin 7–9 g/dl
- Currently no consensus recommendations exist regarding the management of thrombocytopaenia or coagulopathy in VH
- Prophylactic antibiotics and intravenous vasoactive agents introduced pre-endoscopy improve patient outcome

VH remains a medical emergency with high rates of complications and a 20% mortality at six weeks. Treatment must be methodical and start as soon as VH is clinically suspected, before confirmation with upper gastrointestinal endoscopy, which should take place within 12 hours of presentation.

Initial therapy should aim to restore intravascular volume with intravenous fluids. Packed red blood cells can be used to improve tissue oxygen delivery, but a restrictive transfusion strategy is adequate in most patients with a haemoglobin threshold for transfusion of 7 g/dl and a target range after transfusion of 7–9 g/dl. A more liberal transfusion strategy may be considered in individual cases after considering cardiovascular comorbidities, hemodynamic status, and ongoing bleeding. Given the paucity of data, currently no consensus recommendations exist regarding the management of thrombocytopaenia or coagulopathy in VH. Furthermore, prothrombin time is a poor indicator of coagulopathy in cirrhotic patients, and correction with recombinant factor VII has demonstrated no benefit on control of bleeding compared with standard care.

Bacterial infection is observed in up to 50% of cirrhotic patients with upper gastrointestinal (GI) bleeding and is independently associated with re-bleeding and death. Prophylactic antibiotics in patients with cirrhosis and upper GI bleeding (variceal and non-variceal) improve control of bleeding and overall survival, and should be started at presentation and continued for up to seven days.

Intravenous vasoactive drugs (terlipressin, somatostatin, octreotide) introduced before endoscopy and continued for 3–5 days decrease the incidence of active bleeding during endoscopy, facilitate endoscopic therapy, and improve bleeding control and potentially survival. Sodium should be monitored after starting terlipressin because it can precipitate clinically significant hyponatraemia, including seizures, by reducing renal excretion of solute-free water through vasopressin-2 receptor activation.

de Franchis et al. Report of the Baveno VI Consensus Workshop: stratifying risk and individualizing care for portal hypertension. *J Hepatol*. 2015 Sep;63(3):743–752. Doi: 10.1016/j.jhep.2015.05.022.

## 8. A. Cirrhosis

- The three main causes of ascites are cirrhosis (~85%), peritoneal malignancy (~8%), and heart failure (~3%)
- A serum-ascites albumin gradient (SAAG) >11 g/L indicates underlying portal hypertension (from cirrhosis or heart failure)
- When SAAG >11 g/L, an ascitic fluid protein <25 g/L or ≥25 g/L suggests cirrhosis and heart failure, respectively

In the West, the three main causes of ascites are cirrhosis (~85%), peritoneal malignancy (~8%), and heart failure (~3%) with the remainder accounted for by rarer conditions (e.g. nephrotic syndrome, tuberculosis, malnutrition). Five per cent will have more than one cause. Diagnostic paracentesis is a crucial diagnostic test in patients with new ascites, and initial laboratory investigations should include fluid cell count and differential, total protein, and albumin for calculation of the SAAG (serum albumin concentration minus ascitic albumin concentration). The SAAG in this case is 15 g/L. A SAAG >11 g/L indicates ascites related to portal hypertension derived either from cirrhosis or from heart failure, whereas SAAG <11 g/L indicates a non-portal hypertensive cause. Ascitic fluid protein can be used in cases where SAAG >11 g/L to help determine whether the cause is cirrhosis or heart failure. In heart failure, compliant hepatic sinusoids allow protein-rich fluid to leak into the abdominal cavity, often leading to elevated ascitic fluid protein (≥25 g/L), whereas, in cirrhosis, vascular permeability is limited by fibrous tissue deposition leading to lower protein level (<25 g/L). However, this distinction can be complicated over time as congestive hepatopathy progresses to fibrosis.

Ca 125 is expressed by healthy mesothelial cells as well as ovarian cancers, and serum levels are frequently elevated in male and female patients with ascites of any cause. Peritoneal stretch seems to be important as serum levels fall following large volume paracentesis.

Patel YA, Muir AJ. Evaluation of new-onset ascites. *JAMA*. 2016 Jul 19;316(3):340–341. Doi: 10.1001/jama.2016.7600.

## 9. E. Request computed tomography (CT) abdomen and pelvis

- Secondary bacterial peritonitis occurs when ascites becomes infected from an intra-abdominal source (e.g. a perforated viscus or abscess)
- Polymicrobial infection is characteristic of secondary peritonitis
- Early cross-sectional imaging should occur in cases of suspected secondary peritonitis to help with consideration for surgery

Spontaneous bacterial peritonitis (SBP) is a common complication of cirrhosis occurring in ~10% of hospitalized patients and results from translocation of enteric gram-negative bacteria. In contrast, secondary bacterial peritonitis consists of infected ascitic fluid from an intra-abdominal source, such as GI tract perforation/abscess, and represents <5% of all peritonitis in patients with cirrhosis.

Secondary peritonitis tends to occur in patients with less severe liver disease, and presents with a greater degree of abdominal pain compared with SBP. It also causes a more intense local inflammatory response reflected in ascitic fluid analysis that yields a higher neutrophil count, total protein, and lactate dehydrogenase, and lower glucose levels (Runyon's criteria). Polymicrobial infection, as in this case, is characteristic of secondary bacterial peritonitis occurring in two thirds of patients compared with <1% of patients with SBP. Suspicion of secondary peritonitis should lead to early radiological investigation and swift consideration for surgery. Inpatient mortality is significantly higher in patients with secondary peritonitis than in patients with SBP (66.6% vs 26.4%).

Soriano G, Castellote J, Alvarez C et al. Secondary bacterial peritonitis in cirrhosis: a retrospective study of clinical and analytical characteristics, diagnosis and management. *J Hepatol*. 2010 Jan;52(1):39–44. Doi: 10.1016/j.jhep.2009.10.012.

## 10. E. Twenty per cent human albumin solution (1 g/kg) for two consecutive days

- AKI in cirrhosis is defined as a rise in serum creatine ≥26.5 μmol/L in <48 hours, or a rise of ≥1.5-fold from baseline in <7 days
- When there is no identifiable precipitant, human albumin should be administered at 1 g/kg for two consecutive days

AKI is common in patients with decompensated cirrhosis and is defined as an increase in serum creatinine of ≥26.5 μmol/L within 48 hours or by a percentage increase in serum creatinine of more or equal to 50% (1.5-fold from baseline) in less than seven days. Using baseline creatinine is particularly important in patients with cirrhosis as many will be sarcopenic and have lower serum creatinine. Precipitants of AKI include infections, diuretics, gastrointestinal bleeding, nephrotoxic drugs, and raised intra-abdominal pressure secondary to tense ascites.

Management of AKI in cirrhosis should include withdrawal of diuretics and beta-blockers, identification of precipitating factors and the replacement of clear fluid losses (e.g. diarrhoea, excessive diuresis) with crystalloid and/or packed red cells in suspected blood loss. In cases where no obvious cause for AKI can be identified, as in this case, recent guidelines advocate the use of 1 g/Kg of 20% albumin solution (maximum of 100 g of albumin) for two consecutive days. In patients with AKI and tense ascites, therapeutic paracentesis should be performed alongside human albumin infusion. A diagnosis of HRS should only be considered if there is no response to 2-days of diuretic withdrawal and plasma expansion with albumin.

EASL Clinical Practical Guidelines for the management of patients with decompensated cirrhosis. *J Hepatol*. 2018 Aug;69(2):406–460. Doi: 10.1016/j.jhep.2018.03.024.

## 11. C. Increase terlipressin to 2 mg every six hours and continue 40 g human albumin daily

- Terlipressin administered with albumin may improve renal function and short-term survival in patients with HRS-AKI
- In non-responders to 48 hours of 1 mg terlipressin, the dose should be uptitrated in steps to a maximum of 12 mg/day

The original criteria below are still widely used for diagnosing HRS. Those with HRS and AKI (creatinine rise ≥26.5 μmol/L in <48 hours or rise ≥1.5-fold from baseline in <1 week) are deemed to have HRS-AKI (formerly HRS type-1). Those with HRS and no AKI have HRS-nAKI (formerly HRS type 2).

- International Ascites Club (IAC) guidelines: criteria for the diagnosis of hepatorenal syndrome (2005) cirrhosis with ascites
- serum creatinine >133 μmol/L
- absence of hypovolaemia or shock – no improvement in serum creatinine levels (decreased to < 133 μmol/L) after at least two days with diuretic withdrawal (if on diuretics) and volume expansion with albumin.
- no current or recent treatment with nephrotoxic drugs
- absence of parenchymal kidney disease as indicated by proteinuria >500 mg/day, microhaematuria, (> 50 red blood cells per high power field), and/or abnormal renal ultrasound)

Data from International Ascites Club (IAC) Guidelines. Criteria for the diagnosis of hepatorenal syndrome criteria (2005). http://www.icascites.org/about/guidelines

HRS-AKI should initially be treated with terlipressin 1 mg 4–6 hourly alongside 20–40 g/d 20% albumin solution. Terlipressin should only be commenced after careful clinical screening (including electrocardiogram) for risk of ischaemic events. Initial non-response to 1 mg terlipressin (defined as a decrease in serum creatinine <25% from peak value after 48 hours) should prompt stepwise dose escalation to a maximum of 12 mg/day. Relapse of HRS-AKI after cessation of terlipressin occurs in 20%.

Noradrenaline may be beneficial in HRS-AKI. However, data is limited and patients require central venous monitoring. There is limited data for the role of renal replacement therapy but it carries high mortality. LT represents the best treatment for HRS-AKI.

EASL Clinical Practical Guidelines for the management of patients with decompensated cirrhosis. *J Hepatol.* 2018 Aug;69(2):406–460. Doi: 10.1016/j.jhep.2018.03.024.

### 12. D. Splanchnic arterial vasodilation

- Splanchnic arterial vasodilation, caused by vasodilator mediators in patients with cirrhosis and portal hypertension, represents the earliest pathogenic feature of HRS-AKI
- Compensatory activation of vasoconstrictor mechanisms then leads to renal vasoconstriction and reduced glomerular filtration
- Systemic inflammation in increasingly recognized in HRS-AKI pathogenesis with bacterial infection and/or systemic inflammatory response syndrome (SIRS) present in >75%

Circulatory dysfunction is the primary mechanism involved in the pathophysiology of HRS-AKI. In cirrhosis and portal hypertension, increased production of various vasodilators, including nitric oxide, leads to marked splanchnic arterial vasodilation. This leads to decreased vascular resistance and a reduction in effective arterial blood volume and arterial pressure. In the compensated stages of cirrhosis, this arterial hypotension is modest and counterbalanced by increased cardiac output. However, in advanced cirrhosis, splanchnic arterial vasodilation is profound with marked decrease in systemic vascular resistance. In this state, cardiac function, which is often impaired by cirrhotic cardiomyopathy, can no longer compensate, leading to arterial hypotension. This subsequently leads to activation of vasoconstrictor mechanisms including the RAAS, sympathetic nervous system, and vasopressin release. While these processes help maintain arterial blood pressure, they are detrimental to the kidney, causing sodium retention, impaired solute-free water excretion and marked renal vasoconstriction, ultimately culminating in HRS-AKI.

Accumulating evidence suggests that systemic inflammation plays a contributory role in HRS-AKI with >75% of patients having bacterial infection and/or SIRS. In patients with cirrhosis, this inflammation is propagated by pathogen-associated molecular patterns and damage-associated molecular patterns, derived from bacterial translocation and liver damage respectively, which have a further impact on circulatory dysfunction and may also directly cause kidney tissue damage.

Ginès P, Solà E, Angeli P et al. Hepatorenal syndrome. *Nat Rev Dis Primers.* 2018 Sep 13;4(1):23. Doi: 10.1038/s41572-018-0022-7.

### 13. D. Urinary muddy brown casts

- Differentiating between HRS-AKI and acute tubular necrosis–acute kidney injury (ATN-AKI) is important because they require different approaches to treatment
- The significant renal tubular damage in ATN-AKI leads to a high fraction of excreted sodium (FENa) and urea (FEUrea)

AKI is common in patients with cirrhosis (20% of hospitalized patients) yet establishing the underlying cause can be difficult. Because pre-renal AKI usually responds to plasma volume expansion, and post-renal AKI is rare and can be identified by urinary tract imaging, the major challenge is differentiating between HRS-AKI and intrinsic kidney damage, principally ATN-AKI. Hypovolaemia or septic shock often precede ATN-AKI, whereas HRS-AKI commonly occurs with severe alcoholic hepatitis (AH) or in patients with advanced cirrhosis and SBP. While these two conditions often have overlapping triggers, they do require different approaches to treatment (e.g. vasoconstrictive agents and albumin with HRS-AKI and renal replacement therapy with ATN-AKI).

Laboratory investigations can be used to help make a distinction. ATN is caused by ischaemic or nephrotoxic injury to renal tubular epithelial cells, which may slough and form pathognomonic 'muddy brown' casts on urine microscopy. This structural damage impairs sodium and urea reabsorption leading to an elevated FENa (typically >2%–3%) and FEUrea. In AKI-HRS, renal tubular integrity is better maintained and FENa and FEUrea remain low. Recently, there has been interest in urinary neutrophil gelatinase-associated lipocalin (NGAL) as a marker of tubular damage, which may help differentiate AKI-HRS and AKI-ATN although it has not yet moved into routine clinical practice. Both ATN and HRS do not affect the glomerulus and therefore should not cause significant proteinuria.

Despite these distinctions, HRS and ATN are increasingly considered a continuum with direct tubular damage now acknowledged in the pathogenesis of HRS, thus shifting the paradigm away from it being a truly functional disease.

Angeli P, Garcia-Tsao G, Nadim MK. News in Pathophysiology, Definition and Classification of Hepatorenal Syndrome: a step beyond the International Club of Ascites Consensus document. J Hepatol. 2019 Oct;71(4):811–822. Doi: 10.1016/j.jhep.2019.07.002.

## 14. B. An elevated blood ammonia has no prognostic significance in patients with cirrhosis

- Hyperammonaemia alone has no diagnostic, staging, or prognostic value in patients with cirrhosis and HE
- However, a normal value in a patient with cirrhosis considered to have overt HE calls for diagnostic re-evaluation
- Elevated blood ammonia in ALF predicts the risk of developing cerebral oedema

Ammonia is a gut-derived toxin produced by bacterial metabolism of urea from dietary protein. In cirrhosis, liver dysfunction and portal hypertension cause impaired ammonia metabolism and increased shunting to the brain respectively. Ammonia then causes astrocyte swelling and generation of reactive oxygen species. Despite the central role for hyperammonaemia in HE pathogenesis, blood ammonia levels cannot reliably detect HE and its use in isolation results in misdiagnosis of HE in up to 40% of patients with cirrhosis. Joint European and American guidelines therefore emphasize that hyperammonaemia alone does not have any diagnostic, staging, or prognostic value in cirrhosis patients with HE. However, when an ammonia level is checked, a normal value in a patient considered to have overt HE calls for diagnostic re-evaluation. Delay in laboratory measurement of ammonia in a venous sample leads to high false-positive rates. Rifaximin alters colonic bacterial composition and reduces circulating ammonia levels. Blood ammonia has greater clinical significance in ALF with elevated levels predicting the risk of cerebral oedema and intracranial hypertension.

Romero-Gómez M, Montagnese S, Jalan R. et al. Hepatic encephalopathy in patients with acute decompensation of cirrhosis and acute-on-chronic liver failure. J Hepatol. 2015 Feb;62(2):437–447. Doi: 10.1016/j.jhep.2014.09.005.

## 15. B. Approximately half the cases of NASH-related HCC arise in non-cirrhotic patients

- One third of patients with cirrhosis will develop HCC over their lifetime
- The risk of HCC is not eliminated in patients with HCV cirrhosis achieving SVR
- There is a high rate of HCC recurrence post-treatment with curative intent in patients with HCV cirrhosis who achieve SVR

Cirrhosis is an important risk factor for HCC with 1%–8% of patients developing HCC per year and one third developing HCC during their lifetime. In HCV cirrhosis, successful antiviral therapy with SVR reduces but does not eliminate the risk of HCC development, and therefore these patients should continue HCC surveillance. Furthermore, there is a high rate of HCC recurrence post-treatment with curative intent in patients with HCV cirrhosis achieving SVR with DAA regimens, and therefore this group should be closely monitored. Whether recurrence is related to the inherent risk of advanced cirrhosis or due to a direct impact of DAA therapy remains to be completely elucidated. Patients with CHB are at risk of HCC development even in the absence of cirrhosis, but the exact degree of risk is ill-defined and has wide geographical variation. HBV e antigen seropositivity, high viral load, and genotype C are all independent predictors of HCC development. Half the cases of NASH-induced HCC arise in non-cirrhotic patients. However, the incidence of HCC in these patients with non-advanced disease is insufficiently high to currently recommend universal surveillance, particularly given the high prevalence of NAFLD in the general population.

EASL Clinical Practice Guidelines: management of hepatocellular carcinoma. *J Hepatol.* 2018 Jul;69(1):182–236. Doi: 10.1016/j.jhep.2018.03.019.

## 16. A. LT

- The modified BCLC staging system is used as the primary treatment strategy guide for HCC
- Characteristics to consider regarding treatment include tumour factors (nodule size and number, alpha-fetoprotein [AFP] level), liver factors (Childs-Pugh score and portal hypertension) and patient factors (performance status and co-morbidity)

The modified BCLC staging system considers the most appropriate treatment for HCC. This patient would be early stage (A) for which curative intent would be appropriate. Surgical resection (hemi-hepatectomy) would be technically feasible, given the lesions in segment 5 and 7, but the presence of portal hypertension carries a high risk of decompensation (>30%) and liver-related mortality (25%). LT would therefore be the preferred option. Bridging loco-regional therapies (e.g. transarterial embolization or radiofrequency ablation) should be considered in all patients listed for LT with HCC.

Several criteria (including the Milan, University of California San Francisco and AFP-French criteria) are validated for selecting HCC patients suitable for transplantation. Macrovascular invasion and extrahepatic spread are absolute contraindications. Elevated AFP >1,000 ng/ml indicates adverse tumour biology, and in most criteria is a further contraindication to transplantation.

EASL Clinical Practice Guidelines: management of hepatocellular carcinoma. *J Hepatol.* 2018 Jul;69(1):182–236. Doi: 10.1016/j.jhep.2018.03.019.

## 17. B. Lifestyle changes and repeat MRI in six months

- Hepatocellular adenoma (HCA) carries a 25% risk of haemorrhage and 5% risk of malignant transformation

- Surgical resection is recommended in all male patients with HCA because of the increased risk of malignancy.
- In women, six-months observation with repeat MRI is appropriate because many will respond to lifestyle advice (e.g. stopping OCP and weight loss)

This patient has HCA which is a rare, benign hepatic neoplasm carrying a 25% risk of haemorrhage and 5% risk of malignant transformation. It is most frequently diagnosed in younger women taking the OCP. The incidence of HCA in males is increasing due to more widespread use of anabolic steroids and the rising prevalence of obesity and metabolic syndrome. Abdominal pain is the most common symptom although >50% HCAs are asymptomatic and identified incidentally. MRI is the modality of choice for diagnosis and can allow subtype characterization to further stratify the risk of haemorrhage and malignancy.

Surgical resection is recommended in all male patients with HCA because of the higher incidence of malignant transformation. In women, six months' observation with repeat MRI is appropriate because many will respond to lifestyle advice (e.g. stopping OCPs, weight loss). Resection is indicated in lesions persistently >5 cm or increasing in size, whereas a conservative approach with interval imaging can be adopted with smaller lesions.

EASL Clinical Practice Guidelines on the management of benign liver tumours. *J Hepatol.* 2016 Aug;65(2):386–398. Doi: 10.1016/j.jhep.2016.04.001.

### 18. A. Nasogastric feeding

- Patients with AH require 35–40 kcal/kg/day, which is often difficult to achieve orally in clinical practice
- Nasogastric feeding is strongly recommended in patients unable to maintain adequate oral intake
- Protein restriction offers no clinical advantage in patients with AH and/or cirrhosis, with or without encephalopathy, and should be avoided

Protein-energy malnutrition is found in virtually all patients with severe AH. Given the marked catabolic state of AH, the European Society for Clinical Nutrition and Metabolism recommends a target daily energy intake of 35–40 kcal/kg. This is often extremely difficult to achieve in clinical practice and therefore nasogastric feeding is strongly recommended in patients unable to maintain adequate oral intake. While trials demonstrate nasogastric feeding to be equivalent to corticosteroids in AH, their combined use has not been shown to improve survival, although interpretations are limited by half of patients prematurely removing their feeding tube. Nevertheless, patients with severe AH and low calorific intake (<21.5 kcal/kg/day) have double the mortality compared with those with higher intake (≥21.5 kcal/kg/day) and therefore strong expert consensus exists for early consideration of nasogastric feeding.

While parenteral nutrition might circumvent the complications of nasogastric feeding, there is currently insufficient evidence to support a recommendation, particularly given that parenteral feeding is associated with a high risk of line sepsis.

The historical dogma that protein restriction may improve encephalopathy is outdated, and many trials have now shown that this approach offers no clinical advantage and may increase protein catabolism.

EASL Clinical Practice Guidelines: management of alcohol-related liver diseases. March 2018

### 19. B. Start treatment with tenofovir

- Patients with HBV DNA >20,000 and ALT >2 × ULN can be treated without need for liver biopsy or TE
- In patients with CHB, a LSM of >9 kPa or >12 kPa indicates advanced fibrosis/cirrhosis in those with normal and elevated ALT respectively

All patients with HBV cirrhosis require treatment regardless of ALT and viral load because it reduces the rate of decompensation and liver-related complications. Patients without cirrhosis should be considered for treatment when they have HBV DNA >2,000 IU/ml, ALT >ULN (40 IU/L), and moderate necroinflammation and/or moderate fibrosis traditionally assessed by liver biopsy. Patients with HBV DNA >20,000 IU/ml and ALT >2 × ULN, as in this case, should be treated without need for liver biopsy. EASL recommends treatment for patients >30 years with HBeAg-positive CHB with normal ALT and high HBV DNA levels (formerly immune-tolerant phase) because of the correlation between HBV DNA and risk of HCC. This contrasts with American guidelines, which advocate against treatment in immune-tolerant CHB citing lack of prospective outcome data. For those not meeting treatment criteria, the intervals for follow-up are determined by HBeAg status and viral load.

LSM with TE can non-invasively assess for liver fibrosis and LSM <6 kPa reliably excludes significant fibrosis in CHB. TE performs best in patients without significant liver necroinflammation indicated by normal ALT. In these patients, LSM >9 kPa indicates advanced fibrosis/cirrhosis with LSM 6-9 kPa deemed intermediate. In those with elevated ALT, a higher LSM value of >12 kPa is required to diagnose advanced fibrosis/cirrhosis with LSM 6-12 kPa as intermediate. Patients with intermediate values may require liver biopsy.

EASL Clinical Practice Guidelines on the management of hepatitis B virus infection. *J Hepatol.* 2017 Aug;67(2):370–398. Doi: 10.1016/j.jhep.2017.03.021.

### 20. E. Suppression of HBV DNA

- Suppression of HBV DNA is the cornerstone endpoint in the treatment of chronic HBV infection
- Loss of HBsAg can be regarded as a functional cure but it is unrealistic to expect this outcome with the current treatment regimens available

Suppression of HBV DNA is the cornerstone endpoint in the treatment of CHB and represents the best chance of reducing necroinflammation, fibrosis, and the risk of HCC. The target level of HBV DNA suppression in order to achieve these benefits is not well defined but it is generally accepted that the lower the better. LSM does have a role in identifying severe liver disease in CHB but this patient's measurement is below the cut-offs of 9 kPa (with normal ALT) or 12 kPa (with elevated ALT) needed to diagnose advanced fibrosis. Loss of HBeAg correlates with HBV immune control and often leads to normalization of ALT. However, this is a less reliable endpoint compared with suppression of HBV DNA levels particularly as HBeAg seroreversion can occur following treatment cessation. Although loss of HBsAg can be regarded as a functional cure, it is unrealistic to expect this outcome with the current treatment regimens available. Furthermore, cccDNA and integrated HBV still persist, suggesting that HBsAg loss may not add to the prevention of the long-term complications of CHB beyond what can be achieved by the suppression of HBV DNA replication alone.

EASL Clinical Practice Guidelines on the management of hepatitis B virus infection. *J Hepatol.* 2017 Aug;67(2):370–398. Doi: 10.1016/j.jhep.2017.03.021.

## 21. E. Prophylaxis with entecavir throughout R-CHOP treatment and for 18 months after its discontinuation

- HBV reactivation can occur in HBsAg-positive patients and in HbsAg-negative, HBcAb-positive patients on starting immunosuppression
- Rituximab chemotherapy carries a particularly high risk of reactivation

Patients with either chronic hepatitis B (HBsAg-positive) or 'resolved' HBV (HBsAg-negative, HBcAb-positive) who are exposed to immunosuppressive agents can develop reactivation of HBV (HBVr). This can manifest with an acute rise in HBV DNA levels, which in turn can lead to severe acute hepatitis and liver failure. Therefore, all candidates for chemotherapy should be tested for HBV markers prior to their use. The B-cell depleting medication Rituximab carries a particularly high risk of HBVr.

Patients with no evidence of past infection (HBsAg-negative, HBcAb-negative) should receive HBV vaccination. HBsAg-positive patients should be referred to hepatology and receive nucleoside analogues (NAs) as treatment (if evidence of active inflammation or fibrosis) or prophylaxis. Prophylaxis should continue for duration of immunosuppression plus 12 months after its withdrawal, extended to 18 months for Rituximab-based regimens.

Patients who are HBsAg-negative, antiHBc positive ('resolved' infection) should only receive prophylaxis when there is either detectable HBV DNA (when they should be treated similarly to HBsAg-positive patients), or if they require Rituximab. Prophylaxis with NA should continue for 18 months after stopping immunosuppression. HBsAg-negative, antiHBC-positive patients on Rituximab-free immunosuppressive regimes are deemed medium- or low-risk of HBVr (depending on chemotherapy agent) and pre-emptive therapy rather than prophylaxis is preferred. In this group, serology should be monitored every 1–3 months and therapy introduced in the case of detectable HBV DNA or HBsAg seroconversion.

EASL Clinical Practice Guidelines on the management of hepatitis B virus infection. *J Hepatol.* 2017 Aug;67(2):370–398. Doi: 10.1016/j.jhep.2017.03.021.

## 22. D. Sofosbuvir, velpatasvir

- DAA therapy in HCV infection offers SVR in >95% with rates of adverse events and treatment discontinuation <10%
- The new pangenotypic DAA regimens sofosbuvir/velpatasvir and glecaprevir/pibrentasvir provide an opportunity to deliver more widespread treatment with less pre-treatment investigation

Traditionally, HCV treatment centred around the use of interferon and ribavirin regimens that were poorly tolerated and offered disappointing cure rates (40%–75% for non-cirrhotic, treatment naïve patients). Treatment has dramatically evolved over the past ten years with the development of DAA targeting proteins involved in HCV replication. These now achieve SVR in >95% with rates of adverse events and treatment discontinuation <10%. The choice and duration of DAA regimen will depend on genotype, cirrhosis status, co-morbidities, and local drug availability. Barriers to genotype-specific treatment include numbers of infected individuals, the volume of clinical information needed to guide treatment decisions, and the relative complexity of combined treatment strategies. The availability of new pangenotypic regimens (sofosbuvir/velpatasvir and glecaprevir/pibrentasvir) provides an opportunity to deliver simpler, more widespread treatment with less pre-treatment investigation. Twelve weeks' treatment in patients without cirrhosis or with compensated (Child-Pugh A) cirrhosis, including treatment-naïve or treatment-experienced patients, are expected to yield an SVR rate >95%. The only information needed to start treatment with one of these regimens is the presence of HCV replication (as assessed by HCV RNA) and possible drug-drug interactions.

EASL Recommendations on treatment of hepatitis C 2018. *J Hepatol*. 2018 Aug;69(2):461–511. Doi: 10.1016/j.jhep.2018.03.026.

### 23. A. Treat with DAAs post-LT if MELD ≥18–20 and time to transplantation likely to be <6 months

- HCV treatment pre-LT improves MELD scores and survival on the waiting list but can paradoxically worsen outcome through delisting and/or delayed transplantation
- Patients with severe decompensated cirrhosis (MELD ≥18–20) should be treated post-transplantation unless transplant waiting time is likely to exceed 6 months
- Cure rate in decompensated patients may be substantially lower than in post-transplant patients

Decompensated HCV cirrhosis carries a 20% one-year mortality without LT. Allograft HCV infection post-LT occurs universally in those with HCV and can be rapidly progressive requiring retransplantation. Traditionally, the management of decompensated HCV cirrhosis and post-LT HCV was challenging due to low efficacy and tolerability of interferon-based regimes. The era of DAAs has altered the approach to these difficult-to-treat groups and led to debate about whether to treat HCV infection pre- or post-transplantation. While treatment pre-LT improves MELD scores and survival on the waiting list, paradoxically this can worsen outcome through delisting and/or delayed transplantation in up to 20%: a situation labelled 'MELD-purgatory'. A recent North American study combining real-world data and modelling suggests that, above a MELD score of 20, the life expectancy benefit of treating before LT was always less than one year, arguing for transplanting individuals with severe disease prior to HCV therapy. EASL now recommends that patients with decompensated cirrhosis without HCC awaiting LT with a MELD score of ≥18–20 be transplanted first and have their HCV infection treated post-LT. Patients with a MELD score of ≥18–20 can, however, be treated pre-LT if the waiting time is likely to exceed six months.

EASL Recommendations on treatment of hepatitis C 2018. *J Hepatol*. 2018 Aug;69(2):461–511. Doi: 10.1016/j.jhep.2018.03.026.

### 24. D. Treatment with Peg-IFNα for 48 weeks

- Five per cent of patients with chronic HBV have co-infection with HDV; chronic co-infection carries a high rate of progression to cirrhosis and decompensation
- HDV can be acquired at the same time as HBV, or as a superinfection in established HBV carriers
- PegIFNa is the only drug currently available that has proven antiviral efficacy against chronic HDV infection

HDV can only propagate in an individual who has coexistent HBV and occurs in 5% of patients with chronic HBV. HDV can be acquired simultaneously with HBV (co-infection) or via superinfection of established HBV carriers. Acute co-infection is clinically indistinguishable from acute HBV monoinfection and carries the same risk of progression to chronicity (<5%). By contrast, superinfection leads to chronic HDV in >90% of cases. Superinfection can present as acute hepatitis in a previous carrier of HBsAg, as in this case. HDV superinfection accelerates progression to cirrhosis almost a decade earlier than HBV monoinfected persons, although HDV suppresses HBV replication. No clear association between HDV and the risk of HCC has been established.

PegIFNa is the only antiviral agent with proven efficacy against HDV and should be used for at least 48 weeks in co-infected patients with compensated liver disease. If HBV-DNA levels are persistently elevated, concurrent therapy with NAs may also be indicated. Patients with decompensated cirrhosis, where Peg-IFN is contraindicated, should be considered for LT.

EASL Clinical Practice Guidelines on the management of hepatitis B virus infection. *J Hepatol.* 2017 Aug;67(2):370–398. Doi: 10.1016/j.jhep.2017.03.021

## 25. D. Prednisolone 40 mg daily

- Liver biopsy is a prerequisite for the diagnosis of AIH
- Glucocorticoid therapy with prednisolone is the mainstay of induction treatment in AIH
- Budesonide can induce remission in AIH but is contraindicated in patients with cirrhosis, given its high hepatic first pass metabolism

This patient has the classical histological features of AIH. EASL guidelines recommend applying simplified diagnostic criteria, which include histological findings to make a diagnosis of probable/ definite AIH. Liver biopsy is required to make a diagnosis of AIH, and should always be performed prior to starting treatment, which may mask inflammatory activity.

Glucocorticoid induction therapy with prednisolone (0.5–1 mg/kg/day), either as monotherapy or in combination with azathioprine, has been shown to confer survival benefit over placebo and azathioprine monotherapy.

Budesonide in combination with azathioprine has been shown to be effective in the induction of remission in non-cirrhotic AIH. However, budesonide has a high hepatic first pass metabolism (90%), and therefore should not be used in patients with cirrhosis, due to the risk of systemic toxicity. 30% of patients with AIH will have cirrhosis at diagnosis.

The patient also has concomitant steatosis which may be contributing to her liver disease; however, the predominant aetiology is AIH.

Tiniakos DG, Brain JG, Bury YA. Role of histopathology in autoimmune hepatitis. *Dig Dis.* 2015;33 (Suppl 2):53–64. Doi: 10.1159/000440747.

## 26. B. ANA or SMA ≥1:40

- Elevated IgG levels are found in 85% of cases of AIH
- Using the simplified diagnostic criteria for AIH (autoimmune serology, IgG, liver histology, and absence of viral hepatitis), probable AIH is defined as score of ≥6

The varied clinical spectrum of AIH can make the diagnosis challenging, and clinicians have to rely on the interpretation of laboratory and histological findings.

In AIH, a hepatitic pattern of LFTs predominates with normal or modest elevations in cholestatic enzymes. An elevated serum IgG level is found in 85% of cases although, in acute onset disease, levels tend to be lower with up to 40% having an IgG within normal range. Positive ANA and SMA account for 75% of patients but disease specificity is low. Anti-LKM1 and/or anti liver cytosol (anti-LC1) are less common but more specific although anti-LKM1 is also found in 10% of patients with chronic HCV infection. Liver biopsy is essential in diagnostic work-up of AIH with interface hepatitis, lymphoplasmocytic infiltrates in portal tracts extending into the lobule, emperipolesis (penetration by one cell into another), and rosette formation regarded as 'typical' for the diagnosis of AIH. Histology demonstrating chronic hepatitis with lymphocytic infiltration without other typical features is considered 'compatible' with AIH. The simplified diagnosis criteria were developed as a user-friendly tool to assist in diagnosis with a score ≥7 regarded as definite and ≥6 as probable AIH (Table 8.1).

EASL Clinical Practice Guidelines: autoimmune hepatitis. *J Hepatol.* 2015 Oct;63(4):971–1004. Doi: 10.1016/j.jhep.2015.06.030.

**Table 8.1** Simplified diagnostic criteria of the International Autoimmune Hepatitis Group.

| Feature/parameter | Discriminator | Score |
|---|---|---|
| ANA or SMA+ | ≥1:40 | +1* |
| ANA or SMA+ | ≥1:80 | +2* |
| or LKM+ | ≥1:40 | +2* |
| or SLA/LP+ | Any titer | +2* |
| IgG or γ-globulins level | >upper limit of normal<br>>1.1 × upper limit | +1 +2 |
| Liver histology (evidence of hepatitis is a necessary condition) | Compatible with AIH<br>Typical of AIH<br>Atypical | +1<br>+2<br>0 |
| Absence of viral hepatitis | No<br>Yes | 0<br>+2 |

Definite AIH: ≥7; Probable AIH: ≥6.
*Addition of points achieved for all autoantibodies (maximum, two points).

## 27. C. Relapse commonly occurs within the first year of treatment withdrawal

- Biochemical remission in AIH is defined as normalization of transaminases and IgG. Histological remission is defined as normal liver histology or mild histological activity (Hepatitis activity index [HAI]<4)
- Discontinuing treatment should not be considered in those without biochemical remission for more than two years

AIH is a chronic liver disease that can progress to cirrhosis, liver failure, and death if untreated. Treatment of AIH is aimed at obtaining complete biochemical and histological disease resolution to prevent further progression. First-line treatment is prednisolone (0.5–1 mg/kg/day), followed by the addition of azathioprine (1–2 mg/kg) typically after two weeks to allow the opportunity to differentiate between primary non-response and drug-induced hepatotoxicity.

Immunosuppression in AIH improves symptoms, liver function, and survival. It is recommended in all patients with active disease, symptomatic patients, and those with advanced fibrosis and cirrhosis, although there remains debate regarding the benefits in older asymptomatic patients with mild necroinflammation on liver biopsy.

Complete biochemical remission is defined as normalization of transaminases and IgG. Histological remission is defined as normal liver histology or mild histological activity (HAI<4). European guidelines advise that immunosuppression should be continued for at least three years, and for at least two years following normalization of transaminases and IgG. Treatment should not be discontinued in those without biochemical remission for more than two years, at which point a liver biopsy is recommended to confirm histological remission. If there is evidence of histological disease activity (HAI>3), then treatment should not be withdrawn. Only a minority of patients remain in remission without maintenance immunosuppression. Relapses occur most commonly within 12 months of treatment withdrawal but may occur years later, so lifelong surveillance is advised.

EASL Clinical Practice Guidelines: autoimmune hepatitis. *J Hepatol.* 2015 Oct;63(4):971–1004. Doi: 10.1016/j.jhep.2015.06.030.

## 28. D. Primary biliary cholangitis (PBC)

- Antimitochondrial antibody (AMA) is the hallmark of PBC and, together with a raised ALP, is sufficient to make a diagnosis of PBC
- AMA positivity alone with normal liver biochemistry is not enough to make a diagnosis of PBC, but these patients have a 17% chance of developing PBC over the next five years
- AMA is positive in more than 90% of patients with PBC

The hallmark for diagnosis of PBC is a positive AMA in the setting of cholestasis. AMA is positive in more than 90% of patients with PBC and is detected on indirect immunofluorescence. It should be part of the work-up in any patient presenting with cholestatic liver enzymes, particularly if lethargy or pruritis are present.

Patients may occasionally be positive for AMA without abnormal liver biochemistry, and in this setting one in six will develop PBC within five years. However, if patients have cholestatic liver biochemistry and a positive AMA, a definitive diagnosis of PBC may be made without the need for further investigations such as MRCP and liver biopsy.

About 30% of patients with DILI show a cholestatic pattern of liver enzymes with trimethoprim +/- sulfamethoxazole being a common culprit medication. The long-term lethargy, positive AMA and raised IgM level in this case, however, would best support a diagnosis of PBC.

EASL Clinical Practice Guidelines: the diagnosis and management of patients with primary biliary cholangitis. *J Hepatol.* 2017 Jul;67(1):145–172. Doi: 10.1016/j.jhep.2017.03.022.

## 29. D. Start UDCA 13–15 mg/kg/day

- Liver biopsy is not routinely recommended in the diagnosis of PBC except in the case of absence of PBC-specific antibodies or if a coexistent liver disease is suspected
- A diagnosis of AMA-negative PBC can be made in patients with cholestasis and specific ANA immunofluorescence (nuclear dots or perinuclear rims) or assay results (sp100, gp210)
- UDCA 13–15 mg/kg/day is the first-line therapy in PBC

This patient has AMA-negative PBC, with clinical features of lethargy, pruritis, xanthelasma, and hepatomegaly, with cholestatic liver biochemistry, and PBC-specific ANA. PBC is usually a clinical diagnosis and the European Association for Study of the Liver advises against liver biopsy except in specific settings (no PBC-specific antibodies or suspected concomitant AIH or NASH).

ANA is positive in 30% of patients with PBC and the immunofluorescence pattern can sometimes represent a PBC-specific antibody: a nuclear dot pattern for anti-sp100 and perinuclear rim staining for anti-gp210. These antibodies also confer a slightly poorer prognosis. UDCA treatment should be initiated at 13–15 mg/kg/day and confers a LT-free survival benefit. Higher doses are not appropriate. MRCP is only required if there are features suggestive of cholelithiasis or primary sclerosing cholangitis. Autotaxin is possible pruritogen in PBC, but commercially available assays are not available.

EASL Clinical Practice Guidelines: the diagnosis and management of patients with primary biliary cholangitis. *J Hepatol.* 2017 Jul;67(1):145–172. Doi: 10.1016/j.jhep.2017.03.022.

## 30. A. Consider second-line therapy with obeticholic acid (OCA)

- In PBC, the response to UDCA should always be determined one year after starting treatment
- UDCA non-response is associated with increased risk of LT and death

- OCA is a second-line therapy for use in patients with PBC who are either intolerant to UDCA or have an inadequate response with UDCA

Biochemical response to UDCA at one year should always be assessed as those with inadequate response at significantly increased risk of LT or death. There are several different algorithms to assess response although no single scoring system has demonstrated clear superiority. Most revolve around reduction of ALP below certain thresholds such as 1.5–2 × ULN and normalization of bilirubin. This patient's raised ALP would equate to treatment failure.

Male gender and age <45 years also confer a higher risk of UDCA failure and are independently associated with more advanced disease and poorer outcome. Therefore, together with this patient's UDCA treatment failure, it is important that he is initiated on second-line therapy to try and prevent disease progression.

The only licensed second-line therapy in Europe is OCA, a farsenoid X receptor agonist that has shown clinical benefit in PBC in patients who are intolerant to, or have an inadequate response to, UDCA. Unless intolerant, UDCA should be continued on initiation of OCA. Bezafibrate is another potential second-line therapy that has been shown to normalize ALP in PBC, although it is not currently licensed for use in PBC. This patient's UDCA dose is currently 13–15 mg/kg/day, and higher doses are not beneficial.

Corpechot C Chazouillères O, Poupon R et al. Early primary biliary cirrhosis: biochemical response to treatment and prediction of long-term outcome. *J Hepatol.* 2011 Dec;55(6):1361–1367. Doi: 10.1016/j.jhep.2011.02.031.

### 31. C. Poor prognostic group because her ALP is above 2 × ULN and her bilirubin is above the ULN

- ALP >2 × ULN and bilirubin outside normal range are associated with need for LT and/or death in PBC
- PBC patients treated with OCA should be assessed for a biochemical response at one year

This patient was on second-line therapy with maximal dose OCA, and assessment of response and risk stratification should occur one year post-therapy. A response to OCA is classified as attainment of both an ALP value <1.67 ULN (with a ≥15% reduction from baseline) and a normal serum bilirubin level that this patient did not fulfil.

Her ALP was approximately 3 × ULN and bilirubin was over the ULN, which, using all risk-scoring systems (e.g. Barcelona, Paris I and II, UK-PBC risk score) puts her in a high-risk group for progression to death and/or LT. One of the largest studies of PBC outcomes (from the Global PBC Study Group) found that a raised ALP >2 × ULN and an abnormal bilirubin at one year was associated with the highest rate of death and/or LT.

Male gender and younger age (<45 years) are associated with more advanced disease in PBC. This patient had no evidence of decompensated cirrhosis. Therefore, referral for LT was not yet indicated.

EASL Clinical Practice Guidelines: the diagnosis and management of patients with primary biliary cholangitis. *J Hepatol.* 2017 Jul;67(1):145–172. Doi: 10.1016/j.jhep.2017.03.022.

### 32. C. MRCP

- MRCP is the gold standard in making a diagnosis of PSC and has largely replaced ERCP and liver biopsy

- There should be a strong suspicion of PSC in patients with ulcerative colitis (particularly pancolitis) and persistently cholestatic LFTs
- PSC is often asymptomatic at diagnosis and should be screened for with liver biochemistry at routine clinic visits

This patient most likely has PSC. Two thirds of patients with PSC have IBD (75% ulcerative colitis, 15% Crohn's, 10% unclassified, which is usually pancolitis). Typical age at presentation is 30–40 years old, and two thirds are male. Conversely, 7%–12% of patients with ulcerative colitis will have PSC.

The European Association for Study of the Liver recommends MRCP in all patients with chronic cholestasis, after structural abnormalities have been ruled out with ultrasound, and PBC-specific antibodies are found to be negative (AMA, anti-sp100/anti-gp210). The diagnosis of PSC relies on the presence of cholestasis, typical PSC cholangiogram findings (bile duct stricturing and/or beading), and the absence of a secondary cause of sclerosing cholangitis. MRCP has become the cholangiogram of choice given the recent improvement in image quality and the risks of ERCP. PSC patients are particularly susceptible to post-ERCP cholangitis.

Liver biopsy can be useful in the setting of a normal or poor-quality MRCP or when there is a suspicion of overlap with AIH. If MRCP excludes classical 'large duct' PSC but liver biopsy shows histological changes of PSC, then a diagnosis of 'small-duct PSC' may be made, which carries a far better prognosis.

Significant tranaminitis and elevated IgG may indicate AIH (which can overlap with PSC). However, patients with pure PSC frequently have mildly elevated transaminases, immunoglobulins, and often have a positive ANA. WD is not likely in this case, with no evidence of haemolysis and cholestatic versus hepaticliver function tests.

Karlsen TH, Folseraas T, Thorburn D et al. Primary sclerosing cholangitis—a comprehensive review. J Hepatol. 2017 Dec;67(6):1298–1323. Doi: 10.1016/j.jhep.2017.07.022.

## 33. E. Small-duct PSC

- Concentric biliary fibrosis is a hallmark feature of PSC on liver biopsy
- Changes of PSC on liver biopsy with a normal MRCP is termed 'small-duct PSC'
- Small-duct PSC is associated with a good prognosis compared with classical PSC

The liver biopsy shows characteristic features of PSC: concentric fibrosis ('onion skinning') surrounding the hepatic bile duct and a portal inflammatory infiltrate. Together with this patient's cholestatic pattern of liver biochemistry and the typical demographic (young and male), the clinical picture is that of PSC. However, given his normal MRCP, his disease is not affecting the larger bile ducts and he therefore has small-duct PSC.

Given that the biopsy shows no significant plasma cell infiltrate or interface hepatitis and his ALT is not markedly elevated, AIH and PSC/AIH overlap are highly unlikely.

Small-duct PSC occurs in about 10% of PSC cases and carries an excellent prognosis compared with classical PSC with low rates of progression to advanced liver disease and minimal malignant potential. Approximately 25% of patients with small-duct PSC will progress to classical PSC. Therefore, patients should be monitored for a change in their clinical status (such as a sudden rise in ALP or bilirubin, or new symptoms) and if this occurs should be screened for progression to classical PSC with an MRCP.

Karlsen TH, Folseraas T, Thorburn D et al. Primary sclerosing cholangitis—a comprehensive review. J Hepatol. 2017 Dec;67(6):1298–1323. Doi: 10.1016/j.jhep.2017.07.022.

## 34. E. UDCA can cause paradoxical worsening of pruritis in cholestatic liver disease

- An obstructive bile duct lesion should be excluded in new cases of cholestatic pruritis
- Cholestyramine or other resins are regarded as first-line treatment of pruritis but with little evidence base
- LT is effective in managing pruritis but should only be considered when all other available interventions above have proven ineffective

Pruritus can be a feature of any cholestatic disease and can be severe and disabling. Fluctuation is characteristic, both within the day and over longer periods of time. Pruritus can lessen as end-stage liver disease ensues. The European Association for Study of the Liver guidelines provide a comprehensive algorithm for the management of pruritus in cholestasis. An obstructive bile duct lesion must first be excluded.

Topical agents are frequently used but none have proven efficacy. UDCA can cause paradoxical worsening of itch, except in the context of intrahepatic cholestasis of pregnancy. Cholestyramine 4 g up to four times daily is widely used as first-line treatment but with a minimal evidence base. It is limited by poor tolerance and binding with other medications, leading to loss of efficacy. Rifampicin is second line, starting at 150 mg and titrating to 600 mg daily. Drug-induced hepatitis and significant liver dysfunction have been reported in up to 12% of cholestatic patients, typically at 2–3 months. Naltrexone, an oral opiate antagonist, is third line, starting at 25 mg and titrating to 50 mg. An opiate withdrawal-like reaction can occur on initiation. Sertraline is fourth line, although the mechanism of its action remains unclear. LT is effective, but only considered when all other available interventions have proven ineffective.

EASL Clinical Practice Guidelines: management of Cholestatic Liver diseases. *J Hepatol.* 2009 Aug;51(2):237–267. Doi: 10.1016/j.jhep.2009.04.009.

## 35. C. Bilirubin

- ALP, AFP, and clotting factors all increase throughout normal pregnancy
- Bilirubin, aminotransferases, and prothrombin time remain unchanged

An awareness of the normal physiologic, biochemical, and haematological changes found in pregnancy is important to prevent misdiagnosis of liver pathology. For example, several normal clinical findings of pregnancy (e.g. hyperdynamic circulation, palmar erythema, multiple spider naevi) can mimic features of chronic liver disease. Furthermore, in women without liver disease, small clinically insignificant GOV occur in 50% of normal pregnancies due to compression of the inferior vena cava by the enlarging uterus.

Laboratory indices taken during pregnancy need to be interpreted in light of altered normal ranges. ALP increases in the third trimester when it is released both from the placenta and from fetal bone development. AFP level increases up to fourfold in pregnancy due to production by the fetal liver. Other common tests including bilirubin, aminotransferases, and prothrombin time remain unchanged and any elevation of these indices requires further assessment.

*Unchanged*

- Bilirubin, aminotransferases, prothrombin time

*Increased*

- White blood cells, caeruloplasmin, triglycerides, and $\alpha$- and $\beta$-globulins
- $\alpha$-FP
- Cholesterol

- ALP
- Fibrinogen and clotting factors I, II, V, VII, X, and XII

*Decreased*

- Gammaglobulin
- Platelet count (mild reduction but >100 × 10$^9$ in 90%)
- Haemoglobin, in later pregnancy

Westbrook RH, Dusheiko G, Williamson C. Westbrook et al. Pregnancy and liver disease. *J Hepatol.* 2016 Apr;64(4):933–945. Doi: 10.1016/j.jhep.2015.11.030.

## 36. E. UDCA

- Intrahepatic cholestasis of pregnancy (ICP) is characterized by third-trimester pruritis, a moderate ALT rise, jaundice, and elevated bile acids
- It carries an increased risk of preterm labour and intrauterine death
- UDCA is used first line to relieve symptoms

ICP is the most common liver disease in pregnancy affecting 5% of pregnancies. It can present at any stage but usually manifests in the third trimester. Patients first describe pruritis, predominately of the palms and soles, which can become debilitating but resolves quickly following delivery. Risk factors include a personal or family history of ICP, and a history of cholestasis secondary to the OCP. The aetiology is multifactorial with interaction between elevated levels of oestrogen and progesterone, and genetic susceptibility.

The characteristic laboratory finding is elevated maternal serum bile acids (normal range 0–10 umol/L). There is a relationship between serum bile acids and fetal outcome with a threshold of >40 umol/L associated with an increased risk of preterm labour, intra-uterine death, and neonatal respiratory distress. Sixty per cent of patients will have moderate elevations in their ALT (usually × 2 ULN) and ~25% will develop jaundice. In some cases, profound cholestasis can cause steatorrhea and malabsorption of fat-soluble vitamins (A, D, E, and K), which can cause a prolonged prothrombin time.

First-line treatment is with UDCA (10–15 mg/kg), which relieves pruritus in 70%, has no known fetal/neonatal toxicity, and is well tolerated. Its impact on perinatal outcome, however, remains unclear. In refractory cases, UDCA can be used in combination with cholestyramine or rifampicin. Women with ICP should be managed by a consultant-led obstetric service and are usually induced at 37 weeks to reduce the risk of intrauterine death.

Westbrook RH, Dusheiko G, Williamson C. Westbrook et al. Pregnancy and liver disease. *J Hepatol.* 2016 Apr;64(4):933–945. Doi: 10.1016/j.jhep.2015.11.030.

## 37. C. Haemolysis, elevated liver enzymes, and low platelets (HELLP) syndrome

- HELLP syndrome is a subtype of pre-eclampsia
- It typically manifests in the third trimester, but 30% can present post-partum
- The Swansea criteria can be used to help make a diagnosis of AFLP, which can present similarly to HELLP syndrome.

Pre-eclampsia affects 5% of pregnancies and is defined as new onset hypertension and proteinuria after 20 weeks' gestation. Risk factors include past medical history of pre-eclampsia or gestational hypertension, nulliparity, and chronic kidney disease. In pre-eclampsia, placental hypoperfusion leads to a release of vasoactive mediators, triggering endothelial dysfunction and platelet activation.

HELLP syndrome represents a subtype of pre-eclampsia with significant hepatic involvement. It typically manifests in the third trimester although 30% of cases present post-partum. Patients commonly complain of abdominal pain due to liver capsular stretch. Laboratory investigations demonstrate evidence of microangiopathic haemolytic anaemia (schistocytes on blood film and elevated LDH), raised serum transaminases (>2 × ULN) and thrombocytopenia. Severe hepatic complications include liver haemorrhage and rupture. Management is multi-disciplinary with critical care support and prompt delivery.

AFLP is a rare obstetric emergency that typically presents after 30 weeks' gestation. Patients present with abdominal pain, vomiting, and features of liver dysfunction/failure including jaundice, encephalopathy, ascites, and coagulopathy. Cases are associated with foetal enzyme deficiencies resulting in foetal fatty acid accumulation in maternal liver. Diagnosis is aided by applying the Swansea criteria.

Hyperemesis gravidarum is intractable first-trimester vomiting resulting in dehydration and ketosis. A transaminitis occurs in 50%.

Westbrook RH, Dusheiko G, Williamson C. Westbrook et al. Pregnancy and liver disease. *J Hepatol.* 2016 Apr;64(4):933–945. Doi: 10.1016/j.jhep.2015.11.030.

### 38. C. 25%

- NAFLD is the most common liver disease worldwide affecting approximately 25% of the global population
- NAFLD prevalence roughly doubles in those with obesity and type 2 diabetes
- Fewer than 30% of patients with NAFLD will have biopsy-proven NASH and ~40% of NASH patients develop fibrosis

Meta-analysis of studies using imaging modalities for diagnosis has confirmed NAFLD as the most common liver disease worldwide affecting 25% of the global population. NAFLD is most prevalent in the Middle East (32%) and South America (30%), lowest in Africa (13%), and intermediate in Europe (24%), Asia (27%), and North America (24%). The global burden of NAFLD has rapidly increased over time with prevalence increasing from 15% to 25% between 2005 and 2010. The prevalence of NAFLD increases in high-risk groups particularly those with obesity and T2D where prevalence is roughly double that found in the general population.

Six to 30% of patients with ultrasound-proven NAFLD will have biopsy-proven NASH and approximately 41% of NASH patients will have progression of fibrosis over the next five years.

Marjot T, Moolla A, Cobbold JF et al. Non-alcoholic fatty liver disease: current concepts in pathophysiology, outcomes and management. *Endocr Rev.* 2020 Jan 1;41(1). pii: bnz009. Doi: 10.1210/endrev/bnz009.

### 39. C. ELF score of 10.76

- Simple fibrosis markers such as FIB4 and NAFLD scores can be reliably used to exclude advanced liver fibrosis in patients with NAFLD
- ELF score ≥9.8 has high sensitivity and specificity for advanced liver fibrosis in patients with NAFLD

A number of simple fibrosis markers for NAFLD exist, which can be calculated from routinely collected laboratory and clinical data (Table 8.2). At their low diagnostic cut-offs, these tests have

**Table 8.2** Non-invasive fibrosis markers in NAFLD

| Simple fibrosis marker | Constituents | Diagnostic cut-off* |
|---|---|---|
| APRI (AST:platelet ratio) | AST, platelet count | ≥1.0 |
| AST:ALT | ALT, AST | ≥1.0 |
| BARD score | BMI, AST:ALT, diabetes mellitus | ≥2 |
| FIB4 | Age, ALT, AST, platelet count | ≥3.25 |
| NAFLD Fibrosis Score | Age, albumin, ALT, AST, BMI, diabetes mellitus (or impaired fasting glucose), platelet count | >0.675 |

*indicates 'high risk' for advanced fibrosis.

a negative predictive value of more than 90% to rule out advanced liver fibrosis. However, their positive predictive value for advanced fibrosis is relatively poor at 30–50%. They are therefore best utilized to avoid patients unnecessarily undergoing expensive or invasive investigations to stage fibrosis.

The ELF score is a blood test panel of three proteins of extracellular matrix turnover (hyaluronic acid, tissue inhibitor of metalloproteases-1, and amino terminal propeptide of type III procollagen). ELF has been validated in most major aetiologies of liver disease as an accurate predictor of liver fibrosis. Manufacturers recommend that an ELF score of ≥9.8 is consistent with advanced fibrosis. Of note when interpreting ELF score results, advancing age and other causes of tissue fibrogenesis (including osteoarthritis) are associated with elevations in ELF score, independent of liver fibrosis.

McPherson S, Stewart SF, Henderson E et al. Simple non-invasive fibrosis scoring systems can reliably exclude advanced fibrosis in patients with non-alcoholic fatty liver disease. *Gut.* 2010 Sep;59(9):1265–1269. Doi: 10.1136/gut.2010.216077.

## 40. D. N-acetyl-p-benzoquinoneimine (NAPQI)

- Oxidation of paracetamol by cytochrome P450 (CYP) enzymes leads to production of toxic NAPQI, which can be detoxified by glutathione
- In paracetamol overdose, glutathione stores are depleted and hepatotoxicity ensues
- Patients who have upregulated activity of CYP and those with low glutathione stores are predisposed to paracetamol toxicity

Poisoning with paracetamol (also known as acetaminophen) is common and potentially fatal, being the leading cause of ALF in the Western world. At therapeutic doses, paracetamol is mostly metabolized by conjugation to inactive metabolites with a smaller proportion oxidized by CYP enzymes to NAPQI. NAPQI then binds covalently to sulphydyl groups, which are initially provided by hepatic glutathione. With large doses of paracetamol, CYP oxidation is upregulated, leading to increased NAPQI that saturates hepatic glutathione stores and subsequently binds to cellular proteins causing oxidative stress and hepatocyte damage. This initiates a cycle towards SIRS and multiorgan failure.

Factors that increase the risk of liver injury following paracetamol overdose can be separated into those that induce CYP oxidation (e.g. enzyme-inducing drugs or regular excess alcohol consumption) and those that increase the chance of glutathione depletion (e.g. malnutrition, eating disorders, acquired immunodeficiency syndrome, cachexia, and alcoholism).

The mainstay of treatment for patients who have taken a potentially toxic dose of paracetamol is N-acetylcysteine, which is a sulphydryl donor, preventing hepatocyte damage by NAPQI and allowing glutathione stores to replenish.

Ferner RE, Dear JW, Bateman DN. Management of paracetamol poisoning. *BMJ*. 2011 Apr 19;342:d2218. Doi: 10.1136/bmj.d2218.

## 41. D. INR 7

- ALF is characterized by acutely deranged liver blood tests with coagulopathy and HE
- According to King's College criteria for non-paracetamol ALF, patients with INR >6.5 would benefit from emergency liver transplantation (ELT)

ALF is a rare and highly specific syndrome characterized by an acute abnormality of liver blood tests associated with coagulopathy and HE in the absence of chronic liver disease (except *de novo* presentations of AIH, Budd-Chiari syndrome, and WD). Determining aetiology for ALF is important as an indicator of prognosis and to help guide treatment, particularly the need for ELT. ELT may be an option for intrinsic hepatic ALF (e.g. drug related, Budd-Chiari syndrome, AIH, viral hepatitis) but not appropriate for extrahepatic/secondary liver failure (e.g. ischaemic hepatitis, haemophagocytic syndrome, infiltrative disease). The ideal means for selecting patients likely to benefit from ELT remains a subject of some controversy with several validated scoring systems available. Of these, the performance of the King's College criteria remains the best characterized and most widely utilized (Table 8.3).

**Table 8.3** King's College criteria for emergency liver transplantation

| ALF due to paracetamol | ALF not due to paracetamol |
|---|---|
| • Arterial pH <7.3 after resuscitation and >24 hours since ingestion<br>• Lactate >3 mmol/L orthe 3 following criteria:<br>  ♦ Hepatic encephalopathy >Grade 3<br>  ♦ Serum creatinine >300 lmol/L<br>  ♦ INR >6.5 | • INR >6.5 or3 out of 5 following criteria:<br>  ♦ Indeterminate or drug-induced aetiology<br>  ♦ Age <10 years or >40 years<br>  ♦ Interval jaundice-encephalopathy >7 days<br>  ♦ Bilirubin >300 µmol/L<br>  ♦ INR >3.5 |

EASL Clinical Practical Guidelines on the management of acute (fulminant) liver failure. *J Hepatol*. 2017 May;66(5):1047–1081. Doi: 10.1016/j.jhep.2016.12.003

## 42. A. Acetaminophen

- DILI can be classified as intrinsic versus idiosyncratic
- Intrinsic DILI (e.g. acetaminophen) is predictable, dose dependent, and occurs in a high proportion of those exposed
- Idiosyncratic DILI is dose-independent, occurs in a smaller proportion of those exposed, has a longer latency to onset, and is immune mediated

DILI is traditionally classified as either intrinsic or idiosyncratic. Intrinsic DILI is dose related, predictable, occurs in a high proportion of exposed patients, and manifests within a short time frame (hours to days). Acetaminophen (paracetamol) toxicity is the best example of intrinsic DILI. Patients who consume a single dose of acetaminophen yielding plasma concentrations >200 or

>100 µg/L at 4 or 8 hours, respectively, will experience acute liver toxicity. Even acetaminophen intake at the licensed dose of 4 g/day over two weeks results in aminotransferase elevations >3 × ULN in one third of patients. Other medications causing intrinsic DILI include ciclosporin, valproic acid, antimetabolites, and antiretroviral therapy. Conversely, idiosyncratic DILI is dose independent (although >50–100 mg/day is usually required), occurs in a small proportion of exposed individuals and exhibits variable latency to onset (days to weeks). In idiosyncratic DILI, drug-protein activation of the adaptive immune system, alongside genetic susceptibility, plays a major role.

All answer options apart from acetaminophen typically cause idiosyncratic DILI. The clavunalate component of amoxicillin-clavunalate (co-amoxiclav) causes immunoallergic hepatotoxicity predominantly resulting in cholestasis. Halothane, now a little-used anesthetic agent, causes liver damage through production of autoantibodies directed against CYP enzymes. Around 20% of patients taking isoniazid will develop hepatocellular injury; most cases are mild and resolve with immune tolerance but severe injury develops in ~1%. Phenytoin is one of the most common causes of clinically apparent DILI resulting in a hepatocellular or mixed pattern of liver function tests.

Kullak-Ublick GA, Andrade RJ, Merz M et al. Drug-induced liver injury: recent advances in diagnosis and risk assessment. *Gut.* 2017 Jun;66(6):1154–1164. Doi: 10.1136/gutjnl-2016-313369.

### 43. A. Flucloxacillin

- DILI can be classified as hepatocellular (ALT ≥5-fold above ULN or ALT:ALP ratio [R] ≥5), cholestatic (ALP alone ≥2-fold ULN or R ≤2) or mixed (R>2 to <5)
- Cholestatic DILI is most likely to progress to chronic DILI, including vanishing bile duct syndrome

DILI can be classified into three patterns of injury: hepatocellular, cholestatic, and mixed type. Hepatocellular injury is defined by an elevation in ALT alone ≥5-fold ULN or R ≥5, cholestatic injury by an elevation of ALP alone ≥2-fold ULN or R ≤2, and mixed pattern by R >2 to <5.

Cases of hepatocellular DILI tend to be associated with a higher degree of inflammation (particularly eosinophilic infiltrate), necrosis, and apoptosis on histology. Cholestatic DILI is more common with increasing age, and has a greater genetic association (e.g. HLA-A*33:01) and higher propensity to become chronic DILI and vanishing bile duct syndrome.

Important examples of drugs causing cholestatic DILI include amoxicillin/clavulanate, macrolides, trimethoprim/sulfamethoxazole, chlorpromazine, terbinafine, and flucloxacillin. A minority of patients with drug-induced cholestasis will develop ductopenia, which can progress to vanishing bile duct syndrome (>50% bile duct loss) that carries a ~20% liver-related mortality.

The antituberculosis drug, isoniazid, and cancer immunotherapy ipilumumab both typically cause hepatocellular DILI. Physicians must consider herbal and dietary supplements as causative agents of DILI including green tea, which mostly causes hepatocellular injury. Phenytoin is one of the most common causes of clinically apparent DILI and ALF, which most commonly present with a mixed pattern of LFTs.

EASL Clinical Practice Guidelines: drug-induced liver injury. *J Hepatol.* 2019 Jun;70(6):1222–1261. Doi: 10.1016/j.jhep.2019.02.014.

### 44. A. Carbamazepine

- Drug interactions may inhibit or induce the activity of CYP enzymes, posing challenges for dose optimization of CYP-metabolized medications

- Important CYP inhibitors include calcium channel blockers, azole antifungals, macrolide antibiotics, protease inhibitors, and grapefruit juice
- Important CYP inducers include rifampicin, anticonvulsant agents, antiretrovirals efavirenz, nevirapine, and St John's wort

Hepatic drug metabolism involves phase 1 and phase 2 reactions that occur sequentially and ultimately decrease lipid solubility and allow renal excretion. Phase 1 reactions are catabolic (e.g. oxidation, reduction, or hydrolysis) and introduce an active group to allow conjugation (e.g. with glucuronyl, sulphate, methyl) as part of phase 2 reactions, which render the drug inactive. Most phase 1 reactions take place in the smooth endoplasmic reticulum where drug-metabolizing enzymes, including CYP, are embedded. CYP enzymes are a large 'superfamily' of catalytic proteins of which CYP3A is the most clinically important, given its ability to metabolize multiple chemically unrelated drugs and its abundance in both enterocytes and the liver. Significant interindividual variation in CYP enzyme function is influenced by both genetic and environmental factors. In particular, drug interactions may inhibit or induce CYP enzymes, expanding the range of catalytic activity up to 400-fold. As an example, the dosage of cyclosporin often needs reducing by up to 75% in patients concomitantly taking ketoconazole (a CYP inhibitor) whereas the dose may need to be increased up to 3-fold in patients also taking rifampicin (a CYP inducer). Antiretroviral protease inhibitors (e.g. ritonavir, indinavir), grapefruit juice, and macrolide antibiotics (e.g. clarithromycin, erythromycin) are all CYP enzyme inhibitors and would therefore require cyclosporin dose reduction, whereas anticonvulsant agents (e.g. carbamazepine, phenobarbital, phenytoin) are enzyme inducers and may require cyclosporin dose escalation.

Wilkinson GR. Drug metabolism and variability among patients in drug response. *N Engl J Med*. 2005 May 26;352(21):2211–2221.


## 45. C. It is caused by mutations of the ATP7B gene

- In WD, mutations in the ATP7B gene causes copper accumulation in the liver and brain
- WD accounts for 10% of all patients with ALF referred for emergency transplantation
- Treatment is lifelong (e.g. D-penicillamine, trientine, zinc), which should not be discontinued unless LT is performed

WD is caused by mutations in the ATP7B gene on chromosome 13, resulting in defective biliary excretion of copper and accumulation in the liver and brain. Clinical features include liver disease and cirrhosis, neuropsychiatric disturbance, corneal Kayser–Fleischer (KF) rings, and acute episodes of haemolysis often in association with ALF. WD accounts for 6%–12% of all patients with ALF referred for emergency transplantation, and should be suspected in young individuals with jaundice, low haemoglobin, mild elevations in transaminases, and low ALP. Most patients with WD present between the ages of 5 and 35 years, although age alone should not be the basis for eliminating a diagnosis because ~3% present beyond the fourth decade of life.

Traditionally, the combination of KF rings and low serum ceruloplasmin (<0.1 g/L) was sufficient to make a diagnosis of WD. However, KF rings are often absent in hepatic disease and ceruloplasmin levels may be low for other reasons (e.g. AIH, advanced liver disease, familial aceruloplasminemia) or falsely elevated because of its role as an acute phase protein. Many patients therefore require a combination of further diagnostic tests including 24-hour urinary copper, serum-free copper, and hepatic copper content.

Treatment for WD is with lifelong chelating agents, which should not be discontinued unless LT is performed. D-penicillamine has the largest evidence base but is associated with numerous side effects (e.g. lupus-like syndrome, cytopaenias, proteinuria) requiring drug discontinuation in ~30%.

Trientine is an alternative chelating agent that may be better tolerated. Zinc monotherapy appears to be effective and safe in neurologic WD and in asymptomatic siblings.

EASL Clinical Practice Guidelines: Wilson's disease. *J Hepatol.* 2012 Mar;56(3):671–685. Doi: 10.1016/j.jhep.2011.11.007.

## 46. E. Pi*ZZ

- A1ATD is an inherited disorder leading to liver cirrhosis and chronic obstructive pulmonary disease (COPD)
- Ninety-six per cent of pathologies associated with A1ATD occur in Pi*ZZ (<15% alpha-1-antitrypsin [A1AT] level) and 4% in Pi*SZ (35% A1AT level)
- The only approved therapy for A1ATD-associated liver disease is LT, which is curative

A1AT is a serine proteinase inhibitor produced by hepatocytes and the epithelial and inflammatory cells of the lung. A1ATD results from mutations in the SERPINA1 gene inherited in an autosomal co-dominant pattern, indicating that one defective allele results in milder disease than two defective alleles. Protease inhibitor M (Pi*M) is the normal gene product and the most common disease-causing mutations are Pi*S and Pi*Z, which express 50%–60% and 10%–20% of the A1AT protein respectively. A1ATD-associated liver disease results from accumulation of misfolded A1AT in the endoplasmic reticulum of hepatocytes leading to oxidative stress, inflammation, and fibrosis. By contrast, A1ATD-associated lung disease results from inadequate proteinase inhibition, alveolar damage, and COPD. In clinical practice, 96% of pathologies associated with A1ATD occur in homozygous ZZ (<15% A1AT level) and the remaining 4% in heterozygous SZ (35% A1AT level). The PiZZ genotype is also associated with asthma, granulomatosis with polyangiitis, and panniculitis. Genotypes Pi*MZ, Pi*MS and Pi*SS confer a small increased risk of liver disease but usually alongside other liver risk factors (e.g. viral hepatitis, alcohol, metabolic syndrome).

Whereas augmentation therapy (infusion of human plasma-derived A1AT) has a role in the treatment of A1ATD-associated lung disease, the only approved therapy for A1ATD-associated liver disease is LT, which is curative.

Greene CM, Marciniak SJ, Teckman J et al. α1-Antitrypsin deficiency. *Nat Rev Dis Primers.* 2016 Jul 28;2:16051. Doi: 10.1038/nrdp.2016.51.

## 47. D. Metabolic syndrome

- In patients with hyperferritinaemia, genetic HFE testing should only occur once secondary conditions are excluded (e.g. inflammation, metabolic syndrome, malignancy) and after confirmation of elevated transferrin saturations
- Patients with iron overload and C282Y homozygosity can be diagnosed with hereditary HFE-HC without need for liver biopsy

One of the following pathologies can be identified in 90% of outpatients with hyperferritinaemia: chronic alcohol consumption, inflammation, cell necrosis (e.g. rhabdomyolysis), malignancy and NAFLD +/− metabolic syndrome. Investigating for genetic causes of hyperferritinaemia (with HFE testing for C282Y and H63D polymorphisms) should only be performed once these secondary conditions have been excluded and after confirmation of elevated transferrin saturations, which is a prerequisite for a diagnosis of HFE-HC.

In patients with raised ferritin and transferrin saturations who are homozygous for C282Y, a liver biopsy is not necessary to diagnose HFE-HC but could be considered in patients with ferritin >1,000 mg/L, elevated AST, hepatomegaly, or age >40 years who are at high risk of cirrhosis.

Simple C282Y heterozygosity does not cause iron overload and, while C282Y/H63D compound heterozygosity can cause mild iron overload, this usually only occurs alongside other co-factors (e.g. chronic alcoholism or metabolic syndrome).

Genetic testing for rare hemochromatosis genes (e.g. TFR2, SLC40A1, HAMP, HJV) should only be performed in patients with increased iron stores after exclusion of C282Y homozygosity if iron excess has been proven by direct assessment (e.g. liver MRI or biopsy).

EASL Clinical Practice Guidelines for HFE hemochromatosis. *J Hepatol.* 2010 Jul;53(1):3–22. Doi: 10.1016/j.jhep.2010.03.001.

### 48. A. Arthralgia does not improve with phlebotomy

- Despite the absence of RCTs, iron depletion with phlebotomy remains the mainstay of treatment for hereditary haemochromatosis (HH) and improves most clinical features apart from joint disease
- Weekly induction phlebotomy is followed by maintenance venesection around 2–4 × a year aiming to keep serum ferritin at 50–100 µg/L

Phlebotomy remains the mainstay of treatment for HFE-HC. Despite the absence of randomized trials, the mortality benefit of phlebotomy in HFE-HC has been demonstrated by comparing outcomes in historical groups of patients not treated with phlebotomy. Furthermore, there is clear expert consensus that iron depletion can improve fatigue and cardiac function, stabilize liver disease and reduce skin pigmentation. Joint symptoms, however, respond poorly to phlebotomy therapy and can worsen. Phlebotomy can safely be carried out in patients with advanced fibrosis/cirrhosis with histological improvement found in 15%–50% on follow-up liver biopsy.

Phlebotomy typically involves weekly induction venesection of 400–500 ml of blood aiming for a target serum ferritin of 50 µg/L, followed by maintenance venesection 2–4 × a year aiming to maintain ferritin 50–100 µg/L. If anemia is detected, phlebotomy should be postponed until the anaemia is resolved.

Adjunctive oral chelation therapy (e.g. deferoxamine) can be used in severe disease (e.g. juvenile haemochromatosis) and in cases of secondary iron overload (e.g. thalassaemia) but it is expensive, cumbersome, and associated with several adverse effects including blurred vision, tinnitus, and diarrhoea.

Brissot P, Pietrangelo A, Adams PC et al. Haemochromatosis. *Nat Rev Dis Primers.* 2018 Apr 5;4:18016. Doi: 10.1038/nrdp.2018.16.

### 49. B. Aspergillus chest infection

- There are no established age limits for consideration of LT
- Active infection is an absolute contraindication to LT
- PVT and history of curative cancer treatment are not absolute contraindications to LT

All potential LT candidates should undergo extensive work-up before registration on the waiting list. Because of good outcomes of LT in well-selected elderly patients subjected to multi-disciplinary evaluation (including >70 years), there are no established age limits for consideration of LT. All patients should have a cardiovascular assessment including electrocardiogram and transthoracic echocardiography plus consideration of coronary angiography and cardiopulmonary exercise testing in selected cases. Respiratory work-up includes chest X-ray, spirometry, and, when necessary, assessment of hepatopulmonary syndrome (which resolves with LT) and portopulmonary hypertension (which may improve with LT in certain cases [e.g. responders to pulmonary vasodilators]). HRS is usually a reversible cause of renal failure that responds to LT but should be carefully differentiated from other causes of AKI.

Infectious complications are the leading cause of early post-LT mortality, and their prevention includes careful pre-operative screening and treatment of infection alongside post-operative antimicrobial prophylaxis. Active bacterial, fungal, and viral infection represent absolute contraindications to LT, and the potential recipient should first be treated until there is clear radiological, clinical, and microbiological evidence of resolution.

Historically, PVT was considered an absolute contraindication to LT. However, improvements in medical care, surgical techniques, and radiological interventions now mean that patients transplanted with PVT have equivalent outcomes to those without.

A past history of treated cancer should not disqualify candidates from LT although a five-year interval between curative cancer treatment and LT is preferred.

EASL Clinical Practice Guidelines: liver transplantation. *J Hepatol.* 2016 Feb;64(2):433–485. Doi: 10.1016/j.jhep.2015.10.006.

### 50. B. Hepatic artery thrombosis (HAT)

- HAT occurs in 1%–7% of patients after LT
- Early HAT (<21 days post-transplantation) usually presents as graft dysfunction and is a common indication for urgent liver re-transplantation

The HA is reconstructed during LT. Stenotic lesions of the HA can cause significant ischaemic injury of which HAT is the most common cause, occurring in 1%–7% of patients following LT. Early HAT (<21 days post LT) often presents as graft dysfunction with markedly elevated liver enzymes, jaundice, acidosis, and hypoglycaemia. Collateralization is more common in late HAT, which presents more insidiously with bile duct strictures (ischaemic cholangiopathy) and resultant biliary sepsis or abscess formation. Risk factors for HAT include smoking, increasing donor age, low donor weight, multiple arterial anastomoses, and previous HAT. CT angiography is the gold standard for diagnosis. Early diagnosis of HAT reduces septic complications, multi-organ failure and graft loss. Treatment of HAT is centred upon urgent establishment of the arterial circulation (if possible) with surgical revascularization, to reduce complications related to ischaemic cholangiopathy. However, more than 50% of cases of early HAT require urgent re-transplantation. Prevention of HAT post-LT includes the use of long-term antiplatelet agents, smoking avoidance, and tight control of atherosclerotic risk factors.

EASL Clinical Practice Guidelines: liver transplantation. *J Hepatol.* 2016 Feb;64(2):433–485. Doi: 10.1016/j.jhep.2015.10.006.

# chapter 9

# NUTRITION

## QUESTIONS

1. An 89-year old was admitted with a severe community-acquired pneumonia. Their family reported that the patient was struggling to manage at home and they were concerned about ongoing weight loss. The family did not think the patient had eaten properly for the past seven days. The patient used to weigh 75 kg but on this admission weighed 63 kg. Their body mass index (BMI) was 24.6 kg/m$^2$.

   **What is their Malnutrition Universal Screening Tool (MUST) score?**

   A. 0

   B. 1

   C. 2

   D. 4

   E. 6

Best of Five MCQs for the European Specialty Examination in Gastroenterology and Hepatology. Thomas Marjot, Colleen G C McGregor, Tim Ambrose, Aminda N De Silva, Jeremy Cobbold, and Simon Travis, Oxford University Press (2021). © Oxford University Press.
DOI: 10.1093/oso/9780198834373.003.0009

2. **A 67-year-old woman presented to the outpatient clinic with a 14-month history of diarrhoea, nausea, fatigue, and 12 kg weight loss. She had a past medical history of hypertension, chronic kidney disease, type 2 diabetes, osteoarthritis, and hypothyroidism.**

Investigations:

| | |
|---|---|
| Haemoglobin | 116 g/L |
| Mean corpuscular volume (MCV) | 87 fL |
| Serum ferritin | 21 µg/L |
| Serum C-reactive protein (CRP) | <0.2 mg/L |
| Vitamin B12 | 421 ng/L |
| Serum folate | 4.1 µg/L |
| Thyroid-stimulating hormone (TSH) | 2.3 mU/L |
| IgA tissue transglutaminase antibody | <0.2 U/mL |
| Total IgA | 1.26 g/L |
| Human leucocyte antigen (HLA) status | DQ2.5 homozygote |
| Gastroscopy | Scalloped duodenal mucosa |
| Duodenal histology | Marsh 3B villous atrophy and crypt hyperplasia with intra-epithelial lymphocytosis |

**Which of her medications is most likely to be the cause of her symptoms?**

A. Ibuprofen

B. Levothyroxine

C. Metformin

D. Olmesartan

E. Simvastatin

3. **A 46-year-old woman presented with a long history of fullness after eating, nausea, and weight loss with a current BMI of 17.3 kg/m². There was no history of diabetes, previous abdominal surgery, or psychiatric illness. Despite dietary manipulation and a trial of nasogastric feeding, she continued to lose weight.**

Investigations:

| | |
|---|---|
| Gastroscopy | Normal |
| Computed tomography (CT) chest and abdomen | No evidence of bowel obstruction or malignancy |
| Gastric scintigraphy | 85% retention at two hours 40% retention at four hours |

**What is the best next step in management?**

A. Amitriptyline 10 mg once a day and refer for urgent psychiatric assessment

B. Commence parenteral nutrition

C. Long-term metoclopramide 10 mg three times a day

D. Refer for surgical jejunostomy

E. Trial of nasojejunal feeding

4. **A 55-year-old woman with secondary progressive multiple sclerosis developed recurrent lower respiratory tract infections. A percutaneous endoscopic gastrostomy was placed two years ago for long-term enteral tube feeding and to reduce aspiration risk. The patient presented with difficulty flushing the tube and leakage around the gastrostomy site.**

**Which of the following statements is most accurate?**

A. Balloon gastrostomies are more likely to become buried than ones with a silicon disc

B. Buried bumper syndrome is difficult to prevent even with good nursing aftercare

C. Buried bumper syndrome should be suspected if the enteral feed pump alarms regularly

D. Buried bumpers are mostly managed with surgical removal of the gastrostomy

E. Gastrostomy tubes can be safely advanced into the stomach within three days of initial insertion

5. **A 45-year-old man with Crohn's disease presented to the emergency department with unsteady gait, impaired concentration, dysarthria, loose stools, and blurred vision. Following previous operations, he had been left with 80 cm small bowel in continuity with a full colon. His only medications were omeprazole and loperamide. He denied any recreational drug use but admitted to consuming a large amount of beer over the past three days. His diet was poor, largely comprising carbohydrate-based meals. Examination revealed nystagmus and dysmetria on finger–nose testing. Abdomen was soft and non-tender.**

Investigations:

| | |
|---|---|
| Serum sodium | 138 mmol/L |
| Serum potassium | 3.2 mmol/L |
| Serum urea | 2.1 mmol/L |
| Serum creatinine | 66 mmol/L |
| Serum chloride | 106 mmol/L |
| Serum glucose | 6.7 mmol/L |
| Arterial pH | 7.21 |
| Arterial lactate | 1.9 mmol/L |
| Arterial $HCO_3$ | 8 mmol/L |

**What is the most likely diagnosis?**

A. Acute alcohol intoxication

B. Beer potomania

C. Diabetic ketoacidosis

D. D-lactic acidosis

E. Wernicke's encephalopathy

6. **A 45-year-old man with a history of small bowel Crohn's disease had undergone multiple ileal resections for stricturing disease. His current anatomy was 80 cm jejunum anastomosed to full colon with no evidence of active inflammation. He presented with a one-day history of severe left loin pain radiating into his groin with macroscopic haematuria.**

Investigations:

| | |
|---|---|
| CT kidney, ureter, bladder | Large non-obstructing calculus at the left vesico-ureteric junction |

**Which of the following dietary measures would you recommend?**

A. Increasing dietary beetroot

B. Increasing dietary chocolate

C. Increasing dietary fat

D. Reducing dietary calcium

E. Reducing dietary spinach

7. **A 19-year-old being managed for dysmotility and gastroparesis presented with ongoing weight loss and diarrhoea. Feeding via a surgical jejunostomy had not been tolerated due to pain at the insertion site and bloating on increasing rate of feed administration. The patient demanded this be removed. She was commenced on parenteral nutrition but would not allow the rate of feeding to be increased in line with recommendations from the nutrition team. The nursing staff commented that she could be manipulative, and the portering staff frequently saw her running up and down the stairs.**

   Investigations:
   Urinary laxative screen                              Positive

   **What would be the next best step in management?**

   A. Nasogastric feeding

   B. Refer to psychological medicine

   C. Remove jejunostomy and continue current rate of parenteral feeding

   D. Restart jejunal feeding against patient's wishes

   E. Sedate patient and increase rate of parenteral feeding

8. **A 57-year-old was established on parenteral nutrition due to short bowel syndrome. They received 2 500 ml over 12 hours, 7 nights per week (1 400 kcal glucose, 14 g nitrogen, sodium 120 mmol, potassium 60 mmol, magnesium 14 mmol). They were admitted with a suspected central line infection but were haemodynamically stable. Their vascular access was difficult but you were able to insert a 22G cannula.**

   **What is the best option for management over the subsequent 24 hours?**

   A. Encourage the patient to drink water; no intravenous support required

   B. Prescribe 1 litre 0.9% sodium chloride with 40 mmol potassium chloride, 1 litre 0.9% sodium chloride with 14 mmol magnesium sulphate, and 500 ml 5% dextrose to be administered through the 22G cannula

   C. Prescribe 1 litre 0.9% sodium chloride with 40 mmol potassium chloride, 1 litre 5% dextrose with 14 mmol magnesium sulphate, and 500 ml 5% dextrose with 20 mmol potassium chloride to be administered through the 22G cannula

   D. Prescribe usual parenteral nutrition to be administered through the 22G cannula

   E. Prescribe usual parenteral nutrition to be administered through the central venous catheter

9. **A 56-year-old man had undergone small bowel resection with primary anastomosis in the context of small bowel volvulus. Following an anastomotic leak, he developed an enterocutaneous fistula and is now six weeks following his last surgery. He had lost 12 kg in weight and was losing 1200 ml of effluent through the fistula per day. He was haemodynamically stable and CRP had been reducing.**

Investigations:

CT abdomen            Multiple small intra-abdominal abscesses, too small to drain radiologically

**What of the following is most appropriate at present?**

A. Commence octreotide

B. Laparoscopic formation of stoma proximal to fistula

C. Prolonged course of antibiotics

D. Unrestricted oral intake

E. Urgent repeat laparotomy and washout

10. **A 35-year-old woman was reviewed in clinic. She had been on home parenteral nutrition for eight years for short bowel syndrome and had had three central line infections. She had a thrombosed right internal jugular and left subclavian vein.**

Investigations:

| Parameter (units) | 6 months ago | Currently |
|---|---|---|
| Serum bilirubin (µmol/l) | 24 | 94 |
| Serum alanine transferase (ALT) (U/L) | 37 | 153 |
| Serum alkaline phosphatase (ALP) (U/L) | 117 | 326 |

**What is the next most appropriate step in management?**

A. Commence teduglutide

B. Commence ursodeoxycholic acid

C. Inform palliative care

D. Refer for intestinal transplantation assessment

E. Repeat blood tests in six months' time and refer for FibroScan in the interim

11. **A 45-year-old woman with BMI 41 kg/m² was referred to a bariatric surgeon to discuss weight loss surgery. Her preferred option is a laparoscopic adjustable gastric band (LAGB).**

    **Which of the following statements is correct regarding LAGB?**

    A. Anastomotic leak is the most common cause of post-operative 30-day mortality

    B. It induces greater weight loss at one year compared with sleeve gastrectomy (SG) and Roux-en-Y gastric bypass (RY-GBP)

    C. It is better at inducing remission of type 2 diabetes compared with RY-GBP

    D. The long-term re-operation rate is more than 10%

    E. There is a higher post-operative 30-day mortality compared with SG

12. **A 47-year-old woman presented to the outpatient clinic with anaemia. A year ago, she had undergone bariatric surgery for morbid obesity with a RY-GBP at a private clinic abroad. She had lost over 60 kg (45% of her original body weight) since the procedure. She reported recent symptoms of abdominal discomfort and bloating, along with flatulence and loose stool. She also reported fatigue and some hair loss.**

    **Which nutritional deficiency would best explain the patient's anaemia?**

    A. Copper

    B. Folate

    C. Iron

    D. Thiamine

    E. Vitamin B12

13. **A 52-year-old woman was reviewed two months post Roux-en-Y gastric bypass. She complained of abdominal discomfort occurring approximately 45 minutes after meals. This was associated with nausea, watery diarrhoea, drowsiness, palpitations, and sweating. She has also had episodes of collapse an hour after mealtimes on two occasions.**

    **What is the most likely diagnosis?**

    A. Cholelithiasis

    B. Early dumping syndrome (EDS)

    C. Gastro-gastric fistula

    D. Late dumping syndrome

    E. Post-prandial vasovagal syncope

**1. D. 4**

- Identifying patients at risk of malnutrition is a key component of care
- The MUST score is a validated tool for assessing risk of malnutrition and to trigger intervention

Malnutrition is common in health and social care settings, in older people, and in those with disease. It remains underdiagnosed and undertreated, yet is associated with increased healthcare utilization, costs, and poorer outcomes. Approximately one third of patients admitted to hospitals across the UK are at risk of malnutrition.

The MUST is a simple-to-use, validated tool to identify those patients at highest risk of malnutrition and to trigger intervention to reverse further nutritional decline (Table 9.1).

**Table 9.1** Malnutrition Universal Screening Tool (MUST) score

| Score | Body mass index (BMI, kg/m²) | Unplanned weight loss in past 3–6 months (%) | Acute illness score |
|---|---|---|---|
| 0 | >20 | <5 | - |
| 1 | 18.5–20 | 5–10 | - |
| 2 | <18.5 | >10 | if the patient is acutely ill and there has been or is likely to be no nutritional intake for >5 days |

The total score ranges from 0–6 (0 = Low Risk, 1 = Medium Risk, 2 or more = High Risk).

Based on the risk score, patients may receive routine clinical care (Low Risk), observation of dietary intake and reassessment (Medium Risk), or immediate referral to dietitian/Nutrition Support Team (High Risk).

Stratton R, Smith T, Gabe S. Managing malnutrition to improve lives and save money. Malnutrition Action Group, British Association of Parenteral and Enteral Nutrition (BAPEN) October 2018. Available at: https://www.bapen.org.uk/pdfs/reports/mag/managing-malnutrition.pdf (accessed February 2020)

**2. D. Olmesartan**

- Angiotensin II receptor antagonists, such as olmesartan and telmisartan, can cause villous atrophy, leading to severe diarrhoea and weight loss
- Tissue transglutaminase antibodies are likely to be negative, although most will have a predisposing coeliac HLA type (HLA DQ2 or DQ8)

*Best of Five MCQs for the European Specialty Examination in Gastroenterology and Hepatology.* Thomas Marjot, Colleen G C McGregor, Tim Ambrose, Aminda N De Silva, Jeremy Cobbold, and Simon Travis, Oxford University Press (2021). © Oxford University Press.
DOI: 10.1093/oso/9780198834373.003.0009

- Most patients rapidly improve upon discontinuation of the culprit medication

Diarrhoea is a potential side effect of all the listed medications. Olmesartan and telmesartan have both been reported to cause a sprue-like illness with diarrhoea, substantial weight loss, and seronegative villous atrophy, mimicking coeliac disease. Microscopic colitis and lymphocytic gastritis may also be present. Symptoms are often present for years before the drug responsible is identified. Most patients improve clinically, with resolution of the villous atrophy, upon discontinuing the drug.

Non-steroidal anti-inflammatory drugs, such as ibuprofen, commonly cause diarrhoea as well as duodenitis, but would not be expected to cause villous atrophy. Thyroxine in excess can cause diarrhoea. However, the TSH is normal in this case. Metformin and simvastatin can both cause diarrhoea, but not villous atrophy.

Rubio-Tapia A, Herman ML, Ludvigsson JF et al. Severe spruelike enteropathy associated with olmesartan. *Mayo Clin Proc.* 2012;87(8):732–738. Doi:10.1016/j.mayocp.2012.06.003.

## 3. E. Trial of nasojejunal feeding

- Nasojejunal feeding should be strongly considered prior to placement of a surgical jejunostomy for gastroparesis

Gastroparesis is most commonly idiopathic, diabetic, or post-surgical. It affects women more than men and leads to overall shortened survival compared with age- and sex-matched controls. Gastric emptying should be considered delayed if retention on scintigraphy is more than 60% at two hours or 10% at four hours.

Nutritional management is multi-disciplinary and involves close liaison with specialist dietitians. When oral dietary modifications have failed, enteral tube feeding should be considered. This usually entails post-pyloric feeding. A trial of nasojejunal feeding to prove the patient is able to meet their nutritional requirements should be strongly considered prior to placement of a surgical jejunostomy. This is because some patients will have pan-enteric dysmotility and may not tolerate post-pyloric feeding. Parenteral nutrition should not be considered first-line therapy for isolated gastroparesis.

Eating disorders may manifest with similar symptoms, but there is no suggestion in this case that urgent psychiatric evaluation is necessary. The anticholinergic side effects of amitriptyline may worsen the patient's symptoms. Following an alert from the European Medicines Authority, long-term treatment with prokinetics, such as metoclopramide or domperidone, is not advised.

Camilleri M, Parkman HP, Shafi MA et al. Clinical Guideline: Management of gastroparesis. *Am J Gastroenterol.* 2013;108(1):18–37. Doi:10.1038/ajg.2012.373.

## 4. C. Buried bumper syndrome should be suspected if the enteral feed pump alarms regularly

- Buried bumper syndrome is an avoidable complication of gastrostomy placement
- It can be prevented by regular advancement of the tube 5–10 cm and gentle rotation but not within the first seven days of placement
- Endoscopic techniques form the mainstay of management

For patients requiring enteral tube feeding for longer than 4–6 weeks, gastrostomy insertion should be considered. While endoscopic placement is usually preferred, some patients may require radiological or surgical placement—for example, if the stomach is inaccessible endoscopically.

Buried bumper syndrome is a preventable complication whereby the internal fixator becomes buried within the gastric mucosa or at the surface of the skin. It is more common with internal silicon disc than balloon gastrostomies. Signs include leakage around the insertion site, difficulty flushing the tube, regular pump alarms, abdominal pain, or difficulties advancing the tube. It can be avoided by advancing the tube 5–10 cm into the stomach and rotating at least weekly (rotation should be avoided if there is a jejunal extension through the gastrostomy). The distance between internal and external fixators should not be too short. Advancement of the tube into the stomach should not be before one week after tube placement because of the risk of pain and interfering with tract formation.

Management includes endoscopic techniques (needle knife, balloon push, balloon pull, snare, external traction) or radiological/surgical removal. In very high-risk patients, the bumper may be left buried and a jejunal extension passed to permit ongoing feeding.

Bischoff SC, Austin P, Boeykens K et al. ESPEN guideline on home enteral nutrition. *Clin Nutr.* 2020;39(1):5–22. Doi:10.1016/j.clnu.2019.04.022.

## 5. D. D-lactic acidosis

- Short bowel syndrome is a risk factor for D-lactic acidosis
- D-lactic acidosis causes a metabolic acidosis with high anion gap but normal L-lactate
- Treatment includes correcting the acidosis using fluid hydration and intravenous sodium bicarbonate, and decreasing substrate for D-lactate like carbohydrates in meals

D-lactic acidosis is a rare entity with typical clinical features of delirium, slurred speech, ataxia, confusion, and ultimately coma. It should be considered in patients with elevated anion gap metabolic acidosis (27.2 mEq/L in this case), normal L-lactate levels (that measured by standard blood gas machines), and a history of short bowel syndrome. A D-lactate concentration of >3 mmol/L is significant.

The production of D-lactate in the gut is precipitated by two factors:

1. Absence or reduced length of the small intestine, which is normally responsible for the absorption of most simple carbohydrates
2. Presence of colon in continuity where unabsorbed carbohydrates are made available for fermentation by the colonic microbiota

Kowlgi NG, Chhabra L. D-lactic acidosis: an underrecognized complication of short bowel syndrome. *Gastroenterol Res Pract.* 2015;2015:476215. Doi:10.1155/2015/476215.

## 6. E. Reducing dietary spinach

- Oxalate renal stones are more common in patients with short-bowel syndrome and colon in continuity
- Reduction of foods rich in oxalate (e.g. beetroot, chocolate, spinach, kiwi, rhubarb) can be beneficial

Oxalate is absorbed in the colon and precipitates in the renal tubules, resulting in tubular damage. In health, oxalate binds to calcium in the gut lumen reducing the amount available for absorption in the colon. However, in patients with short-bowel syndrome, unabsorbed long-chain fatty acids compete for calcium binding, resulting in more free oxalate entering the colon, increased absorption, and greater risk of renal stone formation. Calcium oxalate renal stones occur in about 25% of patients with short-bowel syndrome and colon in continuity. Some concern has been raised about increased Vitamin C, which is metabolized to oxalate, in parenteral nutrition formulations.

Preventive measures, of varying success, include ensuring adequate hydration and therefore good urinary flow; adopting a low oxalate diet; reduction of dietary fat (to reduce competition for calcium binding); increased dietary calcium (to increase availability for binding to oxalate). Colestyramine, a bile acid sequestrant, has been reported as beneficial in some cases.

Foods high in oxalate include blackberries, blueberries, raspberries, kiwi, rhubarb, spinach, beetroot, aubergine, okra, wheat bran, black tea, chocolate, and almonds.

Pironi L, Arends J, Bozzetti F. ESPEN guidelines on chronic intestinal failure in adults. *Clin. Nutr.* 2016;35:247–307. Doi:10.1016/j.clnu.2016.01.020.

### 7. B. Refer to psychological medicine

- Patients with eating disorders may present atypically to gastroenterology and a high index of suspicion of the diagnosis is essential
- Manipulative and controlling behaviour particularly around intravenous feeding can be a clue

Patients with eating disorders often display gastrointestinal symptoms including pain, distension, early satiety, and nausea. They may meet criteria for irritable bowel syndrome and constipation is not uncommon. Patients may be initially diagnosed and managed for dysmotility, with nutritional support appropriately instituted in the context of weight loss. These patients may develop pain around the site of surgical jejunostomy, and may struggle to meet their full nutritional requirements because of bloating and fullness. Some patients will therefore require parenteral nutrition to be commenced to maintain nutritional state. This can unmask underlying eating disorders, particularly the need to control the amount of nutritional intake. Patients may adjust the pump to reduce the rate of feed, refuse to increase feed rate as guided by the nutrition team, and disconnect/dispose of feed. They may also increase exercise or abuse laxatives in an effort to prevent weight gain. Feeding of patients with eating disorders may require the use of legislation, such as the Mental Capacity Act 2005, Deprivation of Liberty Safeguards, and Mental Health Act 2007 in the UK.

Sato Y, Fukudo S. Gastrointestinal symptoms and disorders in patients with eating disorders. *Clin J Gastroenterol.* 2015;8(5):255–263. Doi:10.1007/s12328-015-0611-x.

### 8. C. Prescribe 1 litre 0.9% sodium chloride with 40 mmol potassium chloride, 1 litre 5% dextrose with 14 mmol magnesium sulphate, and 500 ml 5% dextrose with 20 mmol potassium chloride to be administered through the 22G cannula

- Parenteral nutrition should not be administered through a central venous catheter that may be infected

Managing suspected line infections in patients dependent on parenteral nutrition can be challenging because of resistant organisms or lack of alternative central access. Whether line salvage is attempted or the line is removed, parenteral nutrition should usually not be administered until sterility is confirmed. Peripheral parenteral nutrition can be used in the short term but the formulation may need to be different from this patient's usual prescription. In the short term, matching volume and electrolytes such as sodium, potassium, and magnesium is a pragmatic approach. Knowledge of electrolyte content, particularly sodium, of commonly used intravenous fluids is therefore essential.

Lal S, Chadwick P, Nightingale J et al. Management of catheter related blood stream infections (CRBSIs). British Intestinal Failure Alliance (BIFA) recommendation. British Association of Parenteral and Enteral Nutrition. January 2019. Available at: https://www.bapen.org.uk/pdfs/bifa/recommendations-on-management-of-crbsi.pdf (accessed February 2020)

## 9. C. Prolonged course of antibiotics

- Management of type 2 intestinal failure revolves around the SNAP acronym (Sepsis, Nutrition, Anatomy, Plan)
- Further surgery should be delayed for 4–6 months

This patient has type 2 intestinal failure with a high output (>500 ml per 24 hours) fistula and intra-abdominal sepsis. The approach to management should follow the SNAP acronym (sepsis, nutrition, anatomy, plan). Sepsis is the leading cause of death in this cohort—if collections are amenable to radiological drainage, this should be considered to gain source control. Prolonged antibiotics may be needed to adequately treat infection not amenable to radiological or surgical drainage. In this case, there is no indication for urgent laparotomy and washout due to small abscesses, a reducing CRP, and haemodynamic stability.

This patient will require intravenous nutrition support given the fistula losses. Unrestricted oral intake will increase fluid losses and is not to be advised in this case. Understanding the residual anatomy of this patient is critical prior to attempting definitive reconstructive surgery. Surgery should be delayed for at least 4–6 months following the last operation to reduce the risk of further complication. Surgery before this time should be limited to sepsis control. There is no role for laparoscopic stoma formation here.

Klek S, Forbes A, Gabe S et al. Management of acute intestinal failure: a position paper from the European Society for Clinical Nutrition and Metabolism (ESPEN) special interest group. *Clin. Nutr.* 2016;35:1209–1218. Doi:10.1016/j.clnu.2016.04.009.

## 10. D. Refer for intestinal transplantation assessment

- Referral for transplant assessment should be considered for patients who are developing complications of parenteral nutrition
- Outcomes for liver-containing multivisceral grafts are poorer than for intestine alone and so early referral before the development of irreversible liver fibrosis is desirable

This patient has evidence of intestinal-failure associated liver disease along with other complications of parenteral nutrition (multiple line infections, central venous thromboses) and should be referred for assessment for intestinal transplantation. The development of jaundice is an ominous sign and simply repeating the blood tests in six months and organizing FibroScan is insufficient. Teduglutide is not available in many countries because of cost and in any case may not enable this patient to achieve enteral autonomy—hence the risks of lines and parenteral nutrition would persist here. Palliation of this patient is inappropriate at this stage given there are other treatment options, and ursodeoxycholic acid would not reverse the underlying process.

Usual indications for intestinal transplant assessment include complications associated with parenteral nutrition (whether feed-related or line-related), or for whom evisceration is needed to treat the underlying disease (e.g. desmoid disease). One- and five-year survival for liver-containing grafts is less than intestine alone and so referrals should ideally be made before irreversible liver fibrosis has developed.

Loo L, Vrakas G, Reddy S et al. Intestinal transplantation: a review. *Curr Opin Gastroenterol.* 2017;33(3):203–211. Doi:10.1097/MOG.0000000000000358.

### 11. D. The long-term re-operation rate is more than 10%

- LAGB has a lower post-operative mortality compared with SG and Roux-en-Y gastric bypass but a higher long-term re-operation rate (12%)
- LAGB is inferior to SG and RY-GBP in terms of weight loss and remission of type 2 diabetes

In the UK, bariatric surgery should be considered for patients with a BMI ≥40.0 kg/m$^2$ or with 35–39.9 kg/m$^2$ and comorbidities that are likely to improve following surgically induced weight loss (e.g. type 2 diabetes, cardiorespiratory disease, severe osteoarthritis). To be considered for surgery, patients should have failed to lose weight or to maintain weight loss despite comprehensive medical care. Traditional concepts of restrictive (reducing stomach capacity) and malabsorptive (limiting nutrient absorption) operations are now regarded as too simplistic, and there is a move to refer to all bariatric procedures as 'metabolic operations'. Choice of operation relies on close discussion on a case-by-case basis within the multi-disciplinary team. The average positive metabolic impact increases in the following order: LAGB, SG, RY-GBP, biliopancreatic diversion +/- duodenal switch. However, surgical complexity and potential long-term nutritional complications increase in the same order.

LAGB is the least invasive procedure with very few immediate post-operative complications and low 30-day mortality. However, it is associated with limited metabolic benefit and the highest rate of late complications (25%) and re-operation (12%). Complications include band slippage, band erosion, oesophageal dilation +/- obstruction and gastric necrosis. Post-operative gastro-oesophageal reflux also increases fivefold. These factors have led to a widespread reduction in the use of LAGB over the past 10 years.

Ma IT, Madura JA 2nd. Gastrointestinal complications after bariatric surgery. *Gastroenterol Hepatol (N Y)*. 2015;11(8):526–535.

### 12. C. Iron

- Bariatric surgery can cause a number of nutritional complications, some of which may present months or years after the procedure
- Anaemia is common, with iron deficiency the most likely cause
- Small intestinal bacterial overgrowth (SIBO) can develop following intestinal bypass procedures, further exacerbating vitamin deficiencies

Anaemia is found in a third of patients following RY-GBP. The most common cause is iron deficiency, resulting from the reduction in gastric acid and the bypass of the duodenum and proximal jejunum, the major sites of iron absorption.

SIBO is common following bariatric procedures that alter the anatomy of the small bowel, such as RY-GBP, biliopancreatic diversion and duodenal switch, but not after adjustable gastric banding or SG. SIBO would be consistent with the patient's symptoms of bloating, flatulence, and loose stool, and typically causes an increased serum folate level, but it can lead to severe thiamine deficiency and vitamin B12 deficiency. While vitamin B12 deficiency can cause anaemia, body stores are substantial, and it can take years for deficiency to manifest.

The patient's symptoms of hair loss are most likely due to protein malnutrition, a common problem post-bariatric surgery if patients do not receive tailored help from a dietitian to maintain protein intake above 60 g/day. Copper deficiency is reported post-bariatric surgery and can lead to a microcytic anaemia mimicking iron deficiency as well as neurological complications, but it is much less common.

The complexity of these potential complications highlights the importance of an integrated, multi-professional bariatric service to manage patients before, during, and after surgery.

Bal BS, Finelli FC, Shope TR et al. Nutritional deficiencies after bariatric surgery. *Nat Rev Endocrinol.* 2012;8(9):544–556. Doi:10.1038/nrendo.2012.48.

## 13. B. Early dumping syndrome (EDS)

- EDS is a common post-gastric bypass complication and consists of both gastrointestinal and vasomotor symptoms
- EDS typically manifests six weeks post-operatively with symptoms occurring within one hour of eating
- Late dumping syndrome (LDS) is rare, occurring months to years post-operatively and is characterized by symptoms of hypoglycaemia occurring 1–3 hours after eating

'Dumping' is a symptom complex recognized after gastric surgery. EDS typically develops around six weeks post-operatively with symptoms occurring within the first hour after a meal. It results from the rapid transit of nutrients into the small intestine causing osmotically driven fluid movement into the intestinal lumen. Symptoms are typically gastrointestinal (e.g. watery diarrhoea, nausea/vomiting, abdominal cramps) and vasomotor (e.g. presyncope/syncope, fatigue, drowsiness, palpitations). EDS is common affecting up to 40% of patients after gastric bypass. Dietary changes can be beneficial, particularly reducing meal size, increasing fibre/protein, and reducing carbohydrate. Octreotide or guar gum may be beneficial in some cases.

Conversely, LDS is rare and encountered months to years post-operatively. It is characterized by post-prandial hypoglycaemia in response to hyperinsulinaemia 1–3 hours after eating. This reactive hypoglycemia manifests as autonomic symptoms (tremor, sweating, and palpitations) and neuroglycopenic symptoms (confusion, poor concentration, and altered conscious levels). Gastrointestinal symptoms are not a significant feature of LDS or post-prandial vasovagal syncope.

While bariatric surgery is a risk factor for gallstones because of reduced bile acid secretion and supersaturation with cholesterol, abdominal pain associated with gallstones would be unlikely to be associated with vasomotor symptoms. A gastro-gastric fistula between the proximal gastric pouch and the distal gastric remnant is rarely reported following RY-GBP and presents with abdominal pain and regain of weight.

Nielsen JB, Pedersen AM, Gribsholt SB et al. Prevalence, severity, and predictors of symptoms of dumping and hypoglycemia after Roux-en-Y gastric bypass. *Surg Obes Relat Dis.* 2016;12(8):1562–1568. Doi:10.1016/j.soard.2016.04.017.

1.  **A 69-year-old man with a history of coronary artery disease and atrial fibrillation (AF) is referred with iron deficiency anaemia. He had coronary stent insertion 18 months ago. His current medications include apixaban, aspirin, atorvastatin, and bisoprolol. He agrees to a gastroscopy and colonoscopy. However, he does not wish to return for repeat procedures if this can be avoided.**

    **What advice is most appropriate regarding his medication prior to his planned procedures?**

    A.  Consult a cardiologist

    B.  Stop apixaban 48 hours before, continue aspirin

    C.  Stop apixaban 48 hours before, omit aspirin on morning of procedure

    D.  Stop apixaban 72 hours before, continue aspirin

    E.  Stop apixaban 72 hours before, omit aspirin on morning of procedure

2.  **A 65-year-old man underwent a colonoscopy. A 2.5 cm sessile polyp in the ascending colon was removed by endoscopic mucosal resection with hot snare polypectomy. He was discharged from the endoscopy department the same day. Two days later, he presented with increasing abdominal pain. Clinical examination revealed tachycardia and abdominal tenderness.**

    Investigations:
    | | |
    |---|---|
    | Haemoglobin | 135 g/L |
    | White cell count | $13.0 \times 10$/L |
    | Platelet count | $450 \times 10^9$/L |
    | Serum C-reactive protein | 34 mg/L |

    **What is the best next step in this patient's management?**

    A.  Colonoscopy

    B.  Computed tomography (CT) abdomen

    C.  Erect chest radiograph

    D.  Laparoscopy

    E.  Laparotomy

*Best of Five MCQs for the European Specialty Examination in Gastroenterology and Hepatology.* Thomas Marjot, Colleen G C McGregor, Tim Ambrose, Aminda N De Silva, Jeremy Cobbold, and Simon Travis, Oxford University Press (2021). © Oxford University Press. DOI: 10.1093/oso/9780198834373.003.0010

3.  A patient telephoned the endoscopy department for advice. In the past, they had been given antibiotic prophylaxis for a minor dental procedure and had developed a rash. They wished to know whether antibiotics would be required for their endoscopy.

    **Which of the following scenarios is most likely to require antibiotic prophylaxis?**

    A.  Endoscopic retrograde cholangiopancreatography (ERCP) for jaundice secondary to a hilar cholangiocarcinoma

    B.  Endoscopic ultrasound (EUS) and fine-needle aspiration for a solid lesion in the pancreas seen on a CT scan

    C.  ERCP for stones within the common bile duct without intercurrent sepsis

    D.  Gastroscopy and oesophageal dilatation for a benign oesophageal stricture

    E.  Previous history of an aortic valve replacement undergoing a colonoscopy and polypectomy

4.  A 22-year-old university student presented to the emergency department following a suicide attempt. He reportedly ingested 250 mls of bleach 12 hours earlier. He complained of odynophagia. His background included deliberate self-harm.

    On assessment, his vital observations were normal and his airway was uncompromised.

    Investigations:

    | | |
    |---|---|
    | Gastroscopy | Oesophageal haemorrhage, erosions, blisters, and superficial ulcers |

    **Which Zargar classification is described here?**

    A.  Grade I

    B.  Grade II A

    C.  Grade II B

    D.  Grade IIIA

    E.  Grade IV

5.  A 69-year-old man with Barrett's oesophagus attended for a surveillance gastroscopy. He asked to have sedation for the procedure.

    **Which of the following is the most important risk factor for sedation-related complications?**

    A.  Diabetes mellitus

    B.  Diuretic usage

    C.  Hypokalemia

    D.  Obesity

    E.  Recent hip replacement

6. **Your endoscopy unit is due for its annual appraisal. According to the European Society of Gastrointestinal Endoscopy (ESGE) guidance:**

   **Which of the following is a key performance measure for ERCP?**

   A. Adequate antibiotic prophylaxis before ERCP in at least 95% of procedures

   B. Appropriate stent placement in patients with biliary obstruction below the hilum in at least 90%

   C. Bile duct cannulation rate in at least 90%

   D. Bile duct stone extraction in at least 85%

   E. Post-ERCP pancreatitis in less than 5%

7. **A 48-year-old man with motor neurone disease attended for an elective endoscopic gastrostomy placement. Due to his neurological condition, he was unable to sign his signature during the consenting process.**

   **With respect to valid consent in endoscopy, which statement is best practice?**

   A. Additional consent must be obtained for taking photos or videos as part of standard care

   B. If a patient withdraws consent during an endoscopy, the procedure should be completed as soon as possible

   C. In those lacking capacity, the next of kin may sign consent on their behalf

   D. The formal consent process should be completed before entry into the procedure room

   E. Verbal consent alone may be obtained for patients unable to write and the consenting healthcare professional should sign on behalf of the patient on the Consent Form

8. **A 50-year-old man presented with 48 hours of abdominal pain, distension and vomiting.**

   Investigation:

   | | |
   |---|---|
   | CT abdomen and pelvis | In the distal ileum, there is an intraluminal mass with classic 'target sign' appearance consistent with invaginated bowel. There is moderate proximal small bowel dilatation but no free air to suggest perforation. |

   **Which of the following statements is true regarding this disease in adults?**

   A. It is the third most common cause of bowel obstruction

   B. It most commonly occurs in the colon

   C. Neoplastic lesions account for two-thirds of cases

   D. Ninety per cent of cases are idiopathic

   E. The majority are treated successfully with hydrostatic enema

9. **A 56-year-old man was referred with a history of constipation, tenesmus, pruritis ani, and rectal bleeding. He is otherwise fit and well.**

   Investigation:

   Colonoscopy    Large prolapsing haemorrhoids which have to be manually reduced.

   ### Which of the following would be the next best intervention?

   A. Heater probe coagulation

   B. Injection sclerotherapy

   C. Lord's procedure

   D. Rubber band ligation (RBL)

   E. Stapled haemorrhoidectomy

10. **A 25-year-old girl with constipation-predominant irritable bowel syndrome (IBS-C) was referred to clinic with ongoing anal pain. She described excruciating pain on defecation with hard stools. On rectal examination, her GP had identified an anal fissure. Treatment with warm baths, stool softeners, and topical anaesthetic gels had failed to provide relief.**

    ### What would be the next most appropriate treatment?

    A. Botulinum toxin injections

    B. Lateral sphincterotomy

    C. Topical diltiazem

    D. Topical glyceryl trinitrate (GTN)

    E. Topical hydrocortisone

11. **A 34-year-old teacher was referred to the clinic with a history of rectal bleeding. He had suffered with constipation in the past. A flexible sigmoidoscopy was requested.**

    Investigations:

    Flexible sigmoidoscopy    Insertion to proximal sigmoid. Rectal oedema with superficial ulcerations and mucosal erythema.

    Histology    Fibromuscular obliteration of the lamina propria and surface erosion consistent with solitary rectal ulcer syndrome.

    ### With respect to solitary rectal ulcer syndrome (SRUS), which statement is most accurate?

    A. A minority of patients have associated dyssynergic defaecatory disorder

    B. Rectal bleeding on defaecation is a hallmark feature

    C. SRUS is a misnomer: only 40% of patients have a solitary ulcer

    D. Topical treatments, including sucralfate and mesalazine, are first line

    E. Ulceration is typically deep

12. **A 39-year-old man who had sex with men (MSM) was referred to clinic. He had a three-month history of rectal pain, tenesmus, and a mucopurulent, occasionally bloody, anal discharge. He had lost 6 kg in weight and developed widespread lymphadenopathy. He had had three new sexual partners during the past year.**

    Investigations:
    | | |
    |---|---|
    | Flexible sigmoidoscopy | Distal proctitis, pus in rectum |
    | Colonic histopathology | Consistent with Crohn's colitis |

    **Which of the following most closely resembles Crohn's disease on histopathology?**

    A. *Chlamydia lymphogranuloma venereum* (LGV)

    B. *Cytomegalovirus*

    C. Herpes simplex virus

    D. *Neisseria gonorrhoeae*

    E. *Treponema pallidum*

13. **A 38-year-old accountant was seen in the IBD clinic. He had ileal Crohn's disease for which he had been on azathioprine for several years. His background also included HIV (on HAART). He reported anal discharge and pruritus. Perineal examination revealed a suspicious, pigmented, scaly lesion with associated white plaque.**

    **Which of the following is true for anal intraepithelial neoplasia (AIN)?**

    A. Ablative therapy is preferable to excision of small lesions

    B. Human papilloma viruses (HPV) infection reduces the risk of AIN

    C. Screening is indicated in high-risk groups only

    D. The presence of ulceration in an AIN lesion is pathognomonic

    E. There is an increased incidence of AIN in the immunosuppressed and HIV-positive individuals

14. **A 45-year-old woman is referred to gastroenterology with faecal incontinence (FI). She is normally fit and well. Her general practitioner attempted to manage her symptoms with dietary modifications and anti-diarrhoeal agents with no improvement. Clinical examination, including digital rectal examination, was unremarkable.**

    **Which is the next best investigation to perform?**

    A. Anal electromyography

    B. Anorectal manometry

    C. Endoanal ultrasound

    D. Magnetic resonance imaging (MRI) of pelvis

    E. Magnetic resonance (MR) proctogram

15. **A 45-year-old man presented with abdominal bloating, watery diarrhoea, and flatulence. A glucose-hydrogen breath test was arranged.**

    **Which statement regarding glucose-hydrogen breath testing is correct?**

    A. A double peak in expired breath hydrogen should be considered normal

    B. A rise in breath hydrogen by more than 20 ppm from baseline within 90 minutes would be consistent with a positive test result

    C. Glucose-hydrogen breath testing correlates well with jejunal aspirates

    D. Lactulose is well absorbed across the small intestinal mucosa

    E. The test is not affected by small bowel transit time

## 1. B. Stop apixaban 48 hours before, continue aspirin

- Aspirin is safe to continue prior to routine endoscopic procedures
- Apixaban should be stopped 48 hours prior to high-risk procedures
- Cardiology advice should be sought for patients with high-risk conditions

AF and ischaemic heart disease with long-standing stents are low-risk conditions for stopping anticoagulant and antiplatelet agents. Therefore, consulting a cardiologist is not required. Diagnostic gastroscopy is a low-risk procedure. However, the colonoscopy should best be considered a high-risk procedure to allow for polypectomy, given the patient's preference. Aspirin is safe to continue prior to routine endoscopy.

### High-risk conditions

- <12 months after drug eluting coronary stent
- <1 month after bare metal coronary stent
- AF + prosthetic heart valve
- Prosthetic mitral valve
- AF + mitral stenosis
- <3 months after VTE

### Low-risk conditions

- IHD with no recent stents
- Cerebral vascular disease
- Peripheral vascular disease
- Tissue heart valve
- Prosthetic aortic valve
- Non-valvular AF
- >3 months after venous thromboembolism (VTE)

### Direct oral anticoagulants (apixaban,dabigatran, edoxaban, rivaroxaban)

Low-risk procedures: omit on the morning of procedure
High-risk procedures: stop 48 hours before procedure (72 hours for dabigatran with CrCl 30–50 ml/min)

### Warfarin

Low-risk procedures: continue therapy, check international normalized ratio (INR) does not exceed therapeutic range

*Best of Five MCQs for the European Specialty Examination in Gastroenterology and Hepatology.* Thomas Marjot, Colleen G C McGregor, Tim Ambrose, Aminda N De Silva, Jeremy Cobbold, and Simon Travis, Oxford University Press (2021). © Oxford University Press. DOI: 10.1093/oso/9780198834373.003.0010

High-risk procedures: assess risk of underlying condition
- If low-risk condition, stop five days before procedure, check INR <1.5
- If high-risk condition, stop five days before procedure and bridge with low molecular weight heparin (LMWH)

*P2Y12 receptor antagonists (clopidogrel, prasugrel, ticagrelor)*

Low-risk procedures: continue
High risk procedures:
- If low-risk condition, stop five days before procedure
- If high-risk condition, consult cardiologist

Veitch AM et al. Endoscopy in patients on antiplatelet or anticoagulant therapy, including direct oral anticoagulants: British Society of Gastroenterology (BSG) and European Society of Gastrointestinal Endoscopy (ESGE) guidelines. *Gut.* 2016;65:374–389. Doi: 10.1136/gutjnl-2015-311110.

## 2. B. CT abdomen

Post-polypectomy syndrome:
- Presents similarly to colonic perforation and often requires a CT to differentiate
- Occurs more commonly in larger polypectomies (>2 cm)
- Is managed conservatively in the majority of cases

The most likely diagnosis in this case is post-polypectomy syndrome (or post-polypectomy electrocoagulation syndrome). The electrical current arising from diathermy extends beyond the mucosa and muscularis propria into the serosal surface of the colon. Thermal injury ensues, without evidence of colonic perforation, and results in a localized inflammatory reaction. The syndrome occurs after large amounts of sustained thermal energy have been applied, so it is more commonly seen after larger polypectomies (>2 cm in diameter), or when normal mucosa is inadvertently caught within the snare alongside the polyp. Anecdotal evidence suggests the injection of fluid submucosally prior to polypectomy may reduce the risk of developing post-polypectomy syndrome.

Post-polypectomy syndrome occurs in 0.5%–1% of polypectomies, and in 7%–8% after endoscopic submucosal dissection. Patients can present acutely (within 12 hours) or delayed (up to 5 days post procedure). Clinical presentation includes fever, tachycardia, abdominal pain, and leucocytosis. The main differential is colonic perforation. As such, the definitive investigation to differentiate is a CT scan, which may show focal thickening of the colon and periluminal fat stranding. In contrast to perforation, there will be no evidence of pneumoperitoneum. Therefore, an erect chest radiograph is unhelpful.

Management is conservative and includes nil by mouth, intravenous fluids, and antibiotics until symptoms and inflammatory markers settle. If symptoms and signs are mild, some patients may even be managed as outpatients. There is a very low risk of evolution to frank perforation, and the prognosis is generally excellent.

In this case, repeating a colonoscopy would be inappropriate given the concern of perforation. Equally, surgical intervention would only be indicated if a large perforation were confirmed radiologically.

Cha JM. Clinical outcomes and risk factors of post-polypectomy coagulation syndrome: a multicenter, retrospective, case-control study. *Endoscopy.* 2013;45:202–207. Doi: 10.1055/s-0032-1326104.

## 3. A. Endoscopic retrograde cholangiopancreatography (ERCP) for jaundice secondary to a hilar cholangiocarcinoma

- Some endoscopic interventions may cause bacteraemia; however, complications from bacteraemia are fortunately uncommon
- Antibiotics are no longer routinely required for the prevention of infective endocarditis
- Antibiotics are required in ERCP when adequate biliary decompression is unlikely to be achieved

There are specific situations in endoscopy where antibiotics are indicated. These are summarized in Table 10.1.

Allison MC, Sandow JAT et al. Antibiotic prophylaxis in gastrointestinal endoscopy. *Gut.* 2009;58:869–880. Doi:10.1136/gut.2007.136580.

**Table 10.1** Summary of prophylactic antibiotic regimens recommended for gastrointestinal endoscopy

| Scenario | Rationale | Antibiotics | Dose/route |
|---|---|---|---|
| 1. Patients with valvular heart disease, valve replacement, and/or surgically constructed systemic–pulmonary shunt or conduit or vascular graft | Prevention of infective endocarditis or conduit/graft infection | Not indicated | |
| 2. ERCP in the following: | | | |
| a. Ongoing cholangitis or sepsis elsewhere | Prevention of procedure-related bacteraemia | Guide by culture results. Patients should already be established on antibiotics | Microbiology advice |
| b. Biliary obstruction and/or CBD stones | Prevention of cholangitis | Not indicated unless biliary decompression is not achieved. If biliary decompression is not achieved during the procedure, a full course of antibiotics is indicated | |
| c. When complete biliary drainage is unlikely to be achieved (e.g. PSC, hilar cholangiocarcinoma) (may need to consider alternative antibiotic prophylaxis if repeated procedures are needed) | Prevention of cholangitis | Ciprofloxacin<br><br>or<br>Gentamycin | 750 mg PO 60–90 mins before procedure<br><br>1.5 mg/kg IV over 2–3 mins |
| d. Communicating pancreatic cyst or pseudocyst | Reducing risk of introducing infection into cavity | As (c) | As (c) |
| e. Biliary complications following liver transplant | Prevention of cholangitis | As (c) + amoxicillin<br><br>or<br>vancomycin | 1 g IV single dose<br><br>20 mg/kg IV infused over at least 1 hour |
| 3. EUS in the following: | | | |
| a. FNA solid lesions | Prevention of local infections | Not indicated | |
| b. FNA cystic lesions in or near the pancreas or drainage of a cystic cavity | Prevention of cyst infections | Co-amoxiclav<br><br>or<br>Ciprofloxacin | 1.2 g IV single dose<br><br>750 mg PO single dose |
| 4. PEG | Prevention of peristomal infection<br><br>Possible reduction in risk of other infections, such as aspiration pneumonia | Co-amoxiclav<br><br>or<br>Cefuroxime | 1.2 g IV injection or infusion just before procedure<br>750 mg IV injection or infusion just before procedure |

*(continued)*

**Table 10.1** Continued

| Scenario | Rationale | Antibiotics | Dose/route |
|---|---|---|---|
| | | Teicoplanin can be used if there is a past history of anaphylaxis or angioedema with penicillin/cephalosporin | 400 mg IV for adults |
| 5. Variceal bleeding (not strictly prophylaxis) | Prevention of infections such as spontaneous bacterial peritonitis | Piperacillin/tazobactam | 4.5 g IV 3 times a day |
| | | or<br>Third-generation cephalosporin Seek microbiology or regional liver unit advice in cases of penicillin allergy | e.g. cefotaxime 2 g IV 3 times a day |
| 6. Profound immunocompromise (e.g. neutropenia <0.5 × 10⁹/ L or advanced haematological malignancy) | Prevention of procedure-related bacteraemia | Only indicated in procedures with a high rate of bacteraemia (e.g. sclerotherapy, dilatation, ERCP with obstructed system) | Discuss with haematologist and/or clinical microbiologist |

CBD, common bile duct; PO, by mouth; IV, intravenous; PSC, primary sclerosing cholangitis; ERCP, endoscopic retrograde cholangiopancreatography; EUS, endoscopic ultrasound; FNA, fine-needle aspiration; PEG, percutaneous endoscopic gastrostomy.

## 4. B. Grade II A

- Gastroscopy should be performed between 12 and 48 hours post caustic ingestion
- Zargar's classification is the most common endoscopic tool for assessing caustic injury
- There is a ninefold increase in morbidity and mortality with every increased injury grade

Gastroscopy is an important diagnostic and prognostic tool in the evaluation of a caustic injury, especially during the first 12–48 hours of caustic ingestion. It is contraindicated in patients with haemodynamic instability, severe respiratory compromise, and suspected perforations. In the absence of symptoms, significant lesions are typically not seen endoscopically. Emergent endoscopy is recommended in symptomatic individuals and in those with intentional ingestions of caustic substances.

Endoscopy is the gold standard in diagnosis and prognostication in caustic ingestions. It also guides management. Zargar's classification (Table 10.2) is most commonly used to grade severity of caustic injury. Grades 0–II A generally recover without sequelae. Grades IIB–III eventually develop oesophageal or gastric scarring, which may result in stricture formation. The degree of oesophageal injury endoscopically is a predictor of morbidity and mortality with a ninefold increase with each injury grade.

**Table 10.2** Zargar classification

| Zargar classification | Endoscopic description |
|---|---|
| Grade 0 | Normal mucosa |
| Grade I | Oedema and erythema of the mucosa |
| Grade II A | Haemorrhage, erosions, blisters, superficial ulcers |
| Grade II B | Circumferential lesions |
| Grade III A | Focal deep grey or brownish-black ulcers |
| Grade III B | Extensive deep grey or brownish-black ulcers |
| Grade IV | Perforation |

De Lusong MAA, Tombol ABG, Tuazon DJS. Management of esophageal caustic injury. *World J Gastrointest Pharmacol Ther*. 2017 May 6;8(2):90–98. Doi: 10.4292/wjgpt.v8.i2.90.

## 5. D. Obesity

- Sedation-related complication is the leading factor in endoscopy-related mortality
- Assessment of risk factors for sedation-related complications is paramount
- Opiates and benzodiazepines have a synergistic effect

Conscious sedation is defined as the use of medication to depress the central nervous system without the loss of verbal communication. Sedation is the leading factor in endoscopy-related mortality.

Risk factors for complications of sedation include the following:

- Advanced age
- Obesity
- Comorbidities including cirrhosis, cardiac disease, respiratory disease, renal disease
- Prior administration of sedation or opiates
- Known drug allergies
- Low resting oxygen saturations
- Emergency endoscopy

Complications of sedation include over-sedation, paradoxical excitement, respiratory depression, aspiration, cardiac arrhythmias, acute coronary events, hypertension, hypotension, cerebrovascular events, nausea, vomiting, and flushing (Table 10.3). Risk factors for complications should warrant discussion of un-sedated endoscopy and, if sedation is undertaken, adjustment of doses should be considered.

## 6. C. Bile duct cannulation rate in at least 90%

The ESGE and United European Gastroenterology have identified quality of endoscopy as a major priority. They recommend that endoscopy services adopt the following key performance measures for ERCP and EUS:

1. Adequate antibiotic prophylaxis before ERCP (key performance measure, at least 90%)
2. Antibiotic prophylaxis before EUS guided puncture of cystic lesions (key performance measure, at least 95%)
3. Bile duct cannulation rate (key performance measure, at least 90%)
4. Tissue sampling during EUS (key performance measure, at least 85%)
5. Appropriate stent placement in patients with biliary obstruction below the hilum (key performance measure, at least 95%)
6. Bile duct stone extraction (key performance measure, at least 90%)
7. Post-ERCP pancreatitis (key performance measure, less than 10%)

*Minor performance measure*

8. Adequate documentation of EUS landmarks (at least 90%)

Domagk D, Oppong KW et al. Performance measures for ERCP and endoscopic ultrasound: a European Society of Gastrointestinal Endoscopy (ESGE) quality improvement initiative. *Endoscopy.* 2018;50:1116–1127. Doi: 10.1055/a-0749-8767.

## 7. D. The formal consent process should be completed before entry into the procedure room

- All endoscopic procedures require written consent, except in an emergency

**Table 10.3** Sedatives, analgesics and adjuncts used in endoscopy

| Drug | Effect | Contra-indications | Side effects (SE) | Onset (minutes) | Dose | Reversal agent |
|---|---|---|---|---|---|---|
| **Benzodiazepines** e.g. *Midazolam* | Sedation with amnesia, and no analgesic effect | Neuromuscular respiratory weakness Severe respiratory depression | Confusion Paradoxical excitement or agitation Nausea Vomiting Reduced respiratory effort Hypoxia Hypotension Cardiac or respiratory arrest | Initial: 1 Peak: 1-2 | <70 yrs: 0–2 mg, increment 0–1 mg, max 5 mg >70 years: 0–1 mg, increment 0–0.5 mg, max 2 mg | Flumazenil: 0.2–0.5 mg, increment 0.1 mg, peak effect in up to 1 minute, duration of action 1–2 hours SE: flushing, seizures, and late re-sedation. |
| **Opiates** e.g. *Pethidine*\*, *Fentanyl* | Prevention, reduction, and relief of pain Opiates have a synergistic effect with benzodiazepines Give 3 minutes before benzodiazepines, as doses may need to be reduced by up to fourfold | Acute respiratory depression Phaeochromocytoma | Confusion Nausea Vomiting Decreased responsiveness Reduced respiratory effort Hypoxia Hypotension Cardiac or respiratory arrest | Initial: 1-2 Peak: 3 | <70 years old: Pethidine: initial dose 25 mg, increment 25 mg, max 50 mg Fentanyl: initial dose 50 mg, increment 25 mg, max 100 mg >70 years old: Pethidine: initial dose 12.5 mg, increment 12.5 mg, max 25 mg Fentanyl: initial dose 25 mg, increment 12.5 mg, max 50 mg | Naloxone: Dosage 0.1–0.2 mg, maximum 10 mg, peak effect in 1–2 minutes, duration of action 1–3 hours SE: Pain, agitation, arrhythmias, pulmonary oedema, and late re-sedation. |
| **Buscopan** | Relief of smooth muscle spasm | Myasthenia gravis, acute closed-angle glaucoma | Tachycardia Arrhythmias Anti-muscarinic side effects | Peak: 4 Duration of action (hours): 5 | 20 mg can be repeated every 30 minutes up to a max of 100 mg in 24 hours. | - |
| **Xylocaine Throat Spray (Topical lidocaine)** | Analgesia of oropharynx | Unsafe swallow (Relative) | Risk of aspiration | Peak: 1 Duration of action: 15–60 | Max 20 applications (200 mg lidocaine base) | - |

\*Pethidine is metabolized to fentanyl and therefore has less predictable effects, including a higher risk of hypotension, and hallucinations

Dumonceau JM, Riphaus A et al. European Society of Gastrointestinal Endoscopy, European Society of Gastroenterology and Endoscopy Nurses and Associates, and the European Society of Anaesthesiology Guideline: Non-anesthesiologist administration of propofol for GI endoscopy. Endoscopy. 2010 Nov;42(11):960-74. Doi:10.1055/s-0030-1255728

- A best interest decision should be taken for those who lack capacity
- The consent process should be completed before entry into the procedure room

All endoscopic procedures require written consent, except in an emergency. The endoscopist performing the procedure is ultimately responsible for ensuring that the consent process is appropriate for the procedure being undertaken. The endoscopist performing the procedure should assess capacity to consent. If a patient lacks capacity, delaying the procedure to allow the patient to regain capacity may be appropriate. If the patient is unlikely to regain capacity or the procedure is an emergency, the endoscopist should make a decision to proceed in the patient's best interests. In such instances, where possible, the next of kin should be informed. However, this should not delay emergency treatment. Patients who lack capacity may have a proxy decision maker (e.g. Lasting Power of Attorney) or may require appointment of an Independent Mental Capacity Advocate. In non-emergency cases where the patient lacks capacity, the decision regarding endoscopy is best decided in a multi-disciplinary discussion with best interests in mind. Patients physically unable to sign their consent may have their consent countersigned by a witness (relative or healthcare professional (not the consenting healthcare professional).

All patients should receive written information explaining the procedure, and its intended benefits and risks, in a format that they can understand. Written information should be provided in advance of the procedure. The consent process should be performed by a suitably trained individual before entry into the procedure room. Final validation of the consent process should be completed before the procedure starts. Endoscopic photo- and video-documentation as part of routine clinical care does not require additional consent. If a patient, with capacity, withdraws consent during an endoscopic procedure, the procedure should be stopped. The person's concerns should be explored. If they clearly indicate a wish for the procedure to be discontinued, this must occur without delay unless doing so would result in a risk of serious harm to the patient.

Everett SM, Griffiths H et al. Guideline for obtaining valid consent for gastrointestinal endoscopy procedures. *Gut.* 2016;65(10):1585–1601. Doi: 10.1136/gutjnl-2016-311904.

## 8. D. Neoplastic lesions account for two-thirds of cases

- Intussusception is a rare cause of intestinal obstruction in adults
- It typically occurs in the small bowel and is associated with structural lesions in 90% of which two-thirds are neoplastic

Intussusception is the invagination of one segment of bowel into an immediately adjacent segment. It is most commonly found in children and represents the second most common cause of intestinal obstruction in this group after pyloric stenosis. The majority of paediatric intussusception is idiopathic (90%) and is usually ileocolic. Conversely, adult intussusception is rare, accounting for 1–5% of cases of bowel obstruction and usually occurs in the ileum. Ninety per cent of adult cases will have an underlying structural cause, two-thirds of which will be due to benign or malignant neoplasms. The remainder are caused by infections, adhesions, intestinal ulceration, and congenital abnormalities such as Meckel's diverticulum. These lesions act as a focal area of traction, or 'lead point', which draws the proximal bowel within the peristalsing distal bowel, which can ultimately lead to bowel ischaemia and perforation. Intussusception in adults is usually diagnosed on CT, which classically demonstrates a concentric hyperdense double ring or 'target-sign'. In children, most ileocolic intussusception is successfully managed with ultrasound or fluoroscopy guided pneumatic/ hydrostatic enema. In adults, because of the majority of cases arising from structural pathology in the small bowel, surgery remains the mainstay of treatment.

Marsicovetere P, Ivatury SJ, White B et al. Intestinal intussusception: etiology, diagnosis, and treatment. *Clin Colon Rectal Surg.* 2017 Feb;30(1):30–39. Doi: 10.1055/s-0036-1593429.

## 9. D. Rubber band ligation (RBL)

- RBL is currently the first-line intervention in Grades I–III haemorrhoids, with a long-term success rate of >80%
- Surgical haemorrhoidectomy is associated with the lowest rate of recurrence but should be reserved for when RBL has failed because of higher complication rates (pain, anal stenosis, incontinence)

Haemorrhoids are defined as the symptomatic enlargement and displacement of the anal cushions which are prominences of anal mucosa formed by connective tissue, smooth muscle, and blood vessels. Contributing factors include lack of dietary fibre, chronic straining, excess time on the commode, constipation, and pregnancy. Haemorrhoids can be classified as internal (covered by columnar epithelium) or external (covered by squamous epithelium), and internal haemorrhoids can be graded from I–IV depending on the degree of prolapse during defecation. Conservative management of haemorrhoids includes lifestyle advice (adequate fluid and fibre intake, reduce straining, good anal hygiene), and treatment with laxatives and topical analgesics.

RBL is currently first-line therapy in Grade I–III haemorrhoids with a long-term success rate of >80%. Pain is the most common complication of RBL but can be minimized by proximal placement and single banding at a session. Sclerotherapy and heater probe coagulation can be used in Grade I–II haemorrhoids with variable success and higher complication rates respectively, when compared to RBL. While surgical haemorrhoidectomy is more effective than RBL in the treatment of Grade III haemorrhoids, it is associated with higher rates of complications, pain, and disability, and should therefore be reserved for cases when band ligation has failed. Lord's procedure involves anal dilation to decrease sphincteric pressure but is now an outdated technique because of high rates of post-procedural incontinence.

Ganz RA et al. The evaluation and treatment of hemorrhoids: a guide for the gastroenterologist. *Clin Gastroenterol Hepatol* 2013;11(6):593–603. Doi: 10.1016/j.cgh.2012.12.020.

## 10. C. Topical diltiazem

- Topical diltiazem and GTN have a similar efficacy for chronic anal fissures
- Topical diltiazem has a superior side effect profile
- Surgical options, including sphincterotomy, are reserved for cases refractory to conservative and medical therapy

Following the initial development of an anal fissure, passage of subsequent stool will continue to irritate the area. The internal sphincter may be involved and can go into spasm, causing further pain. It also pulls the edges of the fissure further apart, impairing wound healing, leading to the development of a chronic fissure.

Although conservative treatment may be sufficient for some acute fissures, other patients will need medical or surgical therapy. Stool softeners may reduce the pain and progression of a fissure, warm baths may relax the sphincter, and topical anaesthetic gel can provide pain relief. Topical diltiazem would be the next treatment of choice. This has the same efficacy as GTN—however with a superior side effect profile (30% of patients who use topical GTN suffer from headache). Topical diltiazem has been associated with healing rates of 65%–95%. Fifty per cent of patients treated with topical GTN may experience recurrent fissures. Treatment with botulinum toxin has a similar efficacy to that of GTN and diltiazem. However, it is more expensive and therefore may be used in patients whose fissures do not heal with topical (diltiazem or GTN) therapy or in cases of recurrence.

With regard to surgical treatment, lateral internal sphincterotomy has consistently superior healing rates and less recurrence when compared with medical therapy. However, there is a higher rate of faecal incontinence following treatment. In general, sphincterotomy and the various alternative surgical techniques available should only be used if the patient does not respond to medical treatment.

Stewart D, Gaertner W et al. Clinical Practice Guideline for the management of anal fissures. *Dis Colon Rectum*. 2017;60(1):7–14. Doi:10.1097/DCR.0000000000000735

### 11. B. Rectal bleeding on defaecation is a hallmark feature

- SRUS is a chronic, benign disorder in young adults
- Only 20% of patients have a solitary ulcer
- Patient education and conservative measures, including biofeedback, are the mainstay of treatment

SRUS is a rare, benign disorder characterized by a combination of clinical, endoscopic, and histological findings. Although denoted as a 'solitary rectal ulcer', only 20% of patients have a single ulcer endoscopically. It is a rare and often underdiagnosed disorder, with an annual prevalence of 1 in 100,000 persons. A disorder of young adults, occurring most commonly in the third and fourth decade in men and women respectively. Men and women are affected equally, however. The aetiology is not well understood but is thought to be multifactorial. Characterized by single or multiple ulcerations of the rectal mucosa, symptoms include rectal bleeding and mucus discharge, usually associated with excessive straining or abnormal defaecation. The passage of blood during defaecation is a hallmark feature. However, over a quarter of patients are asymptomatic, diagnosed incidentally.

According to anorectal manometry studies, dyssynergic defaecation is associated with SRUS in 25%–82% of patients. Defaecatory disorders with excessive straining are significantly associated with SRUS. Diagnosis is made on clinical features, endoscopy, and histology. Proctosigmoidoscopy reveals shallow rectal ulcer(s) of varying sizes covered by white or yellow slough. Surrounding rectal mucosa may appear hyperemic. Key histological features include fibromuscular obliteration of the lamina propria, hypertrophied muscularis mucosa, and glandular crypt abnormalities. Defaecatory proctogram and/or anorectal manometry are useful for determining the presence of intussusception, rectal prolapse, or dyssynergic defaecation. Several treatment options include conservative measures (high-fibre diet, patient education), biofeedback, medical therapy (topical sucralfate, mesalazine), and surgery (in presence of prolapse). Conservative measures and biofeedback are the mainstays of treatment.

Zhu Q, Shen R et al. Solitary rectal ulcer syndrome: clinical features, pathophysiology, diagnosis and treatment strategies. *World J Gastroenterol*. 2014;20(3):738–744. Doi: 10.3748/wjg.v20.i3.738.

### 12. A. *Chlamydia lymphogranuloma venereum (LGV)*

- *LGV* proctitis may mimic Crohn's disease
- All patients with *LGV* proctitis should be screened for HIV
- Treatment is with macrolides—doxycycline or erythromycin

All the infections listed can cause proctitis, and often there will be coexisting infections. Patients should be tested for HIV, especially in cases of *LGV*, syphilis, and herpes simplex virus (Table 10.4). Where positive, contact tracing should be instigated.

*LGV* has re-emerged among European MSM in the past decade and is a relatively common cause of proctitis in this population. Anorectal *LGV* is generally a symptomatic infection, although asymptomatic infection does occur. Proctitis is the primary manifestation of *LGV* infection, usually occurring within a few weeks of sexual contact. It is characterized by symptoms of anorectal pain, mucopurulent discharge, bleeding per rectum, tenesmus, and constipation. Endoscopic examination may reveal distal granular or haemorrhagic proctitis with purulent exudate, inflammatory infiltrate, and tumourous masses. *LGV* proctitis mimics inflammatory bowel disease (IBD) such as Crohn's disease, both clinically and on histopathology. Therefore, one should consider *LGV* proctitis in MSM presenting with suspected IBD. Diagnosis of LGV is confirmed by the detection of *C. trachomatis* DNA in rectal specimens from anorectal swabs. Treatment includes oral doxycycline (first line) and erythromycin (second line). Symptoms tend to resolve within 1–2 weeks of antibiotic therapy. Contact tracing, screening for other sexually transmitted infections, and follow-up is conducted by genitourinary medicine staff.

de Vries HJC, Zingoni A et al. 2013 European guideline in the management of proctitis, proctocolitis and enteritis caused by sexually transmissible pathogens. *Int J STD AIDS.* 2014;25:465–474. Doi: 10.1177/0956462413516100.

## 13. E. There is an increased incidence of AIN in the immunosuppressed and HIV-positive individuals

- AIN is the precursor lesion to anal squamous cell carcinoma
- AIN is associated with HPV

**Table 10.4** Sexually transmissible causes of proctitis and proctocolitis

| Causes of distal proctitis | Causes of proctocolitis |
|---|---|
| Neisseria gonorrhoeae | Shigella spp. |
| Chlamydia trachomatis: | Campylobacter spp. |
| Genotypes D-K | Salmonella spp. |
| Genotypes L1-3 (LGV) | Escherichia coli |
| Treponema pallidum | Entamoeba histolytica |
| Herpes simplex virus | Cryptosporidium spp. |
| | Cytomegalovirus[a] |

LGV: lymphogranuloma venereum.
[a]In severely immunocompromised patients (in the context of HIV infection with low CD4 T-cell counts). Sometimes in immunocompetent patients (especially in relation to inflammatory bowel syndromes).
Note: It is important to note that several STIs may co-exist.

- Incidence of AIN is increased in the immunosuppressed and HIV-positive individuals

AIN is a precursor lesion to anal squamous cell carcinoma. Despite lower rates of anal cancer, it is associated with a significant morbidity and mortality most likely due to delay in diagnosis. A high index of suspicion is required for the diagnosis of AIN. Patients may present with perianal symptoms including pruritus and perianal discharge. The perianal skin appears abnormal. However, without a high index of suspicion, lesions may easily be missed. Lesions may be flat and appear white, grey, purple, or brown in colour. Low-grade dysplastic AIN lesions have a similar appearance to anal condyomata. The presence of ulceration in an AIN lesion suggests invasion. Any suspicious anal lesion warrants a biopsy.

AIN is strongly associated with HPV. The prevalence is thought to be <1%. However, a number of groups at high risk for AIN include individuals with HIV, immunocompromised patients (e.g. transplant recipients), long-term corticosteroid users, and those with previous genitourinary condylomata. The prevalence of AIN in HIV is up to 89%. Literature on the risk of AIN in IBD patients is limited.

Risk of progression of AIN to invasive anal cancer is 10% at five years. There is currently no role for screening for AIN. Diagnosis is made by histopathological assessment: grades of AIN are assigned by the depth of epithelial involvement. Treatment may include local and targeted therapies, topical cidofovir or imiquimod, and local ablative therapies. Local excision may be suitable for lesions involving <30% of the anal circumference and are preferable to ablative therapies. Wide local excision or larger lesions are not usually required. Follow-up of patients with AIN is essential given that the natural history remains uncertain.

Siddharthan RV, Lanciault C, Tsikitis VL. Anal intraepithelial neoplasia: diagnosis, screening, and treatment. *Ann Gastroenterol.* 2019;32(3):257–263. Doi:10.20524/aog.2019.0364.

## 14. B. Anorectal manometry

- Anorectal manometry (ARM) is the first-line investigation for faecal incontinence (FI) not responding to conservative measures
- ARM measures rectal sensation, rectal balloon expulsion and anal sphincter resting and squeeze pressures
- In those with weak sphincter pressures additional tests including endoanal ultrasound, pelvic magnetic resonance imaging and electromyography can be considered in the work-up for surgery

The prevalence of FI increases with age and can be debilitating. Causes include traumatic anal sphincter weakness (obstetric or surgical), idiopathic sphincter degeneration, neuropathy (diabetes mellitus), pelvic floor disturbance (rectal prolapse), inflammatory conditions (radiation proctitis, IBD) and central nervous system disorders (dementia, stroke). Patients with urge incontinence have reduced squeeze pressures and experience the desire to defecate but cannot reach the toilet on time. Patients with passive incontinence have lower resting sphincter pressures and are not aware of the need to defecate before the incontinent episode. Nocturnal incontinence is rare but can occur in diabetes mellitus and scleroderma. Anorectal manometry is recommended when local pathology has been excluded (impacted stool, rectal masses) and when conservative measures (dietary modification, anti-diarrhoeal agents) have been unsuccessful. ARM simultaneously assesses rectal sensation, rectal balloon expulsion, and anal sphincter resting and squeeze pressures. For those with weak pressures, sphincter integrity can be further investigated with endoanal ultrasound and/or MRI to help plan for surgery (sphincteroplasty, sacral nerve stimulator). Needle electromyography of the anal sphincter should be considered in patients with suspected neurogenic sphincters who may benefit from sacral nerve stimulation. MR proctography is useful in investigating defecatory disorder (difficulty evacuating stool), which can co-exist with FI. Irrespective of the underlying mechanism of incontinence, pelvic floor retraining including biofeedback may be helpful. Biofeedback allows electronically amplified recordings of sphincter contraction to be visualized by the patient in response to their attempts at sphincter control.

Wald A. ACG Clinical Guideline: Management of benign anorectal disorders. *Am J Gastroenterol.* 2014;109:1141–1157. Doi: 10.1038/ajg.2014.190.

## 15. B. A rise in breath hydrogen by more than 20 ppm from baseline within 90 minutes would be consistent with a positive test result

- Glucose hydrogen breath testing has low sensitivity and specificity for predicting positive small bowel bacterial aspirates
- In patients with a high pre-test probability for small intestinal bacterial overgrowth (SIBO), an empirical trial of antibiotic therapy should be considered
- Abnormal gastric or small intestinal transit time can affect the interpretation of the result

Carbohydrate breath tests indirectly measure the metabolism of a carbohydrate substrate (e.g. glucose or lactulose) by bacterial flora. This leads to production of an analyte (hydrogen or methane), which is measured in breath. For the glucose hydrogen breath test, a peak in breath hydrogen should occur at 2–3 hours from baseline due to glucose metabolism by colonic bacteria in the caecum. In SIBO, an early breath hydrogen peak (≥20 ppm above baseline readings within 90 minutes of glucose ingestion) followed by a second peak due to colonic flora metabolism is considered diagnostic. Compared with measurement of small bowel bacterial colony via aspiration as the reference standard, the sensitivity of glucose hydrogen breath testing is 20%–93% and specificity 45%–86%.

UK guidelines recommend that in patients with high pre-test probability for SIBO (e.g. previous small bowel surgery, or small bowel anatomical abnormalities), an empirical trial of antibiotic treatment is prescribed, rather than investigation with carbohydrate breath testing.

Arasadnam RP et al. Guidelines for the investigation of chronic diarrhoea in adults: British Society of Gastroenterology, 3rd edition. *Gut.* 2018;67(8):1380–1399. Doi: 10.1136/gutjnl-2017-315909.

# chapter 11

# MOCK EXAMINATION

## QUESTIONS

1. **A 50-year-old man with ileocaecal Crohn's disease (CD) in long-term remission had been taking azathioprine monotherapy 200 mg once a day for the last seven years.**

   **Which pattern of drug-induced liver injury is this most likely to have caused?**

   A. Drug-induced autoimmune hepatitis (AIH)

   B. Fibrosis

   C. Granulomatous hepatitis

   D. Nodular regenerative hyperplasia (NRH)

   E. Steatosis

2. **A 59-year-old man underwent small bowel resection for mesenteric infarction. He was seen in clinic and complained of persistent thirst. He had 130 cm small bowel to an end jejunostomy with a stoma output of 1,300 ml per day.**

   **What is the best management advice for this patient?**

   A. Ensure he has long-term parenteral support

   B. Increase oral water intake to at least 1,000 ml per day

   C. Restrict hypotonic fluid intake to less than 500 ml per day and commence a mix of 20 g glucose, 3.5 g salt, and 2.5 g sodium bicarbonate in 1 litre water

   D. Restrict hypotonic fluid intake to less than 500 ml per day and commence Dioralyte™ 5 sachets in 1 litre water

   E. Restrict hypotonic fluid intake to less than 500 ml per day but add no additional fluid

*Best of Five MCQs for the European Specialty Examination in Gastroenterology and Hepatology.* Thomas Marjot, Colleen G C McGregor, Tim Ambrose, Aminda N De Silva, Jeremy Cobbold, and Simon Travis, Oxford University Press (2021). © Oxford University Press.
DOI: 10.1093/oso/9780198834373.003.0011

3. **A 56-year-old man presented with painless jaundice. CT liver and magnetic resonance cholangiopancreatography (MRCP) demonstrated a hilar biliary stricture with subsequent endoscopic retrograde cholangiopancreatography (ERCP) and brushings confirming cholangiocarcinoma.**

   **Which radiological finding is an absolute contraindication to surgical resection?**

   A. Bilateral involvement of the main left and right hepatic ducts

   B. Involvement of the common hepatic duct

   C. Locoregional lymphadenopathy

   D. Tumour abutting hepatic artery

   E. Underlying primary sclerosing cholangitis (PSC)

4. **A 29-year-old dancer presented with persistent abdominal pain, nausea, and constipation. She denied taking opiates or anticholinergics but did smoke cannabis once per month. On examination, her body mass index (BMI) was 17.4 kg/m². She was not diabetic but there was a history of dizziness on standing.**

   Investigations:

   | | |
   |---|---|
   | Gastroscopy | Normal |
   | Ileocolonoscopy | Normal |
   | MR enterography | Normal |
   | Tilt table test | Consistent with postural orthostatic tachycardia syndrome |
   | Beighton score | 6/9 suggestive of hypermobility |

   **What is the most likely cause of her abdominal symptoms?**

   A. Anorexia nervosa

   B. Cannabis excess

   C. Diabetic gastroparesis

   D. Dysmotility associated with hypermobile-type Ehlers-Danlos syndrome (hEDS)

   E. Mitochondrial neurogastrointestinal encephalomyopathy

5. **A 34-year-old man presented with symptoms suggestive of delayed gastric emptying.**

   **With regard to the physiology of gastric emptying, which of the following cells are responsible for controlling the slow-wave phase in the distal stomach?**

   A. Chief cells

   B. Enterochromaffin cells

   C. Interstitial cells of Cajal

   D. Mucous neck cells

   E. Parietal cells

6. **A 19-year-old woman with a history of anorexia nervosa was brought to hospital by her flatmates. She had been withdrawn for several months, eating little and losing weight. Her current weight was 33 kg. She had been running twice daily until the week before, when she had become weaker and had not left her flat since. Physical examination and investigations were performed.**

    **Which finding would indicate that the patient should be deemed high risk in the context of refeeding and rehydration?**

    A. Alanine aminotransferase (ALT) 56 U/L

    B. Blood glucose 4.1 mmol/L

    C. Creatinine 109 µmol/L

    D. Heart rate (HR) 44 beats per minute (bpm)

    E. QT interval 430 ms

7. **The management of a 60-year-old man with a new diagnosis of head of pancreas adenocarcinoma was discussed by the multi-disciplinary team.**

    **Which of the following CT findings makes the tumour most likely to be unresectable?**

    A. Tumour contact with aorta without deformity or stenosis

    B. Tumour contact with the common hepatic artery

    C. Tumour ≥4 cm

    D. Tumour contact with one third of the coeliac axis without deformity or stenosis

    E. Tumour contact with one third of the superior mesenteric vein not exceeding the inferior border of duodenum

8. **A 64-year-old man was admitted with melaena. He had a background of angina and had two drug-eluting coronary stents inserted 10 months previously. His medications comprised aspirin, clopidogrel, bisoprolol, ramipril, and atorvastatin. He had recently been using naproxen for lower back pain.**

    Investigations:

    Gastroscopy                          Duodenal ulcer on the anterior wall of the
                                         duodenal bulb (Forrest classification IIc)

    **How should you manage his antiplatelet therapy following the endoscopy?**

    A. Restart aspirin after three days, stop clopidogrel

    B. Restart aspirin immediately, essential to discuss with cardiology regarding clopidogrel

    C. Restart both aspirin and clopidogrel immediately

    D. Restart clopidogrel after three days, stop aspirin

    E. Stop both aspirin and clopidogrel

9. **A 56-year-old man presented with pruritus ani.**

   **Which of the following statements is true?**

   A. Candida infections are a cause of less than 5% of cases

   B. Capsaicin has good evidence for alleviating the condition through effects on histamine release

   C. Most cases are due to a single identifiable cause

   D. Pinworm is a common cause of the condition in children

   E. The use of soap to clean the perianal area should be encouraged

10. **Regarding gastric acid secretion, which of the following statements is true?**

    A. Enterochromaffin cells are found in abundance in the gastric antrum

    B. Enterochromaffin cells release histamine when stimulated by gastrin or acetylcholine

    C. Gastrin is released from G cells in the body

    D. In the presence of intrinsic factor, pepsinogen is converted to the active enzyme, pepsin, in the stomach lumen

    E. Parietal cells secrete hydrochloric acid only

11. **A 63-year-old lorry driver was referred with a four-month history of bloody diarrhoea 4–6 times per day. He had mild left-sided abdominal pain. There was no history of fevers or weight loss. He denied recent foreign travel. His past medical history included ischaemic heart disease and hypertension.**

    Investigations:

    | | |
    |---|---|
    | Haemoglobin | 129 g/L |
    | Platelet count | 475 × 10⁹/L |
    | Serum albumin | 31 g/L |
    | Serum C-reactive protein (CRP) | 25 mg/L |
    | Flexible sigmoidoscopy | Confluent colitis to point of insertion (50 cm) consistent with ulcerative colitis (UC) |

    **With respect to inflammatory bowel disease (IBD) in the elderly, which statement is most accurate?**

    A. Elderly-onset UC is more common in women

    B. Elderly UC patients have a higher risk of being hospitalized, especially with their first flare

    C. In elderly CD patients, ileal involvement is more common than colonic involvement

    D. Isolated proctitis is most common and left-sided disease is less common in the elderly UC population

    E. Older age is not an independent risk factor for adverse events to medications

12. **A 68-year-old woman was referred with chronic diarrhoea. Her background included hypothyroidism and hypertension for which she took levothyroxine and ramipril. A colonoscopy was indicated but she recalled having had a colonoscopy eight years before and did not tolerate the bowel preparation well.**

    **With respect to bowel preparation, which statement is most accurate?**

    A. All bowel preparations are associated with dehydration and electrolyte imbalances

    B. Extended bowel preparation is recommended in patients with constipation

    C. High-volume polyethylene glycol (PEG) is not safe in the setting of renal impairment

    D. Lower adenoma detection rates correlate with inadequate bowel preparation

    E. Split-dose low-volume PEG is superior to split-dose low-volume PEG preparations

13. **A 45-year-old woman with Child-Pugh C alcohol-related cirrhosis was admitted with a fractured tibia following a fall. She was currently drinking two bottles of wine a day. After 18 hours, she developed severe alcohol withdrawal syndrome (AWS)**

    **Which of the following would be the best treatment option?**

    A. Intramuscular haloperidol

    B. Intravenous diazepam

    C. Intravenous lorazepam

    D. Oral baclofen

    E. Oral chlordiazepoxide

14. **A 45-year-old man with a history of alcohol excess presented with epigastric pain, vomiting, systemic inflammatory response syndrome, and acute kidney injury.**

    Investigations:

    | | |
    |---|---|
    | Serum amylase | 1,200 U/L |
    | Abdominal ultrasound | Normal |

    **Five weeks after presentation, a computed tomography (CT) scan was performed because of ongoing abdominal pain and fevers.**

    | | |
    |---|---|
    | CT abdomen | 10 cm encapsulated homogenous fluid collection around the head of the pancreas |
    | White cell count | $15 \times 10^9$/L |
    | Serum C-reactive protein (CRP) | 145 mg/L |
    | Serum amylase | 205 U/L |

    **What is the most likely diagnosis?**

    A. Acute necrotic collection (ANC)

    B. Acute peripancreatic fluid collection

    C. Interstitial oedematous pancreatitis (IOP)

    D. Pancreatic pseudocyst

    E. Walled-off necrosis (WON)

15. **A 35-year-old woman was referred to clinic with deranged liver function tests. She reported lifelong abstinence from alcohol, which was corroborated by her husband. She had a background of hypertension and type 2 diabetes. She was taking ramipril, metformin, and had completed a course of trimethoprim 2 weeks before for a urinary tract infection.**

Investigations:

| | |
|---|---|
| Serum bilirubin | 10 µmol/L |
| Serum alanine transferase (ALT) | 87 U/L |
| Serum alkaline phosphatase (ALP) | 100 U/L |
| Serum albumin | 42 g/L |
| Serum ferritin | 545 µg/L |
| Anti-smooth muscle antibody | Positive |
| Liver histology | (Fig. 11.1) |

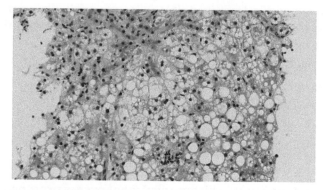

**Fig. 11.1** Liver histology specimen. See also Plate 18

Image courtesy of Dr Eve Fryer, OUH NHS Foundation Trust, Oxford

**What is the most likely diagnosis?**

A. AIH

B. Drug-induced liver injury

C. Haemochromatosis

D. Non-alcoholic steatohepatitis

E. Wilson's disease

16. **A 43-year-old-man is reviewed in clinic with nine months of upper abdominal pain. He has a history of smoking 20 cigarettes a day for the past 15 years.**

    Investigations:

    MRCP                              Marked parenchymal atrophy of the pancreas. Irregular and beaded main pancreatic duct with 6 mm calculi in the mid-pancreatic duct with moderate proximal dilatation

    **What would be the next best management for his pain?**

    A. ERCP and pancreatic duct stenting

    B. ERCP and stone extraction

    C. Extracorporeal shock wave lithotripsy

    D. Pancreatectomy

    E. Pancreatic enzyme supplementation

17. **A 20-year-old man presented to the gastroenterology outpatient clinic. He was an only child whose father was diagnosed with hereditary non-polyposis CRC at the age of 40 years and died of CRC. No other family history was available. The patient was asymptomatic.**

    **What is the next most appropriate step in his management?**

    A. Colonoscopy and gastroscopy

    B. Colonoscopy from age 25 years

    C. Colonoscopy with dye spray

    D. Five-yearly colonoscopy from age 50 to 75 years

    E. Genetic testing

18. **Which statement regarding primary sclerosing cholangitis/inflammatory bowel disease (PSC/IBD) is true?**

    A. CRC incidence in primary sclerosing cholangitis/ulcerative colitis (PSC/UC) is fourfold greater than in UC alone

    B. IBD is detected at colonoscopy in 50% of patients with PSC

    C. Mesalazine is considered an ineffective first-line therapy in PSC/UC

    D. PSC is associated with an increased incidence of small bowel CD

    E. Screening for CRC should begin 8–10 years after PSC/IBD diagnosis.

19. **A 19-year-old student was referred to clinic with persistent non-bloody diarrhoea, abdominal cramps, and bloating. She returned from her gap year a month earlier.**

Investigations:

| | |
|---|---|
| Faecal microscopy and culture | Negative |
| Faecal polymerase chain reaction (PCR) | Positive for *Giardia lamblia* |

**Which statement best describes the *Giardia lamblia* trophozoite cycle?**

A. Trophozoite colonization is limited to the upper small bowel

B. Trophozoites adhere to the mucosal surface, causing cytokine release and consequent fluid and electrolyte loss

C. Trophozoites invade tissues and gain entry to the lymphatic system, facilitating systemic spread

D. Trophozoites invade the epithelium and alter gut hormone balance, resulting in fluid and electrolyte loss

E. Upon entry into the duodenum, intestinal bacteria break down the encapsulating cyst, releasing the trophozoite

20. **A 42-year-old presented with non-specific abdominal discomfort and proceeded to endoscopy.**

Investigations:

| | |
|---|---|
| Gastroscopy | There was a 1 cm, pale yellow, sessile polypoid lesion located at 36 cm from the incisors. The lesion was firm but passable with the endoscope and appeared submucosal. The appearances of the upper GI tract were otherwise normal |
| Endoscopic ultrasound (EUS) | At 36 cm there is a smooth-edged, hypoechoic, homogenous appearing lesion arising from the submucosa |
| Histology of polyp | Polygonal cells with granular eosinophilic cytoplasm |

**What is the most likely diagnosis?**

A. Adenocarcinoma

B. Fibrovascular polyp

C. Granular cell tumour

D. Leiomyoma

E. Lipoma

21. **A 35-year old woman with extensive UC was admitted to hospital with 16 bloody, loose stools per day.**

    Investigations:

    Flexible sigmoidoscopy            Continuous inflammation to 35 cm with deep ulceration, complete obliteration of vascular pattern and free liquid blood in the lumen

    **What is the Ulcerative Colitis Endoscopic Index of Severity (UCEIS) score?**

    A. 4

    B. 5

    C. 6

    D. 7

    E. 8

22. **An 87-year-old man with progressive dysphagia was referred urgently for endoscopy. The endoscope was introduced into the oesophagus with some difficulty, and the view shown in (Fig. 11.2) was seen at 31 cm.**

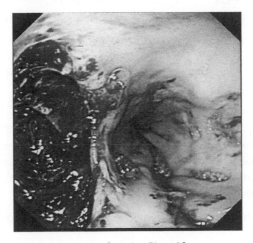

**Fig. 11.2** Endoscopic image of oesophagus. See also Plate 19

**Which of the following is most appropriate?**

A. Covered stent placement

B. Endoscopic clipping

C. Endoscopic gluing

D. Nasogastric tube placement for feeding

E. Urgent thoracotomy

23. **Variants in which gene are the most common cause of hereditary pancreatitis?**
    A. Calcium-sensing receptor (CASR)
    B. Cystic fibrosis transmembrane conductance regulator (CFTR)
    C. Chymotrypsin C (CTRC)
    D. Serine protease 1 (PRSS1)
    E. Serine protease inhibitor Kazal-type (SPINK)

24. **A 45-year-old man was diagnosed with ulcerative pancolitis and concurrent PSC one year ago. He returned for his first annual follow-up appointment. He was asymptomatic.**

    Investigations:

    | | |
    |---|---|
    | Serum bilirubin | 15 µmol/L |
    | Serum alkaline phosphatase (ALP) | 125 U/L |
    | Serum alanine aminotransferase (ALT) | 25 U/L |
    | Serum albumin | 37 g/L |
    | Serum CA 19-9 | 20 U/ml |
    | Colonoscopy | Quiescent UC |
    | Abdominal ultrasound | 8 mm polyp posterior wall of the gallbladder |

    **What is the best next step in this patient's management?**
    A. Cholecystectomy
    B. EUS
    C. MRCP
    D. Repeat ultrasound in six months
    E. Repeat ultrasound in one year

25. **A 36-year-old ex-offender was referred to the gastroenterology clinic with nausea, vomiting, abdominal pain, and early satiety. He reported 6 kg unintentional weight loss recently. He gave a history of previous substance misuse.**

    **Which recreational drug is associated with delayed gastric emptying?**
    A. Amphetamine
    B. Cannabis
    C. Cocaine
    D. Ecstasy
    E. Ketamine

26. **A 48-year-old man with PSC was reviewed in clinic. He had some fatigue but otherwise felt well. He had concomitant UC, which was in clinical remission. His medications were ursodeoxycholic acid (UDCA) 500 mg twice a day and mesalazine 2 g once a day.**

Investigations:

| | |
|---|---|
| Serum bilirubin | 16 µmol/L |
| Serum alkaline phosphatase (ALP) | 195 U/L |
| Serum alanine transferase (ALT) | 285 U/L |
| Serum albumin | 39 g/L |
| Full blood count | Normal |
| INR | 1.0 |
| Antinuclear antibody | Positive |
| Antinuclear cytoplasmic antibody | Positive |
| Anti-mitochondrial antibody | Negative |
| Anti-smooth muscle antibody | Negative |
| IgA | 1.8 g/L |
| IgG | 19 g/L |
| IgM | 1.5 g/L |

**What investigation would you order next?**

A. Anti-sp100 and anti-gp210

B. Liver biopsy

C. Liver elastography

D. MRCP

E. No further investigations required

27. **A 46-year-old female with a history of CD attended clinic. She underwent an ileocaecal resection four years ago and was on no maintenance therapy. She continued to smoke 15 cigarettes/day. She underwent a colonoscopy for symptoms of loose stool.**

Investigation:

| | |
|---|---|
| Colonoscopy | Insertion to neo-terminal ileum. Ileocolic anastomosis patent. Colon normal. Diffuse aphthous ileitis with diffusely inflamed mucosa. No evidence of stenosis or large ulcers. |

**What is her Rutgeerts score?**

A. i0

B. i1

C. i2

D. i3

E. i4

28. **A 37-year-old male presented with a five-week history of fevers, non-productive cough, bloody diarrhoea, and myalgia. Four weeks ago, he returned to the UK from travelling in rural India where he had been in contact with fresh water lakes. On close questioning, he had developed an itchy rash at the start of his symptoms, which had resolved within 3–4 days.**

Investigations:

| | |
|---|---|
| Haemoglobin | 130 g/L |
| White cell count | $7.0 \times 10^9$/L |
| Platelet count | $180 \times 10^9$/L |
| Eosinophil count | $0.6 \times 10^9$/L |
| Serum C-reactive protein (CRP) | 30 mg/L |
| Serum alanine transferase (ALT) | 34 U/L |
| Serum alkaline phosphatase (ALP) | 110 U/L |
| Serum bilirubin | 10 µmol/L |
| Faecal microscopy and culture | Negative including ova, cysts, and parasites |
| Chest radiograph | Ill-defined nodular pulmonary infiltrates |

**Which is the next most appropriate diagnostic test?**

A. Kato-Katz thick smear technique

B. Rectal biopsy

C. Repeat stool microscopy

D. Serology

E. Urine microscopy

29. **A 65-year-old woman with alcohol-related cirrhosis is seen with her husband in the hepatology clinic. She has been abstinent from alcohol for two years. Her husband is concerned that she is not her usual self. She appears oriented to time and place.**

**Which of the following is correct in the diagnosis of hepatic encephalopathy (HE)?**

A. A rise in blood ammonia level is diagnostic of HE

B. Brain imaging is essential for diagnosis

C. Electroencephalography (EEG) examination is only useful in grade IV HE

D. The Stroop test can be used to help make a diagnosis of HE

E. There is no indication for screening for minimal HE

30. **A 37-year-old man with UC had required multiple courses of oral corticosteroids over the past two years. Bowel symptoms recurred whenever prednisolone was reduced below 15 mg daily. Azathioprine was therefore recommended.**

Investigation:

| | |
|---|---|
| Thiopurine methyltransferase | 16 U/L |

**Which of the following statements about thiopurine methyltransferase (TPMT) levels is most accurate?**

A. Normal TPMT levels predict clinical response to thiopurines

B. TPMT activity is absent in 1% of the population

C. TPMT activity is normal in 50% of the population

D. TPMT levels accurately predict the risk of leucopenia

E. Variants in TPMT account for up to 25% of thiopurine-induced leucopenia

31. **A 65-year-old man with Child-Pugh C (10) alcohol-related cirrhosis presents with Grade 3 ascites. Routine blood tests and a diagnostic paracentesis are performed.**

Investigations:

| | |
|---|---|
| Serum bilirubin | 58 µmol/L |
| Serum creatinine | 105 µmol/L |
| Serum sodium | 129 mmol/L |
| Ascites white cell count | 410 cells/µL |
| Ascites neutrophil count | 220 cells/µL |
| Ascites albumin | 5 g/L |
| Ascites total protein | 9 g/L |

**The patient has been referred for consideration of liver transplantation (LT) or transjugular intrahepatic portosystemic shunt (TIPSS) and in the interim repeated large volume paracentesis is performed.**

**Which of the above would be an indication for long-term antibiotic prophylaxis?**

A. Ascites protein concentration

B. Ascites total white cell count

C. Prospective LT

D. Prospective TIPSS

E. Repeated large volume paracentesis

32. **A 56-year-old man presented with a three-month history of intermittent vomiting and weight loss. He had no past medical history, drank 10 units of alcohol a week, and was a non-smoker.**

    Investigations:
    Gastroscopy              4 cm antral tumour
    Histology                Adenocarcinoma

    **With regard to the initial staging of gastric cancer, which is the most useful modality as an adjunct to CT scanning?**

    A. Barium meal

    B. Endoscopic mucosal resection (EMR)

    C. Endoscopic ultrasound

    D. Laparoscopy

    E. Magnetic resonance imaging (MRI)

33. **A 28-year-old Iranian farmer, who had recently immigrated to the UK, was referred to clinic with persistent diarrhoea. He also complained of hair loss, taste disturbance, and a superficial scaling erythematous patchy rash that was most prominent in intertriginous areas and periorally. There was no cognitive impairment.**

    **Which is the most likely nutrient deficiency?**

    A. Niacin

    B. Selenium

    C. Vitamin A

    D. Vitamin E

    E. Zinc

34. **A 68-year-old woman attended for a gastroscopy having been referred by her GP with anaemia, 4 kg weight loss, and abdominal discomfort. No melaena had been witnessed, although she reported occasional dark stools.**

Investigations:

| | |
|---|---|
| Haemoglobin | 122 g/L |
| White cell count | $4.6 \times 10^9$/L |
| Mean corpuscular volume | 76 fL |
| Platelet count | $209 \times 10^9$/L |
| Serum ferritin | 6 µg/L |
| Serum folate | 2.6 µg/L |
| Serum vitamin B12 | 178 ng/L |
| Serum C-reactive protein (CRP) | 16 mg/L |

**The endoscopic images demonstrated the findings shown in (Fig. 11.3).**

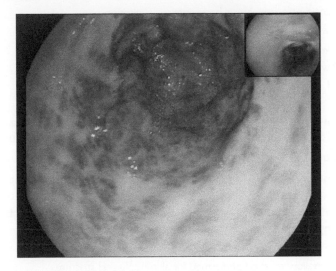

**Fig. 11.3** Endoscopic image of stomach. See also Plate 20

**Which of the following is the most appropriate next step?**

A. Antrectomy

B. Argon plasma coagulation

C. Iron supplementation

D. Propranolol

E. Transjugular intrahepatic portosystemic stent shunt (TIPSS)

35. **A 47-year-old woman presented to the emergency department with recurrent episodes of right upper quadrant pain. She underwent an elective laparoscopic cholecystectomy six months before for similar 'attacks' despite no evidence of biliary calculi found on imaging. Her serum liver enzymes and amylase have always been within the normal limit with each episode.**

    Investigations:

    | | |
    |---|---|
    | Gallbladder histology | Chronic cholecystitis with no gallstones |
    | MRCP | Common bile duct (CBD) diameter 4.9 mm, main pancreatic duct diameter 1.2 mm, no features of chronic pancreatitis |
    | EUS | CBD 4.5 mm, no evidence of biliary microlithiasis or sludge |

    **What is the next most appropriate management strategy?**

    A. Endoscopic intra-sphincteric botulinum toxin injection

    B. ERCP with biliary sphincterotomy

    C. ERCP with manometry

    D. ERCP with pancreatic sphincterotomy

    E. Trial of calcium-channel blocker

36. **A 56-year-old woman presented with progressive dysphagia to solids but not liquids. She took omeprazole 20 mg twice daily for heartburn.**

    Investigations:

    | | |
    |---|---|
    | Gastroscopy | Impassable stricture at 34 cm which appeared endoscopically benign |

    **Which of the following is true with regards to dilatation of benign-appearing peptic strictures?**

    A. Balloon dilatation is more effective than wire-guided bougie dilatation

    B. Barium swallow must be performed for all oesophageal strictures

    C. Biopsies should be taken before proceeding to dilatation

    D. Oesophageal perforation occurs in 4% of procedures

    E. The use of post-dilatation H2 receptor antagonists reduces rates of stricture recurrence

37. **A 78-year-old woman was reviewed in outpatients for dysphagia. She described intermittent difficulties swallowing for several years associated with occasional regurgitation and a sensation of 'bubbling' at the back of her throat. She had a persistent cough and friends had commented that her breath smelt foul. She had a hospital admission with pneumonia a year ago but had fully recovered. Her only medication was amlodipine 5 mg once a day for hypertension.**

Investigation:
   Barium swallow        (Fig. 11.4)

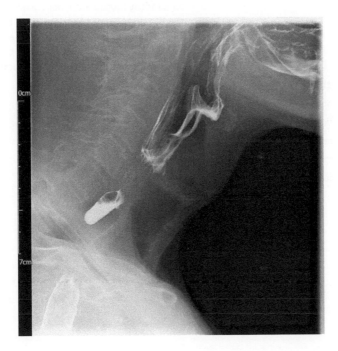

**Fig. 11.4** Barium swallow

Image courtesy of Dr Horace D'Costa, Consultant Radiologist, Oxford University Hospitals NHS Foundation Trust

### Given the diagnosis, which of the following would provide definitive management?

A. Cognitive behavioural therapy

B. Cricopharyngeal myotomy and pouch excision

C. Endoscopic balloon dilatation

D. Endoscopic diverticulectomy

E. Long-term antibiotics

38. **An 18-year-old woman with a three-month history of abdominal discomfort and unintentional weight loss presented with right-sided abdominal pain and vomiting. Her blood pressure was 110/70 mmHg and pulse 110 beats per minute.**

Investigations:

| | |
|---|---|
| Haemoglobin | 104 g/L |
| White cell count | $13.1 \times 10^9$/L |
| Platelet count | $430 \times 10^9$/L |
| Serum C-reactive protein (CRP) | 112 mg/L |
| CT abdomen and pelvis | 12-cm length of terminal ileal stricturing with an adjacent intra-abdominal collection. There are proximal loops of dilated small bowel. Three closely spaced mid-ileal strictures, each about 3 cm, are demonstrated proximal to the dilated loops. Appearances are compatible with active CD. |

## What is the most likely surgical procedure?

A. Defunctioning loop ileostomy proximal to the mid-ileal strictures

B. Defunctioning loop ileostomy proximal to the terminal ileal stricture

C. Ileocaecal resection

D. Ileocaecal resection and en bloc mid-ileal stricture resection

E. Ileocaecal resection and three mid-ileal stricturoplasties

**39.** **A 54-year-old businessman was referred from the rheumatology clinic with a two-year history of migratory arthralgia of the large joints. He had developed episodic non-bloody diarrhoea and crampy abdominal pain. He had lost weight. On examination, a pericardial rub was audible and there was small volume ascites.**

Investigations:

| | |
|---|---|
| Rheumatoid factor | Negative |
| IgA tissue transglutaminase antibody | Negative |
| Thyroid stimulating hormone (TSH) | Normal |
| Faecal microscopy and culture | Negative |
| Faecal ova, cysts, and parasites | Negative |
| HIV | Negative |
| Gastroscopy | Normal |
| Duodenal histology | Mild duodenal villous blunting |
| Colonoscopy | Normal |
| Colonic histology | Normal |
| MR enterography | No evidence of small bowel inflammation |

**What is the diagnostic test?**

A. Carcinoembryonic antigen

B. Faecal calprotectin

C. HLA-DQ2 and DQ8

D. Periodic acid-Schiff (PAS) staining of duodenal biopsies

E. Serology for *Treponema pallidum*

**40. A 48-year-old woman with primary biliary cholangitis (PBC) attended annual clinic follow-up suffering from severe fatigue.**

Investigations:

| | |
|---|---|
| Platelet count | $170 \times 10^9$/L |
| Liver stiffness measurement (LSM) | 10.8 kPa |
| Serum alkaline phosphatase (ALP) | 180 U/L |
| Serum bilirubin | 45 µmol/L |
| Liver ultrasound | Coarse irregular heterogenous liver, no focal lesion, normal portal vein flow, no ascites, spleen size 12 cm |

**Which of the following is true about PBC?**

A. Fatigue is an indication for LT

B. Recurrent PBC following LT often leads to graft loss

C. Severity of symptoms does not correlate with stage of disease

D. This patient should undergo endoscopy for variceal screening

E. Women are at increased risk of hepatocellular carcinoma compared with men

**41. A 40-year-old woman was reviewed on the ward 24 hours after LT for alcohol-related cirrhosis. The organ donor was positive and the recipient was negative for cytomegalovirus (CMV) (D+/R−).**

**What is the most appropriate management regarding CMV infection post-transplantation?**

A. Foscarnet prophylaxis for three months

B. Intravenous ganciclovir for two weeks

C. No prophylaxis and send CMV polymerase chain reaction (PCR) only if clinical suspicion of CMV disease

D. Valganciclovir prophylaxis for three months

E. Weekly CMV PCR during hospitalization and start valganciclovir if persisting viraemia

42. **A 43-year-old female was admitted from the mental health unit having reportedly swallowed a foreign object. She denied any symptoms but refused to say what she had ingested.**

    **Which of the following objects may be safely considered for conservative management?**

    A. 15 mm button battery

    B. 15 mm magnet

    C. 15 mm × 60 mm nail file

    D. 20 mm coin

    E. 25 mm metal toothpick

43. **A 34-year-old man with complex ileocolonic CD developed a secondary loss of response to infliximab. He had evidence of active disease at recent ileocolonoscopy. His background included psoriasis for which he was under the dermatologists.**

    **Which novel therapy is most appropriate to introduce?**

    A. Amiselimod

    B. Mongersen

    C. Tofacitinib

    D. Ustekinumab

    E. Vedolizumab

44. **A 26-year-old-woman attended the IBD clinic. She had left-sided UC diagnosed five years ago, which was confirmed as quiescent on colonoscopy six months earlier. Despite mesalazine 1.2 g twice daily with good compliance, the patient's bowel frequency had increased to five times per day with some rectal bleeding. Her GP had increased the mesalazine to 2.4 g twice daily one week before, but without benefit. She was apyrexial and her pulse was 56 beats per minute.**

    Investigations:

    | | |
    |---|---|
    | Haemoglobin | 134 g/L |
    | White cell count | $9.0 \times 10^9$/L |
    | Platelet count | $320 \times 10^9$/L |
    | Serum C-reactive protein (CRP) | 40 mg/L |
    | Serum alanine transferase (ALT) | 26 U/L |
    | Serum alkaline phosphatase (ALP) | 96 U/L |

    **What should you recommend?**

    A. Azathioprine

    B. Corticosteroid enema

    C. Mesalazine enema

    D. Mesalazine suppository

    E. Oral prednisolone reducing course

**45.** A 50-year-old man with alcohol-related cirrhosis and diuretic-controlled ascites was reviewed in clinic. He complained of several months of worsening shortness of breath that improved when he was lying flat. He had no other past medical history and was a lifelong non-smoker.

Investigations:

| | |
|---|---|
| Chest radiograph | Normal |
| Oxygen saturations on air | 89% |
| Arterial pH on air | 7.35 |
| Arterial $pO_2$ | 7.3 kPa |
| Arterial $pCO_2$ | 4.6 kPa |
| Arterial base excess | 5.1 mmol/L |
| Arterial $HCO_3$ | 28.5 mmol/L |

**What would be the next best investigation?**

A. Lung perfusion scan

B. Spirometry

C. Right-heart catheterization study

D. Transthoracic contrast enhanced echocardiogram

E. Transthoracic echocardiogram

**46.** A 57-year-old man with extensive UC (pancolitis) was admitted to hospital with bloody diarrhoea (15 times per day). On day three of intravenous hydrocortisone, his stool chart showed nine bloody stools in the last 24 hours, his temperature was 37.6°C, and he denied abdominal pain. Abdominal plain film excluded toxic megacolon. His blood pressure was 205/106 mmHg and pulse was 86 beats per minute. His background included treated pulmonary tuberculosis, hypertension, and NAFLD.

Investigations:

| | |
|---|---|
| Haemoglobin | 98 g/L |
| White cell count | $12.0 \times 10^9$/L |
| Platelet count | $455 \times 10^9$/L |
| Serum C-reactive protein (CRP) | 40 mg/L |
| Serum cholesterol | 3.2 mmol/L |
| Serum magnesium | 0.8 mmol/L |
| Serum alanine transferase (ALT) | 35 U/L |
| Serum alkaline phosphatase (ALP) | 104 U/L |

**What is the most appropriate plan?**

A. Continue intravenous steroids for a further 3 days

B. Infliximab 5 mg/kg intravenous induction regime

C. Intravenous ciclosporin at a dose of 4 mg/kg per day

D. Oral ciclosporin at a dose of 2 mg/kg per day in divided doses

E. Subtotal colectomy

47. **A 68-year-old man was admitted with a one-day history of melaena. He had no relevant past medical history and took no regular medications.**

    **What percentage of patients who are admitted with apparent acute upper GI bleeding do not reveal a cause at initial gastroscopy?**
    A. 2%
    B. 9%
    C. 17%
    D. 28%
    E. 44%

48. **Which of the following is a major risk factor for the formation of brown pigment gallstones?**
    A. Cholangitis
    B. Chronic haemolysis
    C. Crohn's disease
    D. Pregnancy
    E. Rapid weight loss

49. **A 64-year-old man presented with large volume melaena. He had a past medical history of type 2 diabetes, peripheral vascular disease with left above-knee amputation, previous endovascular repair of an abdominal aortic aneurysm, and chronic obstructive pulmonary disease. He was a smoker and drank alcohol to excess. On examination, he appeared pale and clammy, pulse 136 beats per minute and blood pressure 86/54 mmHg.**

    Investigations:
    | | |
    |---|---|
    | Haemoglobin | 63 g/L |
    | Serum urea | 23.5 mmol/L (baseline for patient = 11.3) |
    | Serum creatinine | 124 µmol/L (baseline for patient = 108) |

    **After initial resuscitation, what is the most important first investigation?**
    A. Colonoscopy
    B. CT angiography
    C. Gastroscopy
    D. MR angiography
    E. Video capsule endoscopy

50. **A 43-year-old man from Argentina was visiting family in the UK. He presented to the emergency department with a five-month history of abdominal discomfort, anorexia, cough, and shortness of breath.**

Investigations:

| | |
|---|---|
| Haemoglobin | 134 g/L |
| White cell count | 8.7 × 10⁹/L |
| Neutrophil count | 5.1 × 10⁹/L |
| Lymphocyte count | 2.9 × 10⁹/L |
| Monocyte count | 0.3 × 10⁹/L |
| Eosinophil count | 0.6 × 10⁹/L |
| Basophil count | <0.1 × 10⁹/L |
| Platelet count | 453 × 10⁹/L |
| Serum bilirubin | 47 μmol/L |
| Serum alanine transferase (ALT) | 23 U/L |
| Serum alkaline phosphatase (ALP) | 180 U/L |
| CT abdomen | (Fig. 11.5) |

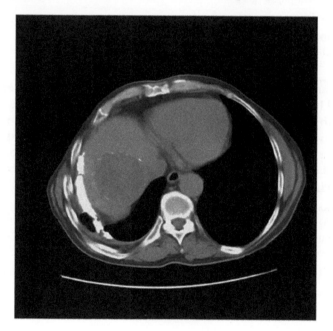

**Fig. 11.5** CT abdomen

Reproduced with kind permission from Dr Paul Burn, Consultant Radiologist

### What is the most likely diagnosis?

A. Amoebic liver abscess

B. Caroli's syndrome

C. Hepatocellular carcinoma

D. Hydatid disease

E. Polycystic liver disease

## 1. D. Nodular regenerative hyperplasia (NRH)

- Thiopurines can cause a transient transaminitis, cholestatic hepatitis, sinusoidal obstruction syndrome, and NRH
- NRH occurs in ~1% of IBD patients treated with azathioprine for 10 years and is characterized by diffuse liver nodularity without annular fibrosis leading to non-cirrhotic portal hypertension

Four patterns of hepatotoxicity are recognized with the use of thiopurines (azathioprine, 6-mercaptopurine, thioguanine):

1. A transient and usually asymptomatic elevation in serum transaminases is the most common, occurring in ~10% of patients. It is usually self-limiting, resolves rapidly on drug discontinuation or dose reduction, and is associated with higher levels of the thiopurine metabolite methyl-mercaptopurine.

2. One in 1,000 develop idiosyncratic cholestatic hepatitis with intrahepatic cholestasis on histology but with only modest elevations in aminotransferases and alkaline phosphatase alongside moderate-to-severe jaundice.

3. Sinusoidal obstruction syndrome (formerly 'veno-occlusive disease') is best recognized with the use of chemotherapy agents or after hematopoietic stem cell transplantation but is rarely reported with chronic thiopurine use. It is characterized by damage to small hepatic vessels causing abdominal pain, jaundice, oedema, and portal hypertension.

4. NRH is a rare liver condition defined by alternating atrophic and hyperplastic areas of liver parenchyma causing diffuse nodulation without annular fibrosis that can progress to non-cirrhotic portal hypertension. The cumulative risk of NRH in patients with IBD treated with azathioprine is 0.5% at 5 years and 1.25% at 10 years. In patients on long-term azathioprine for AIH who develop features of portal hypertension, both NRH as well as fibrosis progression must be considered as an underlying cause.

Drug-induced AIH is associated with minocycline, nitrofurantoin, diclofenac, indomethacin, and infliximab. Hepatic fibrosis can be caused by amiodarone and methotrexate. Steatosis is seen with methotrexate, 5-fluorouracil, corticosteroids, and tamoxifen. Granulomatous hepatitis is associated with allopurinol, carbamazepine, methyldopa, phenytoin, and quinidine.

LiverTox. *Clinical and research information on drug-induced liver injury* [Internet]. Bethesda (MD): National Institute of Diabetes and Digestive and Kidney Diseases; 2012–. Azathioprine. [Updated 21 August 2017]. Available at: https://www.ncbi.nlm.nih.gov/books/NBK548332

*Best of Five MCQs for the European Specialty Examination in Gastroenterology and Hepatology.* Thomas Marjot, Colleen G C McGregor, Tim Ambrose, Aminda N De Silva, Jeremy Cobbold, and Simon Travis, Oxford University Press (2021). © Oxford University Press.
DOI: 10.1093/oso/9780198834373.003.0011

## 2. C. Restrict hypotonic fluid intake to less than 500 ml per day and commence a mix of 20 g glucose, 3.5 g salt, and 2.5 g sodium bicarbonate in 1 litre water

- Oral glucose-electrolyte mixes (e.g. St Mark's solution or double strength Dioralyte™) require a sodium concentration greater than 90 mmol/L to achieve net absorption in the jejunum
- Patients with more than 100 cm jejunum do not usually require parenteral support

The residual small bowel length following resection, together with the presence or absence of colon in continuity, can help predict what hydration and nutritional support patients will require. Radiological estimation (using magnetic resonance (MR)/computed tomography (CT) enterography or barium studies) approximates to bowel length but referral to the operation note is important. Patients with more than 100 cm jejunum, or 50 cm jejunum anastomosed to colon, do not usually require parenteral support.

To achieve net absorption of sodium and water, jejunal contents require a sodium concentration greater than 90 mmol/L. These patients must not be encouraged to drink hypotonic fluids *ad libitum* to quench thirst because this increases stomal losses and worsens hydration. Hypotonic fluids (e.g. water, tea, coffee, fruit juices) should be restricted to less than 500 mL per day. An oral glucose-electrolyte mix, with a sodium concentration greater than 90 mmol/L, aids water/sodium balance. St Mark's solution (20 g glucose, 3.5 g salt, and 2.5 g sodium bicarbonate in 1 litre water) or double strength Dioralyte™ (10 sachets in 1 litre water) are two mechanisms to achieve this. The latter provides a substantial potassium load as well, and should be exercised with caution in patients with a propensity for potassium overload (e.g. renal failure).

Nightingale J, Woodward JM. Guidelines for management of patients with a short bowel. *Gut.* 2006;55(Suppl 4):iv1–12.

## 3. E. Underlying primary sclerosing cholangitis (PSC)

- MRCP and CT are used in the diagnosis and staging of perihilar cholangiocarcinoma (pCCA) to characterize degree of biliary and vascular involvement, respectively
- LT is preferable to resection for pCCA in patients with PSC
- Locoregional lymphadenopathy is not a contraindication to resection but is associated with a poorer outcome

pCCA describes tumours located between the secondary branches of the right and left hepatic ducts, and the common hepatic duct proximal to the cystic duct origin. Tumours more proximal to this are called 'intrahepatic cholangiocarcinomas' and those involving the common bile duct, up to but not including the ampulla, are called 'distal cholangiocarcinomas'. A combination of MRCP and CT is used in the diagnosis and staging of pCCA to characterize degree of biliary and vascular involvement respectively. ERCP also enables detection of strictures and can acquire biliary brushing samples for cytological assessment. Endoscopic ultrasound is associated with high tumour detection but fine needle aspiration should be avoided due to the risk of peritoneal tumour seeding in >80%.

Surgical resection is potentially curative for patients with pCCA without the following exclusion criteria: i) bilateral involvement of the second-order bile ducts; ii) bilateral or contralateral vascular involvement; iii) presence of metastatic disease; iv) underlying PSC. Patients with PSC should preferentially be treated with LT because of the field defect in PSC and frequent underlying advanced fibrosis. The presence of locoregional lymphadenopathy is not a contraindication but is associated with a poorer post-surgical outcome. Abutment (as opposed to involvement) of the vasculature is not a contraindication for resection. Surgery for pCCA involves lobectomy with bile-duct resection, regional lymphadenectomy, and Roux-en-Y hepaticojejunostomy. To maximize post-operative liver function, the ipsilateral portal vein is often embolized pre-operatively to promote contralateral lobe hypertrophy. LT following neoadjuvant chemoradiatherapy offers the best outcomes for patients with unresectable pCCA but only a minority of patients with early stage disease are candidates.

Rizvi S, Khan SA, Hallemeier CL et al. Cholangiocarcinoma—evolving concepts and therapeutic strategies. *Nat Rev Clin Oncol.* 2018;15(2):95–111. Doi:10.1038/nrclinonc.2017.157.

## 4. D. Dysmotility associated with hypermobile-type Ehlers-Danlos syndrome (hEDS)

- hEDS is associated with functional GI disorders and autonomic dysfunction
- These patients often develop more chronic pain and somatization
- hEDS does not have a known genetic basis at present

Approximately one third of patients presenting to gastroenterology clinics have evidence of joint hypermobility. The Beighton score can be used to formalize the degree of hypermobility, with a positive score defined as >6 in prepubertal children, >5 in postpubertal people, and >4 in those over 50 years of age. Patients with both hypermobility and GI symptoms often have evidence of postural orthostatic tachycardia syndrome (POTS) or other autonomic symptoms such as irritable bladder.

hEDS is a clinical diagnosis and there is no known genetic association at present. The 2017 international diagnostic criteria include aspects such as generalized joint hypermobility, positive family history of hEDS, chronic pain, and musculoskeletal pain. The mechanism of GI and autonomic involvement is poorly understood.

Cannabis is known to cause GI upset, including constipation, but usually only when used to excess. The patient is not diabetic and there is no suggestion of an eating disorder causing her symptoms. Mitochondrial disease is unlikely, particularly because there are no visual symptoms.

Fikree A, Chelimsky G, Collins H et al. Gastrointestinal involvement in the Ehlers-Danlos syndromes. *Am J Med Genet C Semin Med Genet.* 2017;175(1):181–187. Doi:10.1002/ajmg.c.31546.

## 5. C. Interstitial cells of Cajal

- Cholecystokinin (CCK) and gastric inhibitory polypeptide (GIP) are gut hormones involved in delaying gastric emptying
- Slow wave stomach contractions are controlled by cells of Cajal whereas phasic contractions of the distal stomach are controlled by the migrating motor complex

The proximal stomach serves as a reservoir for food and, at its maximum relaxation, gastric barostat studies have shown that it can allow over 1L of nutrients to be ingested. In addition, the proximal stomach also helps to regulate the gastroduodenal flow rate and provides the space and time for pepsin and hydrochloric acid to initiate digestion.

The duration of post-prandial motor activity varies according to the volume ingested as well as the chemical characteristics of the ingested foods. The maximum duration of post-prandial motor activity is 120 minutes.

CCK and GIP are hormones involved in producing a negative feedback to slow gastric emptying. CCK regulates gastric emptying and bowel motility to induce satiety, thus delaying gastric emptying. GIP is thought to inhibit gastric acid secretion and reduce the rate at which food is transferred through the stomach, thereby delaying gastric emptying.

Goyal RK, Guo Y, Mashimo H. Advances in the physiology of gastric emptying. *Neurogastroenterol Motil.* 2019 Apr;31(4):e13546. Doi:10.1111/nmo.13546.

### 6. C. Creatinine 109 μmol/l

- Patients with severe weight loss secondary to anorexia nervosa are at risk of refeeding syndrome, but can appear deceptively well on initial assessment
- A structured assessment of a patient's risk of refeeding syndrome is indicated, including physical examination, electrocardiogram (ECG), and laboratory blood tests, in line with the MARSIPAN (Management of really sick patients with anorexia nervosa) guidelines
- Urea and creatinine results should be viewed in context of the patient's weight and protein intake rather than the laboratory normal ranges

Anorexia nervosa is a psychological disorder predominantly affecting adolescent women, characterized by body dysmorphia and severe weight loss. Complications can affect almost every organ system and the condition is associated with increased mortality. In the presence of profound weight loss or high-risk features, a period of inpatient admission for controlled initiation of feeding is needed to establish metabolic stability.

According to the MARSIPAN guidelines, the following features confer higher risk:

- BMI <13 kg/m$^2$
- HR <40 bpm
- Low blood pressure with a postural drop
- Objective severe muscle weakness, as assessed by a Sit Up Squat Stand (SUSS) test
- Raised QTc >450 ms or hypokalaemic changes on ECG
- Sodium <130 mmol/l, potassium <3.0 mmol/l, or glucose <3.0 mmol/l
- Raised urea or creatinine, recognizing that low weight and protein intake may alter the normal range for these investigations

While the ALT rise does suggest severe malnutrition (with increased transaminases likely due to hepatocellular autophagy), this does not confer a particular risk of refeeding in isolation.

Royal College of Psychiatrists, Royal College Physicians, Royal College of Pathologists. 2014. *MARSIPAN: Management of really sick patients with anorexia nervosa* (2nd edn) (College Report CR189).

### 7. A. Tumour contact with aorta without deformity or stenosis

- Only 10%–20% of patients with pancreatic adenocarcinoma have localized, surgically resectable disease at diagnosis
- Pancreatic tumours are deemed unresectable if their removal would theoretically lead to arterial resection and reconstruction
- New international guidelines define tumours deemed borderline resectable when adjuvant chemoradiotherapy may be attempted before resection

In pancreatic adenocarcinoma, surgical resection with adjuvant systemic chemotherapy currently provides the only chance of long-term survival. However, only 10%–20% have localized, surgically resectable disease at diagnosis. Pancreatic cancer is generally deemed to be resectable if it does not involve major blood vessels. Pancreatic cancers are deemed unresectable if they involve the superior mesenteric artery (SMA) or the coeliac axis (CA) to the extent where tumour resection would theoretically lead to arterial resection and reconstruction. Any involvement of the aorta is deemed unresectable disease. The International Association of Pancreatology has further developed the anatomical definition of borderline resectable pancreatic that may be amenable to neo-adjuvant chemoradiotherapy as a bridge to surgery. Borderline resectable tumours can be classified as those with venous involvement alone (not exceeding the inferior border of the duodenum) or arterial involvement (≤180° SMA/CA without deformity, stenosis or common hepatic artery contact alone).

Strobel O, Neoptolemos J, Jäger D et al. Optimizing the outcomes of pancreatic cancer surgery. *Nat Rev Clin Onc.* 2019;16(1):11–26. Doi:10.1038/s41571-018-0112-1.

### 8. C. Restart both aspirin and clopidogrel immediately

- All-cause mortality is lower if aspirin (as secondary cardiovascular prevention) is continued following peptic ulcer bleeding
- Neither aspirin nor clopidogrel impede ulcer healing
- Patients on dual antiplatelet therapy with low-risk stigmata should continue both medications

Five to seven days is sufficient to restore normal platelet aggregation following withdrawal of antiplatelet agents. In patients presenting with non-variceal upper GI bleeding, it is often not practical to stop these medications for five days, and post-procedure management is important in balancing bleeding and vascular risk.

In patients receiving aspirin for primary cardiovascular prevention, it is reasonable to stop this and re-evaluate risks and benefits. Patients receiving antiplatelets as secondary prevention and with low risk endoscopic stigmata (Forrest IIc and III) can safely continue all antiplatelet agents without interruption. Patients with higher risk stigmata (all other Forrest classifications) should resume aspirin by day three if receiving monotherapy. For dual antiplatelet therapy, aspirin should be recommenced immediately with early cardiology consultation regarding timing of restarting the second agent.

In this case, the patient has low risk stigmata and so dual antiplatelet therapy can recommence immediately. It is not essential to discuss the case with cardiology. It would not be appropriate to empirically stop clopidogrel because it is only 10 months since the insertion of drug-eluting stents.

Gralnek IM, Dumonceau JM, Kuipers EJ et al. Diagnosis and management of nonvariceal upper gastrointestinal hemorrhage: European Society of Gastrointestinal Endoscopy (ESGE) guideline. *Endoscopy.* 2015;47:a1–46. Doi:10.1055/s-0034-1393172.

### 9. D. Pinworm is a common cause of the condition in children

- Pruritus ani is often idiopathic in nature
- After excluding secondary causes, management should focus on breaking the itch-scratch-itch cycle and perianal cleanliness
- A sexual history and perianal examination are needed in the assessment of patients

Pruritus ani encompasses any condition that results in itching and irritation of the perianal area. Most cases are idiopathic in nature but in cases where a cause can be found these are often multiple. The itch-scratch-itch cycle, which may become subconscious, can be difficult to break and result in persisting symptoms as the perianal skin become excoriated. Perianal neoplasia and co-existent dermatological conditions should be excluded by a thorough perianal examination.

Local irritation may be due to faecal leakage, excess sweating, and anal fissures, fistulae or tags. Dietary triggers include caffeine, alcohol, tomatoes, and spicy foods. Excessive cleaning and rubbing of the perianal area, often with soap or medicated wipes, causes local trauma and worsening symptoms. Warm water alone should be used to clean the perianal area and the area patted dry with a towel.

Candida infections may be present in more than 10% of cases, particularly in the elderly, obese, immunosuppressed people or those on antibiotics. The presence of erythematous plaques may suggest the diagnosis and fungal skin scrapings can be diagnostic. Antifungal powder or lotion may be helpful but oral fluconazole may be needed for severe infections. Pinworm is a common cause in children and may be treated with anti-helminth agents (e.g. albendazole). A detailed sexual history should be taken to exclude concurrent diseases such as herpes infection.

Treatment should initially focus on secondary causes, local irritation, and managing expectations. Other approaches have included zinc oxide ointment, Berwick's solution, and capsaicin. The latter suppresses histamine release and can help break the itch-scratch-itch cycle but a meta-analysis in 2010 found insufficient evidence to recommend its use for pruritus.

Ansari P. Pruritus Ani. *Clin Colon Rectal Surg.* 2016;29(1):38–42. Doi:10.1055/s-0035-1570391.

## 10. B. Enterochromaffin cells release histamine when stimulated by gastrin or acetylcholine

- Main stimulants of gastric acid secretion are gastrin (G cells), histamine (Enterochromaffin-like [ECL] cells), and acetylcholine (enteric neurons)
- Parietal cells contain multiple membrane-bound receptors stimulating gastric acid secretion

Gastric acid allows the digestion of protein as well as facilitating the absorption of iron, calcium, and vitamin B12. Gastric acid secretion is an important defence against ingested bacteria. Gastric acid secretion is regulated by complex processes dependent on neural, hormonal, and paracrine pathways. The main stimulants of acid secretion are gastrin, histamine, and acetylcholine (ACh).

The body of the stomach contains oxyntic mucosa, richly supplied with gastric glands. Gastric glands are also present in the fundus. Various cells within the gastric glands have specific functions:

### G cells

- Located in the gastric antrum
- Produce and secrete gastrin in response to food in the stomach lumen and gastrin-releasing peptide (neuronal)
- Gastrin stimulates parietal cells directly and indirectly (via release of histamine from ECL cells)

### Parietal cells

Parietal (oxyntic) cells secrete both hydrochloric acid and intrinsic factor
Contain membrane-bound receptors for ACh (muscarinic, M3), gastrin (CCK-2) and histamine ($H_2$), which stimulate secretion of gastric acid (via proton pump H/K-ATPase). ACh is released from intramural neurons in the antrum, body, and fundus of the stomach. ACh stimulates parietal cells directly via M3 receptors or indirectly by inhibition of somatostatin (SS), and thus stimulation of gastrin and histamine secretion

### ECL cells

Found in abundance in the gastric body
Release histamine when stimulated by gastrin, ACh or ghrelin

### Chief cells

Produce pepsinogen, the precursor of the active enzyme pepsin
Pepsinogen is converted to pepsin in the presence of hydrochloric acid in the stomach lumen

### Mucous-secreting cells (neck and surface)

Found in the gastric antrum
Surface mucous cells produce a thick alkaline-rich layer of mucus preventing autodigestion

*D cells*

Found in antrum, body, and fundus of the stomach
Release SS, the main inhibitor of acid secretion via inhibition of the parietal cell directly or via inhibition of histamine release from ECLs.
Luminal acid stimulates SS via local feedback mechanisms
Cholecystokinin and GLP-1 also inhibit acid secretion
Schubert ML. Functional anatomy and physiology of gastric secretion. *Curr Opin Gastroenterol.* 2015;31(6):479–485. Doi:10.1097/MOG.0000000000000213.

## 11.  B. Elderly UC patients have a higher risk of being hospitalized, especially with their first flare

- Elderly UC patients have a higher risk of being hospitalized
- Elderly IBD patients receiving tumour necrosis factor (TNF) inhibitors have an increased risk of severe infection compared with younger patients
- Thiopurine use in elderly patients significantly increases the risks of infection, lymphoproliferative disorders, and skin cancers

The rising incidence of IBD, coupled with a growing ageing population, has led to an increasing number of elderly patients with IBD. Elderly-onset IBD is defined as disease onset at ≥60 years old. Incidence rates for UC are higher than CD for those over 60. In UC, there appears to be a male preponderance with increasing years (male to female ratio of 2:1).

Disease presentation may be atypical in some elderly patients: abdominal pain, fever, and weight loss are less of a feature than in younger patients. The differential diagnosis is larger in the elderly: diagnostic work-up should exclude infectious colitis, ischaemic colitis, and diverticular-associated colitis among others.

Elderly UC patients are more frequently hospitalized for their first flare compared with younger patients, whereas elderly CD patients are more likely to undergo surgical resection at index presentation or shortly after. The indications for surgery do not differ for older and younger patients, and surgical outcomes appear to be comparable.

In elderly CD patients, colonic involvement is most common. In UC, left-sided disease is most common and strict proctitis is less common than in the adult population.

Infections are more common in elderly IBD patients, particularly in those receiving corticosteroids and TNF inhibitors. There is an appreciable risk of opportunistic infections, lymphoma, and skin cancers with thiopurine use. There is no difference in efficacy of treatment with advancing age. Risks and benefits have to be balanced with other co-morbidities and polypharmacy in mind.

Sturm A, Maaser C, Mendall M et al. ECCO topical review on IBD in the elderly. *J Crohns Colitis.* 2017;11(3):263–273. Doi:10.1093/ecco-jcc/jjw188.

## 12.  D. Lower adenoma detection rates correlate with inadequate bowel preparation

- Split-dose bowel preparation is recommended for elective colonoscopy
- Hyperosmolar preparations may increase risks of dehydration and electrolyte imbalances in at-risk groups (chronic renal insufficiency, congestive cardiac failure (CCF) or decompensated liver failure)
- PEG-based regimes are recommended in patients with IBD

Inadequate bowel preparation may lead to failure to complete a colonoscopy and missed pathology. In particular, it has been associated with significantly lower adenoma detection rates. Recently a ≥90% minimum standard for adequate bowel preparation has been recommended by the ESGE.

Split-dose regimens, regardless of the type and dose of cleansing agent, provide excellent cleansing more frequently than day-before bowel preparation. There is no additional benefit to adding an enema to standard bowel preparation. Furthermore, it decreases the patient's acceptability of bowel preparation.

The efficacy of different PEG-based preparations have been assessed in multiple randomized controlled trials (RCTs) and meta-analyses. Split-dose high-volume (≥3L) PEG appears to be superior to split-dose low-volume PEG. PEG is well tolerated and considered safe in the renal impairment or pre-existing electrolyte disturbance. Osmotically balanced PEG solutions are preferred in elderly patients. Hyperosmotic preparations may increase risk of dehydration and electrolyte imbalances in at-risk populations (chronic renal impairment, CCF, decompensated liver disease) and are best avoided.

ESGE does not routinely recommend the use of oral sodium phosphate for bowel preparation because of the risk of acute phosphate nephropathy. Finally, as still a fairly evidence-free zone, there are no specific bowel preparation instructions in patients with chronic constipation.

Hassan C, East J, Radaelli F et al. Bowel preparation for colonoscopy: European Society of Gastrointestinal Endoscopy (ESGE) guideline—update 2019. *Endoscopy.* 2019;51(8):775–794. Doi:10.1055/a-0959-0505.

### 13. C. Intravenous lorazepam

- Benzodiazepines (BZDs) are the gold standard pharmacological treatment for AWS being able to control symptoms and prevent progression
- Lorazepam has a preferable side effect profile in patients with advanced liver disease

AWS is a serious medical condition characterized by increased blood pressure and HR, tremors, hyperreflexia, irritability, anxiety, headache, nausea, and vomiting. Symptoms can occur as early as 6–8 hours after sudden discontinuation or reduction of alcohol intake and peak between 10 and 30 hours. Symptoms may progress to more severe forms of AWS including delirium tremens (tremor, confusion, and hallucinations) in 5%, seizures, coma, cardiac arrest, and death. Alongside supportive management (e.g. fluid and electrolyte replacement, and vitamin administration) BZDs are the gold standard treatment for AWS being able to control symptoms and prevent progression.

The Clinical Institute Withdrawal Assessment for Alcohol (CIWA-Ar) helps grade AWS as mild (≤8), moderate (≥8), and severe (≥15). Moderate and severe AWS require pharmacological management with BDZs with intravenous administration recommended for severe disease. Long-acting BZDs such as diazepam (intravenous or oral) and chlordiazepoxide (oral) are the most widely used and may allow a smoother course of withdrawal. However, they do have an unpredictable metabolism and enhanced sedative effects in patients with coexisting liver disease. In patients with advanced liver disease, lorazepam has a preferable safety profile primarily undergoing hepatic glucuronidation, which is largely preserved in the cirrhotic liver.

Early trials of non-BZD, GABA-ergic drugs (e.g. gabapentin, sodium oxybate, baclofen) have shown similar efficacy to BZDs in managing AWS, and may have the additional advantage of preventing alcohol relapse. However, further randomized control data is required.

Addolorato G, Mirijello A, Barrio P et al. Treatment of alcohol use disorders in patients with alcoholic liver disease. *J. Hepatol.* 2016;65(3):618–630. Doi:10.1016/j.jhep.2016.04.029.

## 14. D. Pancreatic pseudocyst

- Acute pancreatitis can be categorized as IOP (90%) or necrotizing pancreatitis (NP) (10%)
- Fluid collections in IOP can initially form acute peripancreatic fluid collections, which can then mature to form pseudocysts
- Fluid collections in NP initially form ANCs, which can then mature to form WON.

Most patients with acute pancreatitis have a purely inflammatory process called interstitial IOP. However, 10% develop NP involving the pancreatic parenchyma and/or peripancreatic tissue. These two subtypes develop different early (<4 weeks) and late (>4 weeks) local complications. In IOP, acute peripancreatic fluid collections (APFC) are common, usually remain sterile, and resolve spontaneously without intervention. When a localized APFC persists beyond four weeks after onset of IOP, it develops into a pancreatic pseudocyst, defined as an encapsulated collection of homogenous fluid within a well-defined inflammatory wall. Pseudocysts are thought to arise due to the non-necrotic disruption of the pancreatic ducts and can usually be diagnosed by radiological criteria although, if aspirated, demonstrate high fluid amylase. In NP, ANCs containing fluid and solid components can subsequently mature and encapsulate to form heterogenous collections termed WON.

Banks PA, Bollen TL, Dervenis C et al. Classification of acute pancreatitis—2012: revision of the Atlanta classification and definitions by international consensus. *Gut.* 2013;62(1):102–111. Doi:10.1136/gutjnl-2012-302779.

## 15. D. Non-alcoholic steatohepatitis

- Histological features of non-alcoholic steatohepatitis (NASH) include lobular inflammation and ballooning of hepatocytes +/− fibrosis, portal inflammatory infiltrate, Mallory-Denk bodies (Mallory's hyaline), and megamitochondria (Fig. 11.6)
- Severity of fibrosis is the strongest predictor of outcome in patients with non-alcoholic fatty liver disease (NAFLD)
- Hyperferritinaemia and positive autoantibodies are common in patients with NAFLD

Liver biopsy is helpful diagnostically when the cause of abnormal LFTs is unclear despite performing a non-invasive liver disease screen. In such cases, in the absence of excessive alcohol intake or steatogenic drugs, the presence of intrahepatocellular lipid droplets in >5% of hepatocytes would be indicative of (NAFLD, formerly simple steatosis). Features of NASH include the presence of lobular inflammation and ballooning of hepatocytes +/− fibrosis, portal inflammatory infiltrate, Mallory-Denk bodies (Mallory's hyaline), and megamitochondria, all of which can also be seen in alcohol-related liver disease. Severity of fibrosis is the strongest predictor of outcome in patients

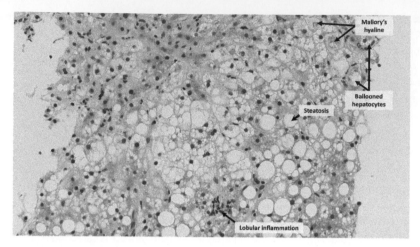

**Fig. 11.6** Liver histology specimen showing features of NASH

with NAFLD, whereas a diagnosis of NASH per se is not important for risk stratification but remains an endpoint in clinical trials.

Hyperferritinaemia is frequently seen in patients with NAFLD and metabolic syndrome. Transferrin saturation should be checked and, if this is normal, goes against iron overload and further investigations for haemochromatosis are not required. Autoantibodies are positive in 20% of patients with NAFLD in the absence of AIH.

Marjot T, Moolla A, Cobbold JF et al. Nonalcoholic fatty liver disease in adults: current concepts in etiology, outcomes, and management. *Endocr Rev.* 2020;41(1). Doi:10.1210/endrev/bnz009.

### 16. C. Extracorporeal shock wave lithotripsy

- Extracorporeal shockwave lithotripsy (ESWL) should be used first line in the management of obstructing main pancreatic duct stones >5 mm
- Painful dominant main pancreatic duct strictures should be treated with plastic stenting
- Pancreatic enzyme supplementation does not improve pain in patients with chronic pancreatitis

In cases of painful chronic pancreatitis with main duct obstruction (in pancreatic head or body), the ESGE recommends duct clearance using ESWL and ERCP for stones >5 mm and <5 mm respectively. ESWL can be followed by ERCP to assist extraction of smaller stone fragments. Meta-analysis has reported that ESWL for stones ≥5 mm leads to complete duct clearance in 70% of patients, with 53% having an absence of pain and 88% having improved quality of life at two years. ESWL is not indicated in patients with extensive calculi or with isolated calculi in the tail area because of increased risk of damage to the spleen. Painful dominant main pancreatic duct strictures should be treated with plastic stenting. If endoscopic therapy and/or ESWL provide no persistent pain relief or technically fail, surgical procedures can be considered including drainage procedures (pancreatico-jejunostomy), partial pancreatic resection, and total pancreatectomy. There is little evidence that pancreatic enzyme supplementation improves pain in patients with chronic pancreatitis.

Dumonceau JM, Delhaye M, Tringali A et al. Endoscopic treatment of chronic pancreatitis: European Society of Gastrointestinal Endoscopy (ESGE) guideline—updated August 2018. *Endoscopy.* 2019;51(2):179-93. Doi:10.1055/a-0822-0832.

## 17. E. Genetic testing

- Immunohistochemistry tumour testing for mismatch repair (MMR)or microsatellite instability (MSI) should be performed in all people when *first* diagnosed with colorectal cancer (CRC)
- Colonoscopic surveillance should be performed at a two-yearly interval
- Colonoscopic surveillance is recommended from 25 years for MLH1 and MSH2 mutation carriers

Lynch syndrome (LS), also known as 'hereditary non-polyposis CRC', is the most common hereditary CRC syndrome accounting for 3%–5% of all CRCs. Autosomal dominant in inheritance pattern, LS is defined by the presence of mutations in any one of the four DNA MMR genes: *MLH1*, *MSH2* (*MSH2* and *MLH1* account for more than 80% of the identified MMR gene alterations in hereditary nonpolyposis colorectal cancer [HNPCC] families), *MSH6* and *PMS2*. Former criteria for diagnosis, Amsterdam or Bethesda criteria, have been superseded by advances in technology that allow for more accurate genetic diagnosis. Guidance recommends the use of colonoscopic biopsies for tumour MMR immunohistochemistry testing.

The onset of GI cancer is early (mean age 44 years). CRCs are commonly right sided (60%–80% proximal to the splenic flexure) and develop more rapidly than sporadic CRCs. Synchronous and metachronous tumours are common. The incidence of extracolonic cancers such as malignancies of the endometrium, ovaries, and urinary tract are significantly raised in LS.

### Surveillance in Lynch syndrome

Colonoscopic surveillance should be performed at two-yearly intervals for all LS patients.
Age of onset of surveillance colonoscopy should be stratified according to the LS-associated gene.
Colonoscopy is recommended from age 25 years for *MLH1* and *MSH2* mutation carriers, and 35 years for *MSH6* and *PMS2* mutation carriers.
Gastric, small bowel, and pancreatic surveillance is not routinely recommended.

### Surgery

The decision to perform segmental versus total colectomy in LS patients with *MLH1* or *MSH2* mutations who develop colon cancer should balance the risks of metachronous cancer, functional consequences of surgery, and the patient's age and wishes.

Monahan KJ, Bradshaw N, Dolwani S et al. Guidelines for the management of hereditary colorectal cancer from the British Society of Gastroenterology (BSG)/ Association of Coloproctology of Great Britain and Ireland (ACPGBI)/ United Kingdom Cancer Genetics Group (UKCGG). *Gut.* 2020;69(3):411–444. Doi:10.1136/gutjnl-2019-319915.

## 18. A. CRC incidence in primary sclerosis colitis/ulcerative colitis (PSC/UC) is fourfold greater than in UC alone

- Overall, 80% of patients of PSC have co-existent IBD
- CRC risk is significant and fourfold greater than patients with UC alone
- Patients should be offered colonoscopy at diagnosis of PSC and then yearly if there is evidence of IBD.

PSC/IBD is a distinct phenotype of IBD. Among patients with PSC, there is an increased prevalence of both UC (seen in approximately 60%–70% of patients with PSC, and more common in males) and Crohn's colitis, but not small bowel CD. It is less common in patients of Asian or Southern European ancestry. Patients are often asymptomatic, highlighting the importance of colonoscopy at diagnosis of PSC. Rectal sparing is common, with predilection for right-sided colitis.

Subsequently, the risk of colorectal dysplasia and cancer is significant. Patients with PSC/UC have a fourfold increased risk of CRC compared with patients with UC alone. Yearly surveillance colonoscopy is therefore imperative from diagnosis of PSC/IBD and should continue even in those patients who have undergone LT. CRC risk is thought to be heightened because of exposure of the colonic mucosa to toxic secondary bile acids (e.g. deoxycholic acid, which promotes carcinogenesis). Medical and surgical treatment of colitis is in line with standard IBD guidelines. Of note, the incidence of stomal and peristomal varices after colectomy for patients with PSC and advanced liver fibrosis is significant.

Annese V, Daperno M, Rutter MD et al. European evidence based consensus for endoscopy in inflammatory bowel disease. *J Crohns Colitis*. 2013;7(12):982–1018. Doi:10.1016/j.crohns.2013.09.016.

## 19. B. Trophozoites adhere to the mucosal surface, causing cytokine release and consequent fluid and electrolyte loss

- Giardiasis is caused by the protozoa, *Giardia lamblia*
- Protozoal cysts are ingested and adhere to the mucosal surface of the small intestine, stomach, or biliary tree
- Treatment is usually with 5-nitroimidazoles (e.g. tinidazole)

*Giardia lamblia* is a flagellate protozoan that exists worldwide and is spread by the faecal–oral route. Cysts are ingested and then excystate in the stomach in response to gastric acid releasing flat, teardrop-shaped trophozoites. The trophozoites undergo asexual reproduction in the gut and colonize the upper small bowel using a sucking disc to adhere to, but not invade, the mucosa. In patients with achlorhydria, they may colonize the stomach, and some patients have biliary involvement. Adherence disrupts the brush border, causing cytokine release and water and electrolyte loss. The trophozoites encyst as they pass through the large intestine, and are passed in the faeces. The cysts are infectious and can survive outside the host. Importantly, chlorination does not eradicate the cysts, so water must be boiled or filtered.

The incubation period can vary from a few days to several months. Symptoms of giardiasis include non-bloody diarrhoea, bloating, flatulence, and abdominal pain, and colonization can lead to malabsorption and weight loss. Treatment is with a single dose of tinidazole or a short course of metronidazole.

Minetti C, Chalmers RM, Beeching NJ et al. Giardiasis. *BMJ*. 2016;355:i5369. Doi:10.1136/bmj.i5369.

## 20. C. Granular cell tumour

- A granular cell tumour is a rare, benign oesophageal lesion usually found as an incidental finding in the lower oesophagus
- Typical presentation is of a pale yellow sub-mucosal polypoid lesion in the distal oesophagus
- Characteristic histological features include polygonal cells with granular eosinophilic cytoplasm

The endoscopic and histological descriptions of the polyp are classical of a granular cell tumour. Benign oesophageal tumours are usually slow growing and are typically seen as incidental findings at endoscopy. While the lesion described has a similar endoscopic appearance to a lipoma, histologically a lipoma has a core of well-circumscribed adipose tissue with normal overlying mucosa.

Leiomyoma is the most common benign oesophageal tumour, usually occurring in men. They arise from the muscularis layers (-propria or -mucosae) and are histologically typified by whorls of long spindle-like smooth muscle cells with eosinophilic cytoplasm.

Fibro-vascular polyps can become very large (up to 20 cm) and in some cases have been reported to regurgitate into the mouth. They typically present in older men. Histologically, they are folds of normal squamous mucosa containing blood vessels, adipose cells, and stroma. Adenocarcinoma is the most common malignant oesophageal tumour. It is typically seen in the distal oesophagus with adjacent Barrett's oesophagus. Histologically, it consists of intestinal (mucin producing) mucosa with variable degree of differentiation.

Choong CK, Meyers BF. Benign esophageal tumors: introduction, incidence, classification, and clinical features. *Semin Thorac Cardiovasc Surg.* 2003;15(1):3–8.

## 21. D. 7

- The Ulcerative Colitis Endoscopic Index of Severity (UCEIS) score is defined by the vascular pattern, degree of bleeding, and ulceration (Table 11.1)
- UCEIS scoring strongly correlates with patient-reported symptoms
- Eighty per cent of acute severe colitis (ASC) patients with a score ≥ 7 will require colectomy irrespective of medical therapy

This patient has a UCEIS of 7/8 due to complete obliteration of vascular pattern, small amounts of free, liquid blood in the lumen, and deep ulceration with raised edges. The validated UCEIS score (Table 11.1) was developed as a tool to reliably measure the endoscopic activity of UC. UCEIS scoring is minimally affected by clinical information of disease activity and strongly correlated with patient-reported symptoms. UCEIS outperformed the Mayo Endoscopic Score as a predictor for

**Table 11.1** Ulcerative colitis endoscopic index of severity (UCEIS) score

| Descriptor (score most severe lesions) | Likert scale anchor points | Definition |
|---|---|---|
| Vascular pattern | None (0) | Normal vascular pattern with arborization of capillaries clearly defined or with blurring or patchy loss of capillary margins |
| | Patchy obliteration (1) | Patchy obliteration of vascular pattern |
| | Obliterated (2) | Complete obliteration of vascular pattern |
| Bleeding | None (0) | No visible blood |
| | Mucosal (1) | Some spots or streaks of coagulated blood on the surface of the mucosa ahead of the scope that can be washed away |
| | Luminal mild (2) | Some free liquid blood in the lumen |
| | Luminal moderate or severe (3) | Frank blood in the lumen ahead of the endoscope or visible oozing from the mucosa after washing the intraluminal blood, or visible oozing from the haemorrhagic mucosa |
| Erosions and ulcers | None (0) | Normal mucosa, no visible erosions or ulcers |
| | Erosions (1) | Tiny (≤5 mm) defects in the mucosa of a white or yellow colour with a flat edge |
| | Superficial ulcer (2) | Larger (≥5 mm) defects in the mucosa, which are discrete fibrin-covered ulcers when compared with erosions but remain superficial |
| | Deep ulcer (3) | Deeper excavated defects in the mucosa with a slightly raised edge |

colectomy in ASC patients. Eighty per cent of ASC patients with UCEIS ≥ 7 subsequently required colectomy, irrespective of medical therapy.

Travis SP, Schnell D, Krzeski P et al. Reliability and initial validation of the ulcerative colitis endoscopic index of severity. *Gastroenterology*. 2013;145(5):987–995. Doi:10.1053/j.gastro.2013.07.024.

## 22. A. Covered stent placement

- Diagnostic gastroscopy is rarely associated with oesophageal perforation
- Early recognition and prompt management are required to optimize outcome
- Endoscopic clip placement, stent insertion or surgery may be needed

The image demonstrates a full-thickness oesophageal perforation (Matull et al. 2008). This is an uncommon complication of diagnostic gastroscopy (0.03%). Most cases occur in the context of therapeutic intervention including dilatation and EMR. Conditions favouring successful management include early recognition and treatment (within 24 hours), small defect, and management by an experienced multi-disciplinary team. Cervical oesophageal perforations have a more favourable outcome because there is less risk of mediastinal contamination. Mortality after oesophageal perforation is high despite intervention—11.9% with a mean hospital stay of 32.9 days.

General management involves broad spectrum antibiotics, proton pump inhibition, fluid resuscitation, and avoiding all oral intake for at least five days. Endoscopic clip placement can be helpful for smaller defects, and self-expanding metal stents for larger mid/lower oesophageal perforations (or in the context of oesophageal malignancy). Nasogastric tube drainage (inserted under direct endoscopic vision) can help divert luminal contents. Surgery is indicated in the case of patient instability following perforation, late recognition (more than 24 hours), or radiology demonstrating free perforation or collections in the mediastinum of pleural cavity.

In this case, the defect is too large for endoscopic closure, there is no role for endoscopic gluing, surgery would be high risk for this patient, and a nasogastric tube should only be inserted for drainage, not feeding.

Paspatis GA, Dumonceau JM, Barthet M et al. Diagnosis and management of iatrogenic endoscopic perforations: European Society of Gastrointestinal Endoscopy (ESGE) position statement. *Endoscopy*. 2014;46(8):693–711. Doi:10.1055/s-0034-1377531.

## 23. D. PRSS1

- Mutations in PRSS1 account for 65%–80% of cases of hereditary pancreatitis, and lead to increased trypsin 1 activation and pancreatic autodigestion
- A range of other gene variants are associated including SPINK, CTRC, CASR and CFTR, the latter which accounts for the chronic pancreatitis phenotype seen in cystic fibrosis

Hereditary pancreatitis is a rare cause of chronic pancreatitis occurring in approximately 0.3/100,000 individuals in Western countries. It is most commonly due to mutations of PRSS1 (65%–80%) which are inherited in an autosomal dominant pattern. Over 35 mutations in PRSS1 have been associated, which increase the conversion of inactive trypsinogen to active trypsin 1 causing injury and inflammation through autodigestion of pancreatic proteins. Variants in other genes have been found to increase susceptibility to chronic pancreatitis, with either familial or sporadic patterns including in SPINK1 and CTRC which both encode inhibitors of trypsin 1. CFTR is a crucial anion channel used by the pancreatic duct cells to secrete bicarbonate, which flushes pancreatic digestive enzyme out of pancreas. This accounts for chronic pancreatitis and exocrine insufficiency seen with mutations leading to cystic fibrosis. Mutations in the genes encoding CASR are also associated with a small increase in the risk of developing chronic pancreatitis triggered by an unfolded protein response independent of trypsin activation.

Kleeff J, Whitcomb DC, Shimosegawa T et al. Chronic pancreatitis. *Nat Rev Dis Primers.* 2017;3:17060. Doi:10.1038/nrdp.2017.60.

### 24. A. Cholecystectomy

- Gallbladder polyps >10 mm, symptomatic polyps, polyps 6–9 mm with additional risk factors for malignancy, and polyps of any size in PSC are all indications for cholecystectomy
- Risk factors for gallbladder malignancy include age >50 years, Indian ethnicity, and sessile polyps
- Surveillance interval and duration for polyps <10 mm depend on polyp size and the presence of risk factors

Gallbladder polyps are detected in 0.3%–9.5% of abdominal ultrasound scans. They can be classified as true neoplastic polyps or non-neoplastic pseudopolyps. Seventy per cent of gallbladder polyps are pseudopolyps and include cholesterol polyps (accumulation of intramural lipid), adenomyomatosis (muscle thickening and diverticula), and inflammatory polyps. These non-neoplastic polyps do not increase the risk of gallbladder cancer. True polyps can be benign (most commonly adenomas) or malignant (most commonly adenocarcinoma).

Gallbladder cancer is rare but early detection is important because it carries a grave prognosis with a five-year survival of 5% in the presence of serosal perforation or regional lymph node involvement. Predicting which polyps are likely to undergo malignant transformation is difficult and management strategies remain contentious. The European Society of Gastrointestinal and Abdominal Radiology has recently released updated recommendations: polyps >10 mm, symptomatic polyps or polyps 6–9 mm with additional risk factors are indications for cholecystectomy. All other polyps should be followed up with interval ultrasounds, the timing and duration of which are guided by size and risk factors.

Gallbladder abnormalities are present in up to 40% of patients with PSC and frequently represent adenocarcinoma (14%–57%), irrespective of size. The European Association for the Study of the Liver (EASL) therefore recommend annual ultrasound in all PSC patients with subsequent cholecystectomy for any gallbladder mass even if <1 cm, if underlying liver disease permits.

Wiles R, Thoeni RF, Barbu ST et al. Management and follow-up of gallbladder polyps: Joint guidelines between the European Society of Gastrointestinal and Abdominal Radiology (ESGAR), European Association for Endoscopic Surgery and other Interventional Techniques (EAES), International Society of Digestive Surgery—European Federation (EFISDS) and European Society of Gastrointestinal Endoscopy (ESGE). *Eur Radiol.* 2017;27(9):3856–3866. Doi:10.1007/s00330-017-4742-y.

### 25. B. Cannabis

- Cannabinoid agents significantly affect gastric and colonic motility
- $CB_1$ receptors are located throughout the GI tract
- Frequent use of hot showers or baths to relieve symptoms is stereotypical of cannabis hyperemesis syndrome (CHS)

Cannabis is the only option associated with delayed gastric emptying. CHS is defined by symptoms of cyclical nausea, vomiting, and abdominal pain with chronic cannabis use. Compulsive showering or bathing to relieve symptoms is a cardinal feature. Symptoms generally last 24–48 hours, but may last up to 7–10 days.

The pathophysiology of CHS is not fully elucidated. Two main cannabinoid receptors have been identified: $CB_1$ and $CB_2$. $CB_1$ receptors are located throughout the GI tract, predominantly expressed in myenteric and submucosal neurons. Activity at the $CB_1$ receptor is thought to account for the clinical effects of cannabis use. Studies postulate that disruption of the $CB_1$ receptors in the enteric nerves results in delayed gastric motility and therefore hyperemesis. $TRPV_1$ is a G-protein coupled receptor that interacts with the endocannabinoid system. This receptor is activated by heat (T>41°C) as well as capsaicin, and may correspond with relief of symptoms with hot showers or baths.

CHS is primarily associated with inhalation of cannabis. However, symptoms can be seen with other formulations. Delayed gastric emptying may be confirmed with a gastric emptying study. Blood tests are not diagnostic. If an individual denies cannabis use but clinical suspicion is high, a urinary drug screen should be considered.

Cessation of cannabis use improves symptoms. The mainstay of treatment is symptomatic relief, patient education, and, most importantly, cannabis cessation.

Camilleri M. Cannabinoids and gastrointestinal motility: pharmacology, clinical effects, and potential therapeutics in humans. *Neurogastroenterol motil.* 2018;30(9):e13370. Doi:10.1111/nmo.13370.

## 26. B. Liver biopsy

- Liver biopsy should be performed in patients with known PSC if transaminases and/or IgG are significantly elevated in order to identify overlap with AIH
- Around 10% of patients with PSC have overlap with AIH and may benefit from immunosuppressive therapy

Overlap syndrome with AIH is present in around 10% of patients with PSC and should be suspected in patients with PSC who have significantly raised transaminases or IgG. There are no established definitions of the required degree of elevation of transaminases or IgG levels but ALT at >5 × upper limit of normal (ULN) and IgG at >2 × ULN may serve as a guide. However, patients with PSC usually have mildly elevated transaminases and IgG levels, which can make the diagnosis difficult. If patients do have overlap with AIH, they may benefit from immunosuppressive therapy.

The histological pattern of PSC/AIH overlap is ill-defined and complicated by the fact that coincidental biliary injury is often found in AIH and that interface hepatitis can be part of the disease spectrum of a range of hepatic conditions including PSC. A PSC/AIH overlap diagnosis therefore requires the combination of biochemical, serological, and histological features of AIH.

Liver elastography is being increasingly used in PSC and a large international study is underway to establish clear cut-offs for identifying advanced fibrosis which is not currently well-defined. Repeated MRCP in PSC is not routine, unless there is worsening cholestasis and/or signs of cholangitis. Finally, anti-sp100 and anti-gp210 are PBC-specific antinuclear antibodies, but the possibility of PBC is not raised in this setting.

Boberg KM, Chapman RW, Hirschfield GM at al. Overlap syndromes: The International Autoimmune Hepatitis Group (IAIHG) position statement on a controversial issue. *J Hepatol.* 2011;54(2):374–385. Doi:10.1016/j.jhep.2010.09.002.

## 27. D. i3

- The Rutgeerts score was developed in 1990 to predict post-surgical CD recurrence (Table 11.2)
- The score is defined by the severity of the endoscopic findings at the anastomotic site and neoterminal ileum
- Endoscopic recurrence is defined as a score of ≥2

**Table 11.2** Rutgeert's score

| Rutgeerts' score | Endoscopic description of findings |
| --- | --- |
| i0 | No lesions |
| i1 | ≤5 aphthous ulcers |
| i2 | >5 aphthous ulcers with normal intervening mucosa, skip areas of larger lesions, or lesions confined to |
| i3 | Diffuse aphthous ileitis with diffusely inflamed mucosa |
| i4 | Diffuse inflammation with larger ulcers, nodules, and/or narrowing |

Rutgeerts P, Geboes K, Vantrappen G et al. Predictability of the postoperative course of Crohn's disease. *Gastroenterology*. 1990;99(4):956–963.

### 28. D. Serology

- Katayama syndrome is a hypersensitivity reaction to schistosoma eggs found in travellers exposed to fresh water in endemic areas
- In the returning traveller, schistosoma serology is the best diagnostic test

Schistosomes are blood-dwelling trematodes that infect freshwater molluscs as intermediate hosts and the bloodstream of humans as definitive hosts. Exposure of infection-naïve travellers to schistosoma-containing water can lead to migrating schistosomula, egg deposition, and a systemic hypersensitivity reaction called 'Katayama syndrome'. Acute infection is often asymptomatic but can present with a typical 'swimmers itch': an urticarial, maculopapular rash, and progress weeks later to high-grade nocturnal fevers, cough, myalgia, headache, diarrhoea, and abdominal pain. Eighty per cent of patients have eosinophilia and those with respiratory symptoms may have patchy infiltrates on chest radiograph. While microscopic examination of stool/urine for schistosoma eggs remains the diagnostic gold standard, it takes 6–12 weeks for these to be produced and excreted, and the examination is less sensitive in returning travellers where the parasite count is generally low. For diagnosis in this group, serum antischistosomal antibodies perform better. Returning travellers to endemic areas with fresh water exposure should be screened routinely with serological testing even in the absence of symptoms. Rectal biopsy is useful as a diagnostic tool for hepatic forms of schistosomiasis in the absence of positive laboratory tests. The Kato-Katz method is a quick test used in epidemiological studies in endemic settings using 5 mg of stool examined with low-power microscopy. Schistosomiasis can usually be treated with a short course of praziquantel.

Ross AG, Vickers D, Olds GR et al. Katayama syndrome. *Lancet Infect Dis*. 2007;7(3):218–224.

### 29. D. The Stroop test can be used to help make a diagnosis of HE

- HE comprises a wide range of neuro-psychiatric abnormalities caused by liver dysfunction and/or porto-systemic shunting
- A range of neurophysiological and psychometric tests including Stroop testing have been validated in the diagnosis of HE although none are specific

HE is characterized by a wide spectrum of non-specific neurological and psychiatric abnormalities that can make diagnosis challenging. When suspecting HE, clinicians must consider whether the degree of hepatic failure and/or portosystemic shunting is severe enough to cause HE and exclude other causes of brain dysfunction that are often more common in patients with cirrhosis (e.g. nutritional encephalopathy, alcohol-related dementia, cerebrovascular disease). Thirty to forty per cent of patients with cirrhosis will experience at least one episode of overt HE. Minimal or covert HE occurs in ~50% of patients with cirrhosis and is characterized by the presence of brain dysfunction in patients who do not display asterixis and are oriented on clinical assessment. Minimal HE can still have a significant impact on patients and carers, and is a prognostic marker for future overt HE. While brain imaging is not essential for diagnosis, it should be considered because patients with cirrhosis have a fivefold increased risk of intracranial haemorrhage, which can mimic HE. EEG abnormalities can be detected at every grade of encephalopathy but, as with all neurophysiological testing, it is non-specific and should be used in patients without confounding psychiatric disorders, psychoactive medications, and alcohol use.

The Stroop test evaluates psychomotor speed and flexibility by measuring the reaction time to a coloured field and a written colour name. A Stroop smartphone application has also been shown to detect cognitive dysfunction in cirrhosis with good discriminative validity and test-retest reliability.

Vilstrup H, Amodio P, Bajaj J et al. Hepatic encephalopathy in chronic liver disease: 2014 practice guideline by the EASL and AASLD. *J Hepatol.* 2014;61(3):642–659. Doi:10.1016/j.jhep.2014.05.042.

### 30. E. Variants in TPMT account for up to 25% of thiopurine-induced leucopenia

- Leucopenia most commonly occurs in individuals with normal TPMT
- TPMT does not predict clinical response or drug toxicity
- 0.3% of the population is a homozygous carrier for a TPMT variant resulting in low or absent TPMT activity

Azathioprine use in TPMT deficiency can result in higher levels of thioguanine nucleotide cytotoxic metabolites and myelotoxicity. Prior to treatment, TPMT genotype assessment may help to identify patients at risk of myelosuppression. However, studies report that up to 75% of cases of azathioprine-induced myelosuppression have no TPMT mutation, and leucopenia most commonly occurs in individuals with a normal TPMT. The prospective randomized controlled TOPIC trial of pre-treatment TPMT screening demonstrated a 10-fold reduction in myelotoxicity in heterozygote variant carriers who were given a reduced thiopurine dose compared with equivalent carriers treated with a standard dose. The utility of measuring thiopurine metabolites (6-thioguanine nucleotides [6-TGN] and 6-methylmercaptopurine ribonucleotides [6-MMPR]) was assessed in a subset of patients from the TOPIC trial. In approximately 80%, thiopurine-induced leucopenia could be predicted from week one 6-TGN and/or 6-MMPR elevations.

TPMT does not predict clinical response or drug toxicity. The level of TPMT relates to genetic polymorphisms as per Table 11.3.

**Table 11.3** TMPT gene variants and enzyme activity

| Population percentage* | Genetics | TPMT activity |
|---|---|---|
| 90% | Homozygote wild type | High/normal |
| 10% | Heterozygote | Low |
| 0.3% | Homozygote variant type | None |

*Caucasian population

Wong DR, Coenan MJ, Vermeulen SH et al. Early assessment of thiopurine metabolites identifies patients at risk of thiopurine-induced leukopenia in inflammatory bowel disease. *J Crohns Colitis.* 2017;11(2):175–184. Doi:10.1093/ecco-jcc/jjw130.

## 31. A. Ascites protein concentration

- Advanced cirrhosis and low protein ascites (<15 g/L), and previous spontaneous bacterial peritonitis, are all indications for prophylactic antibiotics

Studies have demonstrated that prophylactic antibiotics are effective in preventing spontaneous bacterial peritonitis in patients with advanced cirrhosis and low-protein ascites. European guidelines currently advocate for use of primary prophylaxis in patients with Child-Pugh score ≥9 and serum bilirubin level ≥50 μmol/L, with either impaired renal function or hyponatraemia, and ascitic fluid protein <15 g/L. Prior spontaneous bacterial peritonitis is itself an indication for secondary antibiotic prophylaxis in ascites in the context of portal hypertension. In this case, neither the total white cell count nor the neutrophil count is suggestive of spontaneous bacterial peritonitis: a cut-off of ≥250 neutrophils per μL (or alternatively ≥500 total white cells per μL) is used to diagnose spontaneous bacterial peritonitis by cell count alone. Spontaneous bacterial peritonitis may also be diagnosed by culture of ascites. Repeated large-volume paracentesis, prospective LT, and prospective TIPSS are not indications for prophylactic antibiotics.

Angeli P, Bernardi M, Villanueva C et al. EASL clinical practice guidelines for the management of patients with decompensated cirrhosis. *J Hepatol*. 2018;69(2):406–460. Doi:10.1016/j.jhep.208.03.024.

## 32. D. Laparoscopy

- Diagnostic laparoscopy accurately stages for local and metastatic disease in gastric cancer
- MRI has similar rates of accuracy to CT in TNM staging
- EUS is useful in detecting local spread or nodal disease

There is good evidence indicating that laparoscopy should be considered in patients with gastric tumours and in those with oesophageal tumours extending to the proximal stomach.

European Society of Medical Oncology (ESMO) guidance recommends all patients with resectable gastric cancer to undergo a diagnostic laparoscopy in order to accurately stage for local spread and metastatic disease.

Barium studies are sensitive in diagnosing malignancy. However, they have been shown to be less sensitive than endoscopy for identifying cancer in situ or T1 cancers. MRI has similar rates of accuracy to CT in TNM staging, and therefore will not add anything in this case. Positron emission tomography (PET)-CT scanning can also be helpful In staging. ESMO suggests its utilization in oesophageal and oesophagogastric junctional tumours, because it provides additional functional and anatomical data to optimize M and N staging pre-treatment. EUS is often useful in detecting local spread or nodal disease. EMR can be used to accurately stage the depth of invasion in small, early disease.

The presence or absence of metastatic disease will be critical in this patient's management. Therefore, laparoscopy is likely to be more discriminatory.

Smyth EC, Verheij M, Allum W et al. Gastric cancer: ESMO clinical practice guidelines for diagnosis, treatment and follow up. *Ann Oncol*. 2016;27(Suppl 5):v38–49.

## 33. E. Zinc

- Zinc deficiency is rare in the Western world but dietary deficiency can occur in low-resource settings
- A characteristic skin rash develops with zinc deficiency, also seen with the genetic condition acrodermatitis enteropathica
- Symptoms usually resolve with zinc supplementation

Zinc deficiency in adults was first recognized in 1961 in an Iranian farmer with a diet high in cereals but low in animal produce. It is an essential trace element, actively absorbed in the small intestine, and largely excreted through the GI system. Meat, chicken, nuts, and lentils are good sources of dietary zinc. Some food products in the Western world are also fortified with zinc. Dietary deficiency still exists in lower-income countries.

Zinc deficiency can lead to growth retardation, hypogonadism, dysgeusia, and characteristic skin rashes (mainly affecting the intertriginous and perioral areas). Zinc deficiency used to be seen in patients on total parenteral nutrition until zinc was routinely incorporated into intravenous nutrition prescriptions. Pregnancy increases the risk for zinc deficiency and patients with alcohol-related cirrhosis may have low hepatic stores of zinc. Acrodermatitis enteropathica is an autosomal-recessive disorder affecting zinc absorption. Features include the characteristic periorificial rash with nail changes, secondary skin infections, alopecia, and diarrhoea. Zinc supplementation tends to result in resolution of symptoms. High zinc intake can interfere with copper absorption and lead to copper deficiency.

Niacin deficiency can cause dermatitis and diarrhoea but typically also causes cognitive impairment. Selenium deficiency results in thyroid dysfunction and cardiac complications. Vitamin A deficiency causes night blindness, and Vitamin E neuromuscular conditions.

Roohani N, Hurrell R, Kelishadi R et al. Zinc and its importance for human health: an integrative review. J Res Med Sci. 2013;18(2):144–157.

## 34. C. Iron supplementation

- Gastric antral vascular ectasia (GAVE) is characterized by a classical 'watermelon stomach' appearance endoscopically
- Portal hypertensive gastropathy (PHG) is differentiated from GAVE by its diffuse distribution and localization to the fundus and body
- Argon plasma coagulation is an endoscopic therapy in symptomatic individuals

The image illustrates GAVE, a capillary-type vascular malformation predominantly affecting the gastric antrum. Endoscopic appearances are characterized by red areas. These often appear as streaks, hence the term 'watermelon stomach'. Histology is rarely necessary, but can demonstrate dilated capillaries in the lamina propria. The aetiology has not been established. GAVE is most common in women over 70 years of age. It is associated with autoimmune disease (commonly systemic sclerosis), renal failure, and heart disease. Less than 30% of GAVE cases are associated with liver cirrhosis. In cirrhosis, GAVE can be mistaken for PHG.

Cases of GAVE often present with chronic blood loss resulting in anaemia, although up to 4% of acute bleeds may relate to GAVE. Iron deficiency anaemia should be corrected with iron supplementation. If the anaemia is associated with significant bleeding or unresponsive to supplementation, treatment should be considered. Treatment of GAVE is often endoscopic, involving treatment with argon plasma coagulation at endoscopy. This may have to be performed repeatedly. Antrectomy can be considered in severe cases that are unresponsive to endoscopic management.

Treatment of portal hypertension is not helpful. PHG is differentiated from GAVE by its diffuse distribution, rather than streaks, and its location predominantly in the fundus and body of the stomach. PHG improves with reduction in portal pressures with non-selective beta blockers (e.g. propranolol, carvedilol) or TIPSS.

Hsu WH, Wang YK, Hsieh MS et al. Insights into the management of gastric antral vascular ectasia (watermelon stomach). Therap Adv Gastroenterol. 2018;11:1756283X17747471. Doi:10.1177/1756283X17747471.

### 35. E. Trial of calcium-channel blocker

- Type III sphincter of Oddi dysfunction (SOD) no longer exists and has been replaced with the term 'functional biliary-type pain'
- There is no role for ERCP in functional biliary-type pain

Dysfunction of the biliary sphincter is considered in patients who present with biliary-type pains post-cholecystectomy, once biliary calculi and other structural lesions have been excluded. Earlier recommendations were that type I SOD (with a dilated bile duct and elevated liver enzymes) patients should undergo biliary sphincterotomy without manometry, and that type II SOD (dilated duct or elevated liver enzymes) and type III SOD (no abnormalities) patients should be considered for manometry-directed sphincterotomy. This classification is now outdated and has been revised in the Rome IV criteria. Most patients with prior type I SOD have organic stenosis rather than functional pathology, and they are best treated with biliary sphincterotomy. For patients with post-cholecystectomy pain and some objective findings (previous type II SOD), the term suspected 'functional biliary sphincter disorder' is used. They may undergo further investigations with hepatobiliary scintigraphy or ERCP with manometry, although the majority would be treated directly with biliary sphincterotomy. Functional biliary-type pain replaces the term Type III SOD. The EPISOD trial showed that patients with Type III SOD do not respond to sphincter ablation better than sham intervention. The patients are therefore managed medically. Nifedipine, amitriptyline, and duloxetine are frequently used to manage symptoms. Intra-sphincteric botulinum toxin injection has been used successfully by some groups but remains controversial.

Cotton PB, Elta GH, Carter CR et al. Rome IV. Gallbladder and sphincter of Oddi disorders. *Gastroenterology*. 2016. Doi:10.1053/j.gastro.2016.02.033.

### 36. C. Biopsies should be taken before proceeding to dilatation

- Perforation rates for benign strictures are approximately 1%
- Proton pump inhibitor (PPI) therapy reduces the need for dilatation and rates of stricture recurrence for peptic strictures
- Both bougie and balloon dilatation are equally effective in managing benign strictures

Symptomatic narrowing of the oesophagus may be caused by acid reflux, eosinophilic oesophagitis, ingestion of corrosive substances, or following endoscopic therapy and is an indication for oesophageal dilatation. Characteristically, dysphagia is to solids but not liquids, unlike motility disorders where dysphagia is often for both. Biopsies should be taken from all strictures to exclude malignancy and eosinophilic oesophagitis, ideally before dilatation is attempted. Not only does this allow diagnosis but also estimation of perforation risk (1% benign strictures, 6% malignant strictures). Barium swallow should be considered for suspected complex strictures to establish length, diameter, and number of strictures. Cross-sectional imaging is advised if malignancy is suspected.

RCTs have confirmed no difference in efficacy between wire-guided bougie dilatation and through-the-scope balloon dilatation. The choice of technique should be based on endoscopist preference and expertise, availability of equipment, and cost. Strictures should be dilated using no more than three successively larger dilators in a single session. Further sessions may be needed every 2–4 weeks to achieve adequate dilatation. For peptic strictures, PPI therapy, but no H2 receptor antagonists, reduce the need for dilatation and rates of stricture recurrence.

Sami SS, Haboubi HN, Ang Y et al. UK guidelines on oesophageal dilatation in clinical practice. *Gut*. 2018;67(6):1000–1023. Doi:10.1136/gutjnl-2017-315414.

### 37. D. Endoscopic diverticulectomy

- Zenker's diverticulum, also called 'pharyngeal pouch', is a common oesophageal diverticulum particularly in older individuals
- Aspiration pneumonia may be the presenting symptom, but halitosis and dysphagia may also be described
- Endoscopic diverticulectomy is associated with lower complication rates and shorter hospital stay than open surgery

Zenker's diverticulum (black asterisk in Fig. 11.7), first described in 1877, is a prolapse of the mucosal and submucosal layers of the oesophagus through Killian's triangle. Prevalence is between 0.01% and 0.11% and occurs typically in middle-aged and elderly patients, but the pathogenesis is not well understood. It has been proposed that discoordination between pharyngeal contraction and upper oesophageal relaxation may be relevant. Many patients are asymptomatic but aspiration of food and resultant pneumonia can be the presenting feature. Oropharyngeal dysphagia, regurgitation of food, and halitosis may also occur. Most patients should be offered treatment but particularly if symptomatic. Cricopharyngeal myotomy forms the mainstay of management and may be offered surgically or endoscopically (usually with a stapling technique). A meta-analysis of 11 studies (596 patients) demonstrated that endoscopic diverticulectomy results in shorter length of procedure, shorter hospital stay, shorter time to reintroduction of oral diet, and lower risk of complications (cervical leak, aspiration pneumonia, chest pain, oesophageal perforation). The surgical approach demonstrated reduced risk of symptom recurrence.

Long-term antibiotics would not provide definitive management of the underlying diagnosis in this case, and balloon dilatation is not indicated because there is no stricture. Cognitive behavioural therapy has no role in the definitive management of Zenker's diverticulum.

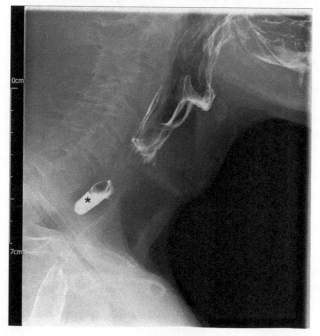

**Fig. 11.7** Barium swallow showing pharyngeal pouch

Image courtesy of Dr Horace D'Costa, Consultant Radiologist, Oxford University Hospitals NHS Foundation Trust

Albers DV, Kondo A, Bernardo WM et al. Endoscopic versus surgical approach in the treatment of Zenker's diverticulum: systematic review and meta-analysis. *Endosc Int Open*. 2016;4(6):E678–686. Doi:10.1055/s-0042-106203.

### 38. D. Ileocaecal resection and en bloc mid-ileal stricture resection

- Active small bowel CD with obstruction and concomitant abdominal abscess requires surgical intervention
- When there are multiple strictures in a short segment, resection is preferable to strictureplasties

The patient has an apparent perforation with raised inflammatory markers. Therefore, surgery rather than medical therapy is indicated. The mid-ileal strictures are causing symptomatic subacute small bowel obstruction. Although medical management post-ileocaecal resection is a possibility, the strictures should be treated surgically in this case. Strictureplasty would be recommended if the strictures were separated. However, it is not possible with such closely spaced strictures.

Symptomatic small bowel disease and perianal disease are the most common reasons for surgery in CD. Bowel-preserving surgery is advised to avoid short bowel syndrome. Most surgeons limit conventional strictureplasties to small bowel strictures <10 cm in length.

Colonic resections for Crohn's colitis can be segmental. Colonic resections are usually for strictures in CD and only rarely for toxic megacolon.

Perianal disease should only be managed surgically if it is symptomatic, with the purpose to drain and control sepsis rather than cure disease. Sepsis must be drained before contemplation of treatment with biological agents.

Gionchetti P, Dignass A, Danese S et al. Third European evidence-based consensus on the diagnosis and management of Crohn's disease 2016: Part 2: surgical management and special situations. *J Crohns Colitis*. 2017;11(2):135–149. Doi:10.1093/ecco-jcc/jjw169.

### 39. D. Periodic acid-Schiff (PAS) staining of duodenal biopsies

- Whipple's disease classically presents with arthralgias, weight loss, diarrhoea, and abdominal pain
- PAS-positive staining of duodenal biopsies is diagnostic
- Treatment is with long-term antibiotics such as co-trimoxazole

Whipple's disease is caused by the gram-positive bacteria, *Tropheryma whipplei*. Most patients are males with a mean age at diagnosis of approximately 50 years. The spectrum of symptoms is wide but classically comprises joint and GI involvement. The former may precede the latter by many years, with some patients initially receiving treatment for a seronegative inflammatory arthritis. Joint symptoms are typically, but not exclusively, migratory arthralgias of the large joints. Watery diarrhoea and abdominal pain may progress to chronic malabsorption resulting in weight loss and ascites. Cardiac manifestations include endocarditis, pericarditis, and myocarditis, and neurological involvement is also seen, commonly presenting with cognitive impairment. The diagnosis can be made by demonstrating (PAS)-positive macrophages in small intestinal biopsies. Alternatively, polymerase chain reaction for *T whipplei* from a relevant body site can also be performed. Treatment is with prolonged antibiotic therapy, often intravenous initially and then oral with co-trimoxazole commonly used.

Coeliac disease is unlikely to cause this symptom profile and human leucocyte antigen (HLA) testing, while excluding coeliac disease definitively, would not provide a positive diagnosis. Faecal calprotectin is of no benefit because endoscopic and radiological evaluations have demonstrated no evidence of IBD. Syphilis would not cause this presentation and a serum carcinoembryonic antigen is unhelpful given that a colonic malignancy has been excluded at colonoscopy.

Marth T, Moos V, Müller C et al. Tropheryma whipplei infection and Whipple's disease. *Lancet Infect Dis.* 2016;16(3):e13–22. Doi:10.1016/S1473-3099(15)00537-X.

## 40. C. Severity of symptoms does not correlate with stage of disease

- In PBC, pruritus refractory to medical therapy, but not fatigue, is an indication for LT in highly selected patients
- Recurrence of PBC after LT occurs in ~20% over 10 years but rarely leads to graft loss

Patients with PBC should be offered structured lifelong follow-up. Clinicians should determine the presence of symptoms, particularly fatigue and pruritus, but acknowledge that their severity does not correlate with the histological stage of disease.

In contrast to other liver chronic diseases, patients with PBC may rarely develop portal hypertension in the pre-cirrhotic stage of the disease, although this tends to occur in those with high-risk markers (male sex, low albumin, elevated bilirubin). Screening, prophylaxis, and treatment approaches to varices in PBC should be applied in the same way as other chronic liver diseases according to Baveno VI guidelines. This includes avoiding variceal screening endoscopy in patients with platelets >150 × 10$^9$ and LSM <20 kPa, although it is acknowledged that patients with PBC were not well represented in studies to date.

LT is an effective treatment for advanced PBC and should be considered in all patients with hepatic decompensation or bilirubin >50 µmol/L. Pruritus refractory to medical therapy, but not fatigue, is an indication for LT in highly selected patients regardless of disease stage. Recurrent PBC after LT is well recognized (~20% by 10 years) but graft loss is rare. Recurrent PBC often requires histological confirmation as anti-mitochondrial antibody persists post-transplant and a range of post-transplant complications (immunologic, vascular, biliary) can present with cholestatic LFTs. Men who are PBC patients with cirrhosis are at particularly increased risk of hepatocellular carcinoma.

Hirschfield GM, Beuers U, Corpechot C et al. EASL clinical practice guidelines: the diagnosis and management of patients with primary biliary cholangitis. *J Hepatol.* 2017;67(1):145–172. Doi:10.1016/j.jhep.2017.03.022.

## 41. D. Valganciclovir prophylaxis for three months

- Donor positive/recipient negative for CMV (D+/R−) are at highest risk of developing CMV disease and require three months' valganciclovir prophylaxis post-LT
- D+/R+ and D−/R+ patients should have regular CMV PCR with valganciclovir only introduced in the event of persisting viraemia

CMV infection remains the most common and significant opportunistic infection in LT recipients. Direct effects include CMV syndrome (fever and myelosuppression) and tissue-invasive CMV disease (e.g. hepatitis, retinitis, colitis) whereas indirect effects include increased risk of acute and chronic rejection, vanishing bile duct syndrome, post-transplant lymphoproliferative disorder, and hepatitis C virus recurrence.

The incidence of CMV disease varies according to donor and recipient CMV serologic status with the highest risk of *de novo* infection in D+/R−; so-called 'CMV mismatch'. In this group of patients, valganciclovir prophylaxis for at least three months is recommended. D+/R+ and D−/R+ patients are at intermediate risk and a pre-emptive approach to treatment is preferred with regular CMV

PCR and introduction of valganciclovir in the event of persisting viraemia despite trial of reduced immunosuppression. D−/R− patients are at low risk of infection and only require CMV PCR when CMV disease is clinically suspected. CMV disease should be treated with at least two weeks of oral valganciclovir or intravenous ganciclovir with foscarnet reserved as a second-line agent given its nephrotoxicity.

Lee SO, Razonable RR. Current concepts on cytomegalovirus infection after liver transplantation. *World J Hepatol.* 2010;2(9):325–336. Doi:10.4254/wjh.v2.i9.325.

### 42. D. 20 mm coin

- Blunt and small (≤2 cm) objects in the stomach may be managed conservatively
- Large objects (>20 mm diameter or >50 mm length), sharp objects, batteries, magnets, and all oesophageal objects should be endoscopically retrieved
- Endoscopic retrieval should not be attempted on illicit drug 'body packers'.

Sharp objects, magnets, and batteries in the stomach should be retrieved endoscopically <72 hours because of their risk of mucosal injury and perforation. Objects >2 cm in diameter or longer than 5 cm rarely pass the pylorus and duodenal bend, respectively, and should be removed non-urgently (<72 hours). Conservative outpatient management may be appropriate for asymptomatic patients with blunt objects in the stomach that are smaller than ≤2 cm in diameter because these usually pass spontaneously within a week.

Endoscopic retrieval should not be attempted in those who have ingested concealed illicit drugs ('body packers'), because of the risk of packet rupture and systemic intoxication. Symptomatic patients should be urgently assessed for signs of bowel obstruction or intoxication because surgery may be required in these situations. Asymptomatic patients should be given whole-bowel irrigation or laxatives and closely observed.

Birk M, Bauerfeind P, Deprez PH et al. Removal of foreign bodies in the upper gastrointestinal tract in adults: European Society of Gastrointestinal Endoscopy (ESGE) clinical guideline. *Endoscopy.* 2016;48(5):489–496. Doi:10.1055/s-0042-100456.

### 43. D. Ustekinumab

- Ustekinumab is licensed for use in both CD and psoriasis
- Ustekinumab targets the shared p40 subunit of pro-inflammatory cytokines IL-12/-23

Increasing understanding of the immunopathogenesis of IBD at a cellular and molecular level has led to the development of novel therapies. The most appropriate answer here is the interleukin-12/23 (IL-12/23) antagonist, ustekinumab. IL-12 and -23 have been implicated in the pathophysiology of CD. IL-12 and -23 share a common p40 subunit, to which ustekinumab is directed against. The UNITI-1, UNITI-2, and IM-UNITI trials demonstrated the clinical efficacy of ustekinumab in moderate-to-severe CD in anti-TNF naïve and exposed groups. In this case, ustekinumab is an appropriate second-line option for CD and a well-established treatment option for psoriasis. Although currently only licensed for use in CD, a recent RCT has demonstrated the efficacy of ustekinumab over placebo for inducing and maintaining remission in patients with moderate-to-severe UC.

Vedolizumab, an anti-α4β7 integrin, is licensed for use in both UC and CD. The GEMINI-2 trial demonstrated clinical efficacy in inducing (14.5% vs 6.8%) and maintaining (39% vs. 21.6%) clinical remission in CD when compared with placebo. As a gut-selective biologic, vedolizumab has the advantage of use in patients where systemic immunosuppression carries significant risk, such as in elderly patients or those with previous malignancy. Its gut selectivity precludes its sole use in patients with extra-intestinal manifestations. Currently administered intravenously, subcutaneous preparations are being developed. Ustekinumab has a good safety signal with lower rates of active tuberculosis than anti-TNFs.

Many inflammatory cytokines signal through the JAK family of receptors triggering inflammatory cascades in IBD. Tofacitinib is an orally administered selective inhibitor of mainly JAK1 and JAK3 receptors. It is currently licensed for use in UC only following successful completion of the Phase 3 study, OCTAVE, which demonstrated that tofacitinib was superior to placebo in achieving clinical and histological remission.

Amiselimod and Mongersen are a sphingosine 1-phosphate receptor modulator and Smad7 inhibitor respectively. Both have entered Phase 3 clinical trials for use in CD.

Hindryckx P, Vande Casteele N, Novak G et al. The expanding therapeutic armamentarium for inflammatory bowel disease: how to choose the right drug[s] for our patients. J Crohns Colitis. 2018;12(1):105–119. Doi:10.1093/ecco-jcc/jjx117.

### 44. C. Mesalazine enema

- Topical therapy should be added to all UC patients with an incomplete response to oral 5-aminosalicylate (5-ASA)
- Combination of oral and topical 5-ASA therapy is superior to monotherapy

Combined therapy has been shown to work more rapidly and effectively than oral or topical mesalazine therapy alone. In left-sided disease, enemas are more appropriate; in proctitis, suppositories may be sufficient. If combination 5-ASA treatment fails to resolve rectal bleeding within 10–14 days, treatment with systemic corticosteroids should be considered. Azathioprine and mercaptopurine are thiopurines indicated in steroid-refractory disease or steroid-intolerant patients. They have a slow onset of action and are therefore not useful in inducing remission.

Probert CS, Dignass AU, Lindgren S et al. Combined oral and rectal mesalazine for the treatment of mild-to-moderately active ulcerative colitis: rapid symptom resolution and improvements in quality of life. J Crohns Colitis. 2014;8:200–207. Doi:10.1016/j.crohns.2013.08.007.

### 45. D. Transthoracic contrast enhanced echocardiogram

- Hepatopulmonary syndrome (HPS) is common in patients with advanced liver disease occurring in 5%–32% of LT candidates.
- Diagnosis requires a triad of liver dysfunction, impaired oxygenation, and presence of intrapulmonary vascular dilatations (IPVD), which are best identified on contrast echocardiogram.

The patient in this case is highly likely to have HPS, which is the most common cause of respiratory insufficiency in patients with advanced liver disease, occurring in 5%–32% of LT candidates. The diagnosis should be suspected in all breathless patients with cirrhosis, particularly those with orthodeoxia and platypnoea, multiple telangiectasia, clubbing, and oxygen saturations <96%.

HPS is characterized by a triad of liver dysfunction, abnormal oxygenation defined by elevated alveolar-arterial oxygen gradient, and the presence of IPVD caused by increased circulating nitric oxide in patients with cirrhosis. IPVD are best identified by transthoracic contrast enhanced echocardiogram (a 'bubble' echocardiogram) where microbubbles contained in peripherally injected agitated saline are able to shunt through the lung into the left chambers of the heart.

Spirometry values are usually within the normal range in HPS. Nuclear lung perfusion scanning can help identify IPVD but has an inferior sensitivity compared with contrast echocardiography.

Therapeutic options in HPS include long-term oxygen therapy or LT, which leads to complete resolution.

Fuhrmann V, Krowka M. Hepatopulmonary syndrome. *J Hepatol.* 2018;69(3):744–745. Doi:10.1016/j.jhep.2018.01.002.

## 46. E. Subtotal colectomy

- Subtotal colectomy with end ileostomy is the operation of choice in acute colitis
- Pouch formation may be delayed in young women wishing to have children

This case meets the Travis criteria and needs consideration of second-line therapy. Therefore, there is no role for prolonged steroids. Ciclosporin is contraindicated in uncontrolled hypertension. Infliximab is relatively contraindicated in patients with prior tuberculosis, because of the risk of reactivation. Of the options that are given, surgery is the safest.

Indications for emergency surgery in acute severe ulcerative colitis include the following:

- Toxic megacolon
- Perforation
- Massive haemorrhage
- Obstruction

Surgeons experienced in ileoanal pouch reconstruction should ideally perform emergency cases in order to preserve anatomy for future restorative surgery. The initial operation is a subtotal colectomy with end ileostomy, and closure of the rectal stump (or mucous fistula formation). If the stump is left without a mucous fistula, a large rectal catheter should be sutured in place for about five days. The next stage is a completion proctectomy and ileal pouch–anal anastomosis (IPAA) at least three months later. An ileoanal pouch is a neo-rectum fashioned from ileum, creating a larger lumen, which is often referred to as a 'J-pouch', although it may be J-, W-, or S-shaped. A stapled anastomosis is preferable because it results in decreased nocturnal incontinence.

IPAA is done in one or two stages. In the two-stage procedure, pouch construction with a temporary loop ileostomy is performed, and the ileostomy is then closed about two months later. In women of reproductive age, pouch formation may be delayed to avoid the risk to fertility.

Øresland T, Bemelman WA, Sampietro GM et al. European evidence based consensus on surgery for ulcerative colitis. *J Crohns Colitis.* 2015;9(1):4–25. Doi:10.1016/j.crohns.2014.08.012.

## 47. C. 17%

- The most common cause of upper GI bleeding in all age groups is peptic ulcer bleeding
- Seventeen per cent of patients have a normal gastroscopy despite compatible symptoms

A nationwide audit across the UK of 5,004 patients with symptoms of upper GI bleeding identified the following pathologies:

- Peptic ulcer           36%
- Oesophagitis           24%
- Gastritis/erosions     22%
- Erosive duodenitis     13%
- Varices                11%
- Mallory-Weiss tear     4.3%

- Malignancy                                      3.7%
- Other (e.g. vascular ectasia, haemobilia)       2.6%
- No abnormality seen                             17%

Some variation in frequencies is seen with different age groups. For instance, peptic ulcer disease and malignancy are more common in older patients, whereas variceal bleeding and Mallory-Weiss tears are less common.

Hearnshaw SA, Logan RF, Lowe D et al. Acute upper gastrointestinal bleeding in the UK: patient characteristics, diagnoses and outcomes in the 2007 UK audit. *Gut.* 2011;60:1327–1335. Doi:10.1136/gut.2010.228437.

## 48. A. Cholangitis

- Ninety per cent of gallstones are cholesterol gallstones, which have a large number of genetic and environmental risk factors including female gender, pregnancy, metabolic syndrome, and rapid weight loss
- Ten per cent of gallstones are pigment stones that form secondary to altered bilirubin metabolism
- Black pigment stones occur in conditions with systemic hyperbilirbinaemia, whereas brown pigment stone formation requires biliary obstruction and infection.

More than 90% of gallstones are composed mainly of cholesterol (cholesterol gallstones) for which a wide range of risk factors have been well established. These include female gender, pregnancy obesity, type 2 diabetes, and physical inactivity. A number of genetic polymorphisms have also been identified through genome wide association studies, the most common of which is the hepatobiliary cholesterol transporter (ABCG8 p.D19H) gene variant. Rapid weight loss from bariatric surgery and/or a very low-calorie diet can also promote cholesterol stone formation through mobilization of cholesterol from adipose tissue and gallbladder hypomotility due to reduced stimulation from dietary lipid.

The remaining 10% of gallstones are represented by black and brown pigment stones that contain excess amounts of unconjugated bilirubin. Black pigment stones form in the gallbladder and biliary tree in the absence of infection, particularly in patients with conditions that increase the concentration of systemic bilirubin, including chronic haemolytic anaemias, ineffective erythropoiesis, or liver cirrhosis. Diseased or resected ileum (e.g. CD) also promotes black pigment stone formation as malabsorbed bile acids in the colon solubilize unconjugated bilirubin, promoting its reabsorption and increasing the rate of bilirubin secretion into bile.

Brown pigment stones form mainly outside the gallbladder in the intra- and extra-hepatic bile ducts as a result of biliary stasis from obstruction and superimposed infection, especially with *Escherichia coli (E. coli). E. coli* produces β-glucuronidase, which converts soluble conjugated bilirubin to insoluble unconjugated bilirubin that combines with calcium to form calcium bilirubinate stones.

Lammert F, Gurusamy K, Ko CW et al. Gallstones. *Nat Rev Dis Primers.* 2016;2:16024. Doi:10.1038/nrdp.2016.24.

## 49. B. CT angiography

- Aorto-enteric fistulae can be rapidly fatal and require prompt investigation and management
- CT angiography is the imaging modality of choice with high sensitivity and specificity
- Aorto-enteric fistulae should be considered in anyone presenting with GI bleeding in the presence of aortic grafts

Although aorto-enteric fistulae may result from untreated aortic aneurysms eroding through the intestine, they are more often secondary to surgical or endovascular aortic repair. Most develop between the aorta and duodenum. 'Herald bleeding' whereby patients experience multiple smaller bleeds before massive haemorrhage is not uncommon. Between 27% and 60% of patients do not present with GI bleeding, instead presenting with sepsis. CT angiography is the imaging modality of choice (sensitivity 94%, specificity 85%) and should be performed before upper GI, lower GI, or small bowel endoscopy. There is no role for MR angiography in acute massive GI haemorrhage with haemodynamic instability. Aorto-enteric fistulae may be treated surgically (excision of graft, and then graft reconstruction or bypass) or via an endovascular approach with stenting, balloon occlusion, or coil embolization. There is a 7% in-hospital mortality rate for endovascular repair (34% for surgical repair), and a risk of infection of 44% at 13 months (25% at 9 months for surgical repair).

Partovi S, Trischman T, Sheth RA et al. Imaging work-up and endovascular treatment options for aorto-enteric fistula. *Cardiovasc Diagn Ther.* 2018;8(Suppl 1):S200–207. Doi:10.21037/cdt.2017.10.05.

## 50. D. Hydatid disease

- Hydatid disease occurs when the eggs of *Echinococcus granulosus* are ingested leading to cystic lesions in the liver and lungs
- Diagnosis is with a combination of serologic tests and imaging alongside a history of possible exposure in an endemic area
- Choice of treatment with medication, surgery, or radiological intervention is guided by staging with ultrasound

Hydatid disease, or 'cystic echinococcosis (CE)', is a widely endemic disease of humans caused by the tapeworm *Echinococcus granulosus*. Dogs are the main definitive host, harbouring worms in their intestines that shed their eggs in faeces. Humans then become infected through ingestion of contaminated food or water, after which larvae encyst predominantly in the liver (70%) and lungs (20%). CE is globally distributed with particularly high prevalence in South America, East Africa, Central Asia, and China. The asymptomatic incubation period of disease can last years but, when the cysts reach sufficient size, abdominal pain, nausea, and anorexia develop with hepatic disease and chronic cough, chest pain, and shortness of breath with pulmonary involvement. In hepatic CE, liver enzymes, particularly ALP, are elevated in 40% and large cysts can compress adjacent bile ducts causing obstructive jaundice. Eosinophilia is present in 40% of patients with CE, unlike in amoebic disease where neutrophilia with fever predominate. Diagnosis is confirmed with a combination of serologic tests and imaging. Ultrasound and CT often demonstrate fluid density cysts with frequent peripheral focal areas of calcification. The complexity of cystic lesions on ultrasound helps guide the treatment, which includes chemotherapeutic agents (e.g. albendazole, mebendazole), surgical cystectomy, expectant management or percutaneous aspiration, injection (of scolicidal agent), and reaspiration (PAIR).

Pakala T, Molina M, Wu GY. Hepatic echinococcal cysts: a review. *J Clin Transl Hepatol.* 2016;4(1):39–46. Doi:10.14218/JCTH.2015.00036.

# INDEX